CHILDREN AND LANGUAGE: DEVELOPMENT, IMPAIRMENT AND TRAINING

CHILDREN AND LANGUAGE: DEVELOPMENT, IMPAIRMENT AND TRAINING

MICHAEL A. REED
EDITOR

Nova Science Publishers, Inc.
New York

For permission to use material from this book please contact us:
Telephone 631-231-7269; Fax 631-231-8175
Web Site: http://www.novapublishers.com

LIBRARY OF CONGRESS CATALOGING-IN-PUBLICATION DATA

Children & language : development, impairment & training / [edited by] Michael A. Reed.
p. cm.
Includes index.
ISBN 978-1-60692-395-5
1. Children--Language. 2. Language acquisition. 3. Language awareness in children. 4. Verbal ability in children. 5. Language disorders in children. I. Reed, Michael A., 1955- II. Title. III. Title: Children and language.
P118.C485 2009
401'.93--dc22

2008045624

Published by Nova Science Publishers, Inc. ✦ New York

CONTENTS

PREFACE

The theory of mind (ToM) is the ability to perceive, interpret and predict behaviors or actions of others based on their underlying mental states. The linguistic influence on the developmental neural basis of ToM is described in this book. Furthermore, the deferential effects of context and isolated word training on reading fluency is explained. Using children's literature to assist in science inquiry and in building knowledge in other subject areas has been on the rise, due to the benefits of supporting children's language and literacy learning. Such developments are explored. In addition, the authors give an overview of the electrophysiological correlates of developmental dyslexia, a reading impairment in childhood.

This book describes the impact of various cognitive functions on language acquisition and language processing in different groups of children. In addition, the effects of bilingual teaching on the development of children's literacy skills during the first six years of school are explored. Furthermore, selective mutism, a disorder characterized by a lack of speech in specific unfamiliar situations or around unfamiliar people, is described.

Crying represents the very first communicative channel infants can use to communicate with their environment and thus, it plays an important role in child development. Studies that have investigated expressions of distress, specifically crying, during early stages of infancy development are reviewed. In addition, studies done to test whether language input strongly influences the development of vocabulary and syntax in children are described. Children with developmental dysphasia were also studied and the outcomes of this study are reviewed.

This book looks at the connection between middle ear effusion (MEE) in the first years of life compared to central auditory processing at age seven. Furthermore, problems and questions with regard to diagnosis and intervention of multilingual specific language impairment (SLI) is examined. Future areas of research in this field are also addressed. Finally, the results from a longitudinal study between apparent pain insensibility and non-verbal communication and symbolisation disorders in autism is explored.

Chapter 1 - Theory of mind (ToM) – ability to perceive, interpret and predict behaviors or actions of others based on their underlying mental states – has been explored with a plethora of paradigms in normally and atypically developing children by many researchers. ToM is fundamental for human social interaction universally. Among ToM researchers it has long been debated whether or not language development constrains ToM development. Recent results from neurological studies suggest that some aspects of language (e.g., grammar) may function merely as a 'co-opted' system, but other aspects of language (e.g., pragmatics and reading communicative intentions) may profoundly affect ToM throughout the development.

Neuroimaging studies of ToM development are still scarce. However, results from a few studies that explored neural correlates of ToM and related socio-cognitive functions revealed age-related differences in ToM/social-cognition-specific brain activity in several language regions. Despite the increasing evidence that supports the developmental relationship between language and various cognitive capacities ToM, current developmental theories of ToM (except one) discount the linguistic effects on ToM. There are four main-stream theories of ToM development; 1) Modular ToM hypothesis, 2) Theory, theory of mind hypothesis, 3) Simulation ToM hypothesis, and 4) Linguistic determinism of ToM hypothesis. In the first part of the chapter, I will discuss both behavioral and neurological evidence that supports or negates the linguistic influence on ToM. In the second part of this chapter, I will discuss those four prominent theories of ToM development and whether or not evidence from the most current neuroimaging studies of ToM in children and adults (including ours) support these theories. Finally, based on the most current results, I will present a new model for the developmental mechanism of ToM.

Chapter 2 - The first priority for novice readers is to understand that the letters they see in written language correspond to the sounds they hear in speech. Once children grasp the letter-to-sound pairings afforded to them by the alphabetic principle, they can begin to identify some of the written words that are contained in their spoken vocabularies. At this point, the question becomes whether reading practice should take place in stories (context) or in lists (isolation). Two camps have emerged with opposing views on this topic. On the one hand, investigators have shown increased long-term word recognition when children practice reading words in isolation.

In contrast, it has also been suggested that reading words in context can act as a secondary self-teaching mechanism. Proponents of this view argue that the added value of context increases reading ability beyond that achieved by other methods of training. At present, then, the evidence on best training practices (context vs. isolation) is mixed. The studies discussed here begin to unify these two differing perspectives by elucidating the circumstances that mediate the utility of each type of training. In brief, during the five training studies reviewed, context training dominated isolated word training with regards to word acquisition. However, after words were learned, retention over an eight-day interval approached ceiling under both conditions. Finally, fluency transfer (reading words quickly and accurately in new texts or new lists) was maximized when the congruency between training and testing was high; words trained in isolation were read more fluently in novel lists, whereas words trained in context were read more fluently in novel stories. To conclude, the decision of which training method to use cannot be made independently from the task to be done after training has ceased. However, if the goal of instruction is to have students who excel during training, remember what they have learned, and who use their learning to read new texts fluently, the research plainly suggests that training in context is a more fruitful method of instruction than isolated word training.

Chapter 3 - Using children's literature to assist in science inquiry and in knowledge building in other subject areas has been on the rise due to the benefits of supporting children's language and literacy learning. However, published research has reported a substantial variation in the methods of utilizing children's literature to support learning and language development. A deficiency in the association between reading and writing, and in the amount of time children are given to write has also been reported. "Writing was not linked to reading, and students seemed to spend relatively little time composing" (Allington, Guice, Li,

Michelson, & Baker, 1995). In some classrooms in the United States, science is separately taught and given relatively less time in comparison with English/Language Arts (Royce & Wiley, 2005). In the real world, however, when it comes to learning science concepts, children do not often separate science from other subject areas that assist them in the inquiry, because the human brain naturally makes meaningful connections when new information is presented (Bredekamp & Copple, 1997). "One of the most important constants throughout human development is that all domains of development are interrelated. Development in one dimension influences and is influenced by development in other realms" (Bredekam & Copple, 1997, p. 144). Furthermore, Allington, et al also found ". . . hardly any art or drama activities linked to the reading children were doing in any of the classrooms" (p. 10). Therefore, the purpose of this study was to examine what might provide a scaffolding to a child's language and literacy competencies when reading was closely connected to writing and when art was linked to reading in the process of acquiring a science concept. The underlying research question is "What does an integrated curriculum provide to facilitate and how does an integrated curricular approach mediate children's language and literacy competencies when they are engaged in acquiring a science concept?"

Chapter 4 - Electrophysiological measurements enabled us to greatly increase our knowledge on the most spread learning disability in childhood represented by the Developmental Dyslexia (DD). The present chapter reviews the most relevant studies, which used either Event Related Potentials (ERPs) or Electroencephalographic (EEG) bands to investigate reading disabilities in developmental age. Several studies are here described, which succeeded in showing processing abnormalities not only in dyslexics, but also in children genetically at risk of dyslexia, through the analysis of both the "classical" electrophysiological components (i.e., MMN, P300, N400) and earlier evoked potentials. The electrophysiological markers of neuronal dysfunctions found in these children, helped scientists to uncover the psychophysiological mechanisms chiefly involved in this language disorder. These are: deficits in speech sound processing and impairment in manipulating the phonological features of grapheme strings. A considerable advance in the field has been recently reached by using EEG bands, traditionally used for detecting group differences in resting state, but currently extended to the measure of cognitive activation obtained through different experimental tasks. Such studies revealed functional differences in both fast and slow EEG rhythms between dyslexics and controls. The use of two functionally distinct EEG rhythms, theta and beta bands, in line with several ERP results, supports the view that dyslexics' reading difficulties are related to a linguistic impairment which is represented essentially at phonological level. Similar conclusions were further supported by the analysis of delta rhythm - a functional marker of cortical inhibition - during the performance of different linguistic tasks. Group differences in delta activation points to a delay in dyslexics' brain maturation. The review of recent literature on electrophysiological correlates of DD, on one hand supports the view that ERPs, with their excellent time resolution, can represent an optimal tool for investigating language disorders mainly along time domain. On the other hand, EEG bands are able to show both functional and maturational aspects of dyslexics' brains, thus representing a distinct measurement with respect to ERPs. These two electrophysiological methods provide complementary information for a better understanding of the neural and cognitive mechanisms involved in DD. In conclusion, electrophysiological measures could represent an effective tool for making early diagnoses of dyslexia or for predictions of future reading problems in infants at risk, but they could also be valuable for testing the efficacy of rehabilitative trainings.

Chapter 5 - The focus of this chapter is on the impact of various cognitive functions on language acquisition and language processing in different groups of children. Empirical data are presented on individual variations of language and cognition in typically developing children, children with specific language impairment, and in young adults with dyslexia. The interaction between flexible cognition (attention switching, working memory, and inhibition control) and language comprehension was examined in English-speaking and Hungarian participants.

The findings suggest that working memory performance and language comprehension are strongly influenced by task complexity, age, and language structure. Working memory storage and processing are affected differently by stimulus complexity.

Children with specific language impairment and young adults with dyslexia showed deficits in flexible cognition and language comprehension (oral and written). Children with SLI performed more poorly than their age-matched and language-matched peers in tasks that measured working memory capacity and inhibition control. In addition to the group effects, participants with language impairment showed different errors and performance patterns than their peers.

Chapter 6 - The study described in the article investigated the effects of bilingual teaching (Content and Language Integrated Learning, CLIL) on the development of children's literacy skills during their first six school years. In the CLIL classes 20–25 per cent of the instruction was given in a foreign language. The results of the study showed that the children in the CLIL classes learned to read and write their first language equally well than their peers in monolingual classes. In addition, bilingual teaching did not have a negative effect on the development of those children who started school with poor learning readiness either. After the two first study years the children in the CLIL classes were more fluent readers and had better reading comprehension and spelling skills than their peers in the other classes.

After four school years it was obvious that the children's creative writing skills had also benefited from bilingual teaching. The students in the CLIL classes had learned to pay attention to languages, as well to their mother tongue as to other languages. Moreover, they had more positive attitudes towards reading, writing and foreign language learning. Especially the boys' attitudes proved to be more positive in the CLIL classes than in the other classes.

After six study years the students in the CLIL classes had achieved significantly better first language spelling skills than the students in the other classes. They made significantly less spelling errors and understood significantly better different texts. Furthermore, they showed more proficiency in deriving the meaning of new words from the written context than the other students. Likewise, they succeeded significantly better in finding the most important facts of the non-fiction text and summarising the text than their peers in the other classes. It is worth mentioning that in the other classes the girls' skills were significantly better than the boys' skills but in CLIL classes the difference was not significant. The students in the CLIL classes enjoyed studying the foreign language and also studying through it. Consequently, their foreign language skills developed very well.

Chapter 7 - Selective mutism is a disorder that is characterized by a lack of speech in specific unfamiliar situations or in the presence of unfamiliar individuals despite speaking normally in other situations (APA, 2000). Although the disorder usually first appears in the preschool years (Black & Uhde, 1995; Cunningham, McHolm, Boyle, & Patel, 2004; Dummit, Klein, Tancer, Asche, Martin, & Fairbanks, 1997; Steinhausen & Juzi, 1996), it is typically not diagnosed until the child is between 6.5 to 9 years of age (Ford, Sladesczek, Carlson, & Krochwell, 1998; Kumpulainen, Rasenen, Raaska, & Somppi, 1998; Remschmidt, Poller, Herpertz-Dahlmann, Hennighausen, & Gutenbrunner, 2001; Standart & Le Couteur, 2003). Given that the disorder manifests itself early in development, the child' limited speaking in select situations and its impact on language development warrants careful consideration.

The purpose of the present chapter is to review the literature on language performance in children with selective mutism. The chapter is divided among three sections. In the first section, the authors provide an overview of selective mutism, including its definition, prevalence, diagnosis, classification, etiology and functional impairment. In section two, the authors review the research that has been conducted to date on language performance in children with selective mutism. The authors conclude the chapter in section three with a review of possible developmental pathways for the association between selective mutism and language performance as well as implications for future research.

Chapter 8 - Crying, which represents the very first communicative channel infants can use to communicate with their environment, plays an important role in child development. Crying is a biological signal that alerts those in the caregiving environment about the needs and wants of the infant and motivates them to respond. Cries act to release specific and appropriate patterns of caregiving actions, thereby ensuring the infant's survival. The aim of this chapter is to review studies that have investigated expressions of distress, specifically crying, during early stages of development in infancy. Emphasized is the importance of cry evaluation in specific psychopathology, particularly Autism Spectrum Disorders (ASD). First the neurobiological activation that takes place during an episode of crying, both in the caregiver and the infant brain, is described. A description of the function of crying episodes and their evolution, starting from the fetal stage through childhood, follows. Finally, how anomalies in the expression of cry can bias the caregiver's perception of them, and how parents' reactions to pathological crying can be qualitatively different from their reactions to typical crying of same-aged children, is described. Such differences can confound parental attempts to share feelings and develop inter-subjectivity with their children.

Chapter 9 - Correlational, quasi-experimental and experimental research conducted with typical children has shown that language input strongly influences the development of vocabulary and syntax. Another approach to this issue, based on the pathological method, is reviewed in the present chapter. This approach consists in studying participants with intellectual disability because they present a "natural" (i.e., unprovoked) dissociation between their general developmental level and their educational experience. Indeed, compared to intellectually average children of the same mental age, children and adolescents with intellectual disability have had more learning opportunities simply because, given their chronological age, they have lived longer. In particular, and all things being equal, they have participated more often in educational or leisure activities and have a far greater language experience, including more verbal interactions with their parents, grandparents, educators, teachers and all their other caregivers. This language experience related to age may well give them, among other things, an advantage with regard to the acquisition of additional vocabulary. Indeed, if interindividual differences in lexical development are caused, at least in part, by differences in language input, then CA-related language experience should give adolescents or children with intellectual disability a vocabulary advantage over typical children of comparable cognitive level. In the present literature review, the classical approaches (i.e., correlational, quasi-experimental and experimental) used to study the relationship between the language learning environment and the acquisition of lexicon are successively presented. The pathological method is then considered and illustrated with the aim of showing that the study of children and adolescents with intellectual disability might be an innovative way to examine the relationship between language experience and language development.

Chapter 10 - This study reports longitudinal follow-up of 300 children with developmental dysphasia. Their expressive disturbances are a manifestation of their auditory decoding impairment. These children were investigated on battery of tests of spoken language, of phonological processing and of different audiometric procedures, in order to register all the information necessary to be able judge the speech-language development. The tests focused on diagnosis of central auditory disorder, confirmed the difficulties in association area in children with developmental dysphasia. In speech perception, the temporal processing is one of the functions necessary for the discrimination of phonemes, and of similar words. The authors results confirmed long-term problems of children with developmental dysphasia with central auditory perception disorder.

Short Communication A - This study examined the relation of middle ear effusion (MEE) in the first three years of life to central auditory processing at age seven. Ears were examined on a regular basis frequently in the home over the first three years and a count of days with bilateral MEE was used to quantify ear status. Central auditory processing was assessed with SCAN, Screening Test for Auditory Processing Disorders. With a sample of 76 children studied prospectively from birth there were significant correlations between MEE and all four SCAN measures. A possible link between SCAN and attention problems was also examined using the Test of Variables of Attention (TOVA). Three of 16 possible correlations were significant, suggesting a weak relation between attention and SCAN.

Short Communication B - Children with Specific Language Impairment (SLI) show a significant language deficit with no obvious accompanying condition such as mental retardation, neurological damage, or hearing impairment. While about 6-8% of all children are affected by SLI, it is therefore logical to assume that 6-8% of all multilingual children are affected by SLI as well. In order to diagnose SLI with certainty, SLI must be diagnosed in both languages. While for many languages diagnostic tools exist, there are a large number of languages for which appropriate tests have not yet been designed. Particularly in children with successive bilingual language development, inadequate acquisition of the second language may mask a clinically relevant language impairment or vice versa.

While diagnosis is difficult, the issue of adequate language training or therapy respectively is just as complicated. This situation may be further exacerbated by a general uncertainty of professionals about the effects of multilingual intervention or parent advising regarding the choice of one or two languages. In addition, little is known about the neurophysiological bases and manifestations of multilingual SLI – making appropriate intervention all the more difficult.

In this short communication, the authors will outline problems and questions with regard to diagnosis and intervention and address future areas of research in the field.

Short Communication C - Numerous clinical reports sustain the hypothesis of the pain insensitivity in autistic children. This insensitivity may be explained by the increase of the opioid activity (in particular the Bêta-endorphin). However, the rates of the plasma beta-endorphin concentrations in autistic children are contradictory. The authors have therefore studied in autism the relationship between the behavioural pain reactivity and the verbal and non verbal communication disorders. This study suggests that the apparent decrease of the behavioural pain reactivity in autistic children can be explained by a different way to express pain, specifically in relation with the communication and symbolisation disorders and other cognitive disorders (learning disabilities; own body image disorders; difficulties for mental representations of sensations and emotions; difficulties in understanding causes and effects relations), rather than a real endogenic analgesia.

RESEARCH AND REVIEWS

In: Children and Language: Development, Impairment … ISBN 978-1-60692-395-5
Editor: Michael A. Reed

Chapter 1

LANGUAGE AND THOUGHT: LINGUISTIC INFLUENCE ON DEVELOPMENTAL NEURAL BASIS OF 'THEORY OF MIND'

Chiyoko Kobayashi
Department of Psychology, Cornell University, Uris Hall, Ithaca, NY 14853

ABSTRACT

Theory of mind (ToM) – ability to perceive, interpret and predict behaviors or actions of others based on their underlying mental states – has been explored with a plethora of paradigms in normally and atypically developing children by many researchers. ToM is fundamental for human social interaction universally. Among ToM researchers it has long been debated whether or not language development constrains ToM development. Recent results from neurological studies suggest that some aspects of language (e.g., grammar) may function merely as a 'co-opted' system, but other aspects of language (e.g., pragmatics and reading communicative intentions) may profoundly affect ToM throughout the development. Neuroimaging studies of ToM development are still scarce. However, results from a few studies that explored neural correlates of ToM and related socio-cognitive functions revealed age-related differences in ToM/social-cognition-specific brain activity in several language regions. Despite the increasing evidence that supports the developmental relationship between language and various cognitive capacities ToM, current developmental theories of ToM (except one) discount the linguistic effects on ToM. There are four main-stream theories of ToM development; 1) Modular ToM hypothesis, 2) Theory, theory of mind hypothesis, 3) Simulation ToM hypothesis, and 4) Linguistic determinism of ToM hypothesis. In the first part of the chapter, I will discuss both behavioral and neurological evidence that supports or negates the linguistic influence on ToM. In the second part of this chapter, I will discuss those four prominent theories of ToM development and whether or not evidence from the most current neuroimaging studies of ToM in children and adults (including ours) support these theories. Finally, based on the most current results, I will present a new model for the developmental mechanism of ToM.

INTRODUCTION

Are our thoughts same as our language? Or, are they different? Whorf (1956) hypothesized that our language constrains our thoughts and reflects our culturally unique world view. Later, Vygotsky (1967) elaborated this hypothesis, positing that human consciousness (or thought) has its basis in linguistic or historical contexts and is enabled only through the internalization of culture-specific symbols (i.e., language). According to the Vygotskyan view, human consciousness never develops independently of language, which is acquired only through intersubjective perspective-taking and communication with other individuals in the society [Tomasello, 2001; Valsiner, 1989; Vygotsky, 1967]. From the late 1960s to mid 1990s, the so-called Sapir-Whorf hypothesis was discredited by cognitive scientists and linguists who emphasized universal and veridical ways of perceiving our world. Throughout these decades a view, which posited that universal linguistic [Chomsky, 1980] and cognitive developmental [Piaget, 1962; Sinclair, 1970] principles determined individuals' thoughts and cognition, dominated.

Following the Chomskyan tradition (and counter to the Whorfian hypothesis), Fodor (1975) argued that humans possess a rich, propositional system which we share with nonhuman primates and infants. Fodor named this innate representational system "language of thought." This primitive computational and symbolic system, he has theorized, exists independently from natural language and governs our preverbal theory of mind (ToM): our ability to perceive, interpret and predict the behaviors or actions of others in terms of their underlying mental states [Fodor, 1975; the definition is by Scholl & Leslie, 1999]. A few years later, Premack and Woodruff (1978) tested this ability in a chimpanzee and found evidence for ToM in this nonhuman primate. Although the validity of their tests and the very capacity of ToM in nonhuman primates are still debated [Cheney & Seyfarth, 1990; de Waal, 2001; Hayes, 1998)], no one questions that the ability to understand others' desires and intentions is important for humans [Frith & Frith, 2003].

Since the first experiment with the chimpanzee [Premack & Woodruff, 1978], various paradigms have been devised to test ToM in humans [Baron-Cohen, 2000]. Among those ToM tasks, a false-belief (FB) task has been the most commonly used for testing normally developing [Wimmer & Perner, 1983] as well as atypically developing children [Baron-Cohen, Leslie, & Frith, 1985; see Baron-Cohen, 2000 for a review]. In a typical FB task, two characters appear (e.g., Sally and Ann) in a scene. When one character, Sally, is present, Ann, the other character, puts a toy into a basket. Sally then disappears from the scene. While Sally is away, Ann takes the toy out of the basket and puts it into a box. The experimenter then asks the child the critical false-belief question, "Where will Sally look for the toy?" Nearly universally observed results are that adults and children over 4 years of age correctly answer "basket" whereas younger children (as well as older children and adolescents with autism) fail the task by answering "box" [Baron-Cohen, Leslie, & Frith, 1985; 1986]. These failures reflect their lack of understanding that Sally's belief about the location of the toy is different from Ann's [Frith, 2003; Happé, 1993].

Several brain imaging studies have examined the neural correlates of ToM using the FB style paradigm in adults [Brunet et al., 2000; Fletcher et al., 1995; Gallagher et al., 2000; Goel et al., 1995; Happé et al., 1996; Kobayashi, Glover, & Temple, 2006; Sabbagh & Taylor, 2000; Saxe & Kanwisher, 2003; Vogeley et al., 2001]. Many of these studies have found significant activity in medial prefrontal cortex (mPFC) during false-belief conditions [Flethcer et al., 1995; Gallagher et al., 2000; Goel et al., 1995; Happé et al., 1996] (**Figure 1**). In addition, the temporo-parietal junction (TPJ) has also been suggested to be important for ToM processing. This area was found to become active during both true- and false-belief conditions and not during false representations in a non-social control condition [Saxe & Kanwisher, 2003; Saxe & Wexler, 2005]. Other brain regions implicated in these and other ToM brain imaging studies include the anterior cingulate cortex (ACC), the middle frontal gyrus, the precuneus/posterior cingulate cortex, the superior temporal sulcus, the orbito-frontal cortex, and the temporal pole. However, these areas have not been implicated as consistently as the mPFC and the TPJ [see Frith & Frith, 2003, and Saxe, Carey, & Kanwisher, 2004 for reviews]. Although brain imaging studies of ToM in children are still scarce, several studies found similar medial frontal and/or TPJ activity using a variety of ToM or related social/cognitive tasks [Dapretto et al., 2006; Kobayashi, Glover, & Temple, 2007a; 2007b; Liu, 2005; Liu et al., 2005; Moriguchi et al., 2007; Ohnishi et al., 2004; Wang et al., 2006a; 2006b] **(Table 1).**

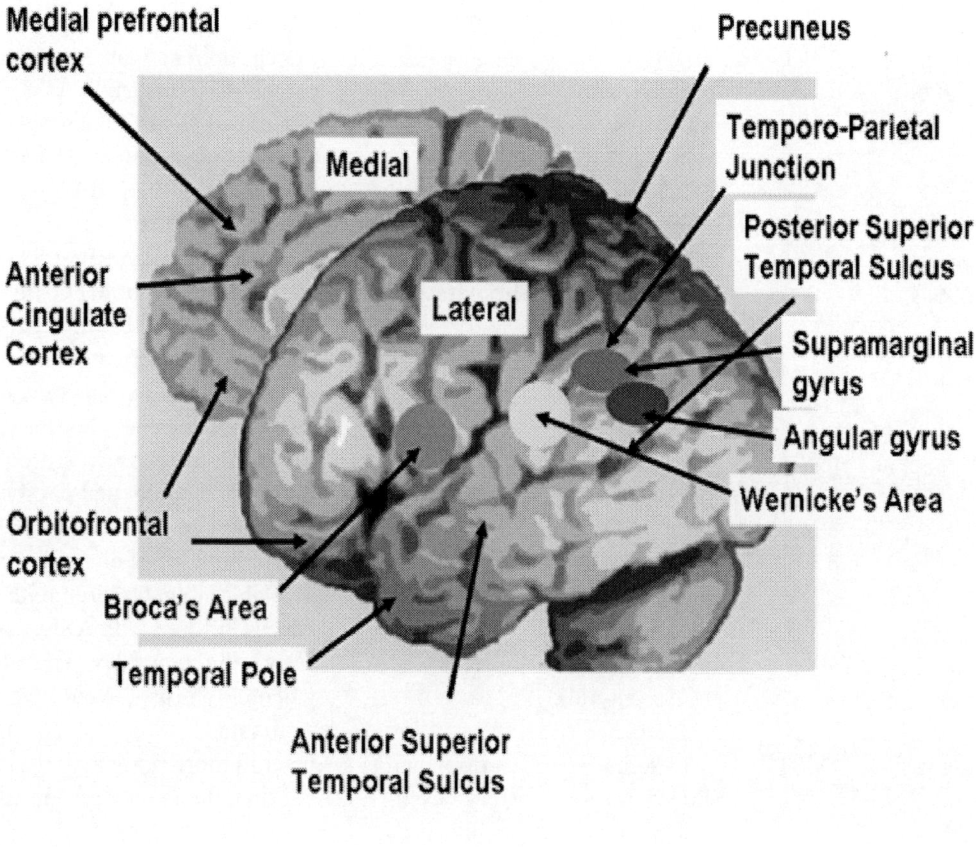

Figure 1.

Table 1. Developmental neuroimaging studies of ToM and related social/ cognitive functions (selected studies in ascending Order by Year of Publication)

Authors (Year)	Imaging Method	Subject	Task	Main Findings
Ohnishi, et al. (2004)	fMRI	11 children (7-13 yrs-old)	Video of hands grasping some objects (imitation). Animation of intentional movement of geometric figures (ToM).	ToM condition activated right mPFC, bilateral STG, right SMG, right MTG, right TP, right FG, bilateral MOG, and left cerebellum. Both imitation and ToM conditions activated bilateral MTG, right STG, bilateral MOG, and bilateral FG.
Liu (2005)	ERP	24 adults and 41 children (5-7 yrs-old)	Animation based first-order TB and FB task	Increasing localization in the left frontal region from child-passers to adults. More diffused bilateral frontal activity in children than in adults.
Dapretto, et al. (2006)	fMRI	10 TD children and 10 children with ASD (12-13 years-old)	Facial imitation task	TD children activated more right precentral gyrus, right ACC, bilateral IFG, insula, amygdala, hippocampus, caudate, putamen, and thalamus than children with ASD.
Wang, et al. (2006a)	fMRI	12 Adults (23-33 yrs-old) and 12 children (9-14 yrs-old)	Cartoon based Irony task	Children activated Right STG, bilateral IFG, right MFG, right STS, and left mPFC more than adults. Adults activated more posterior brain regions (e.g., visual cortex) than children.
Wang, et al. (2006b)	fMRI	18 children/ adolescents with ASD (7-17 yrs-old) and 18 TD children/ adolescents (8-16 yrs-old)	Story-based irony task	TD children activated more right IFG (when contextual cues were available) and bilateral STS (when both types of cues were available) than children with ASD. Children with ASD activated temporal regions more when only prosodic cues were available.
Kobayashi, et al. (2007a)	fMRI	16 Adults (18-40 yrs-old) and 12 children (8-12 yrs-old)	Cartoon and story based second-order FB task	Overall more brain activity in children than adults. Both Adults and children activated right IPL and TPJ. Adults activated ToM areas (e.g., TPJ) during the story condition, but children activated these areas during the cartoon ToM condition.

Table 1. (Continued)

Authors (Year)	Imaging Method	Subject	Task	Main Findings
Kobayashi, et al. (2007b)	fMRI	12 American and 12 Japanese children (8-12 yrs-old)	Cartoon and story based second-order FB task	Both American children and Japanese bilingual children activated bilateral vmPFC.
Moriguchi, et al. (2007)	fMRI	16 children/ adolescents (9-16 yrs old)	Animation of intentional movement of geometric figures.	Age related positive correlation in the dorsal mPFC, and negative correlation in the ventral mPFC.

Abbreviations: ACC = anterior cingulate cortex, FG = fusiform gyrus, IFG = inferior frontal gyrus, IPL = inferior parietal lobule, MFG = middle frontal gyrus, MOG = middle occipital gyrus, mPFC = medial prefrontal cortex, MTG = middle temporal gyrus, OFC = orbito-frontal cortex, SMG = supramarginal gyrus, STG = superior temporal gyrus, STS = superior temporal sulcus, TP = temporal pole, TPJ = temporo-parietal junction, vmPFC = ventro-medial prefrontal cortex; AS = Asperger's syndrome, ASD = autism spectrum disorder, HFA = high functioning autism, TD = typically developing

Despite a long period of obloquy, the Whorfian hypothesis has recently been revived following several new findings from cross-cultural/linguistic studies that have shown some influences of culture/language on people's representations of conceptual properties [e.g., Boroditsky, 2001; Bowerman & Choi, 2003; Brown & Levinson, 1993; Choi & Bowerman, 1991; Lucy, 1992]. Although certain aspects of cognition may precede language, as shown in studies of prelinguistic infants [McDonough, Choi, & Mandler, 2003; Hespos & Spelke, 2004], our cognition or thoughts may be influenced strongly by the language we speak throughout development. However, the biological underpinnings of the linguistic influence on thoughts have been unknown. A few recent neuroimaging studies exploring linguistic influence on arithmetic ability were the first to present evidence that language may influence one's cognition at the neural level [Dehaene et al., 1999; Venkatraman et al., 2006]. Likewise, our group's findings on American and Japanese adults and children have supported the Whorfian hypothesis by demonstrating some influence of language on the neural bases of ToM [Kobayashi, Glover, & Temple, 2006; 2007b]. In addition, several recent neuroimaging studies in children found activity in several "language regions" [Brauer & Friederici, 2007; Price, 2000] including the superior temporal gyrus (STG) and/or inferior frontal gyrus (IFG) while children processed ToM or related social/cognitive tasks [Dapretto et al., 2006; Kobayashi, Glover, & Temple, 2007a; 2007b; Moriguchi et al., 2007; Ohnishi et al., 2004; Wang et al., 2006a; 2006b]. For instance, in our group's study, children activated the STG while they processed verbal FB task, yet adults activated the same region while they processed nonverbal FB task [Kobayashi et al., 2007a]. These results suggest that language influences ToM throughout development.

Despite the increasing evidence that supports the developmental relationship between language and various cognitive capacities (including ToM), current developmental theories of ToM (except one) discount the linguistic effects on ToM and its neural basis. In this chapter, I first discuss some of the prominent theories of ToM development and whether evidence from the neuroimaging studies of ToM (including ours) supports these theories. Especially, my focus is on "Linguistic determinism" hypothesis of ToM [de Villiers, 2000]. I then review literature on the developmental relationship between language and ToM and its neural basis. I then discuss the possible interactions between brain areas associated with language processing and ToM candidate regions. Finally, I present a new model for the developmental mechanism of ToM.

FOUR THEORIES OF ToM DEVELOPMENT

The developmental mechanism of ToM has been investigated with a plethora of paradigms by many researchers. There are four primary theories of ToM development; "Modular", "Theory-theory", "Simulation", and "Linguistic determinism". Each of the four theories was developed mainly to account for the results of the FB task performance; failure in normally-developing 3-year-old children and older children with autism, and successful performance in 4-year-old children.

Modular ToM Theory

Since Fodor's highly influential book, "The Modularity of Mind" (1983) was published, the 'modular' view has become influential in cognitive science. According to Fodor's view, the architecture of each of our sensory (and some of our cognitive) functions can be best described as modular in the sense that it is: (1) informationally encapsulated, (2) unconscious, (3) fast, (4) has shallow outputs, (5) involves obligatory firing, (6) localized, (7) domain specific, and (8) ontogenetically and pathologically universal. This highly nativistic point of view has been supported by several ToM researchers, though not in a purely Fodorian sense. A main advocate of modular ToM, Leslie describes ToM as maturing serially in three steps during the course of development. The first one is termed 'theory of body mechanism' (ToBy), which matures around 4 months of age and embodies the infant's theory of physical objects. At this stage, the infant formulates a primary theory about the mechanical movement of objects, but is not capable of associating the animation with the 'Agent', nor can he/she distinguish the intentionality of the 'Agent' from mere physical force. The next one, 'theory of mind mechanism 1' (ToMM1), matures around 8 months of age and confers upon the infant a new knowledge that the 'Agent' has to have some intention to move the objects. The sequence completes when a more adult-like ToM, dubbed 'theory of mind mechanism 2' (ToMM2), matures around 18 months of age and enables the toddler to formulate 'propositional attitudes' such as "she believes/pretends/thinks that …" [Leslie, 1992; 1994]. According to Leslie, the reason why 3-year-olds fail the FB task is not due to any impairments in the core ToMM module, but due to immature 'selection processing' (SP) mechanism which is domain-general (unlike ToMM which is domain-specific) and functions like an inhibitory control. He argues that older children with autism are impaired in ToM not because of any damage in the SP part, but because of some dysfunction in the ToMM module [Roth & Leslie, 1998] and this component of ToM comprises the specific innate basis of

ToM. Modular hypothesis has recently found some robust support from a series of 'habituation' experiments in infants. These experiments have shown that non-verbal FB tasks can be passed even by 15 month-old infants [Onishi & Baillargeon, 2005, Southgate, Senju, & Csibra, 2007; Surian, Caldi, & Sperber, 2007]. These studies support the main tenet of modular hypothesis; innate basis of ToM. They, however, were criticized because they failed to show why the reality-bias seen in 3 years-olds was not seen in the infants that they tested and that infants may be doing three-way association among agent, object, and place without any FB understanding [Perner & Ruffman, 2005].

In terms of neural bases of ToM, the modular hypothesis of ToM predicts that ToM is represented in a highly circumscribed brain region [Gallagher & Frith, 2003]. However, neuroimaging studies of ToM and autism have presented mixed results regarding this prediction. On the one hand, many ToM imaging studies utilizing a variety of ToM paradigms have consistently implicated the mPFC [Brunet et al., 2000; Fletcher et al., 1995; Gallagher et al., 2000; Gallagher et al., 2002; Goel et al., 1995; Happé et al., 1996; Kobayashi et al., 2006; Vogeley et al., 2001; see also Frith & Frith, 2003, for a review], indicating some modularity in ToM. On the other hand, structural brain imaging studies on autism alone found abnormalities (usually increases/decreases in volume) in more than 14 brain regions that are widely distributed [Brambilla et al., 2003]. Although the amygdala is most often found to be structurally abnormal in individuals with autism [Schultz, Romanski, & Tsatsanis, 2000], only a few functional brain imaging studies of ToM implicated this region for ToM (e.g., Baron-Cohen, Ring, et al., 1999). The increasing evidence suggests that autism is not a modular but a distributed disorder involving functionally connected multiple brain regions [Müller, 2007]. Moreover, it has become increasingly likely that none of the candidate ToM areas are specialized for ToM or *mentalizing* [Frith & Frith, 2003] per se. For instance, it has been shown that the medial prefrontal area is also involved in reading emotional cues [Gusnard et al., 2001; Lane et al., 1997], social norm transgression [Berthoz et al., 2002], and finding coherence in stories [Ferstl & von Cramon, 2002].

Another prediction of the modular ToM hypothesis is that since ToM is relatively unchanging throughout the development (after 18 months), children's neural bases of ToM would be very similar to adults' [Fodor, 1983; Scholl & Leslie, 1999]. However, evidence from several recent brain imaging studies of developmental neural basis of ToM argues against this prediction. For instance, Liu (2005) found more diffused bilateral frontal activity in children than adults who showed more localized left frontal activity during the animation-based FB task. Similarly, in our study, children activated many more brain regions than adults during the ToM condition relative to the baseline [Kobayashi et al., 2007a]. Moriguchi et al. (2007) has also found an age related positive correlation in the dorsal mPFC area, but a negative correlation in the ventral mPFC area. Moreover, examining neural basis of irony in adults and children, Wang et al. (2006a) found more robust activity in the prefrontal areas in children than in adults, who activated posterior brain regions more during the irony relative to the control conditions. These results seem to argue against the main prediction of the 'modular' hypothesis of ToM: ToM is innate and relatively unchanging throughout development, and so, there should be little variation between adults and children in the neural bases of ToM. Thus, the results from the developmental neuroimaging studies of ToM do not seem to lend support to the strict 'modular' theory of ToM.

Nonetheless, one thing that the 'modular' ToM theory (but not others) explains well is the relationship between the executive function (or inhibitory control) and ToM. Although the neuro-functional relationship between the executive function and ToM is still controversial [see Saxe, Carey, and Kanwisher, 2004 and Kain & Perner, 2005 for reviews], several brain imaging studies of ToM (including ours) have implicated the DLPFC (i.e., a brain region often implicated in the neuroimaging studies of executive function) [Baron-Cohen, Ring, et al., 1999; Brunet et al., 2000; Kobayashi, Glover, & Temple, 2006; Sanfey et al., 2003]. Thus, neurological evidence may at least support the domain-general SP part of this hypothesis.

Theory-Theory ToM

The 'Theory-theory' hypothesis of ToM has been developed as an alternative to the 'modular ToM' view, which Wellman and his colleagues describe as being 'anti-developmental' (Wellman, Cross, & Watson, 2001). This hypothesis posits that the adults' version of ToM, *folk psychology*, is drastically different from the children's version because we revise our ToM theory many times throughout life just as a scientist revises his/her theory based upon alternative empirical evidence. They further argue that ToM is essentially a dynamic process: it is subject to revision depending upon our individual experiences [Gopnic and Wellman, 1992]. Although the theory-theorists agree that some innate modules or 'core' structures exist for ToM, they contend that these structures are subject to extensive revisions throughout one's life, whereas the modularists insist that those 'core' modules do not change [Wellman, Cross, & Watson, 2001]. According to this theory, the reason why 2-year-olds fail the FB task is that they do not have the concept of 'belief,' which develops only sometime after the third birthday when other epistemic concepts (e.g., 'knowing' and 'thinking') become available along with lexical expansion [Bartsch & Wellman, 1995]. Evidence from a meta-analysis of more than 100 ToM studies seems to support the 'theory-theory' hypothesis: it has failed to show early ToM competence in children younger than 3 years of age, but has shown instead a significant covariation between age and ToM performance.

Until recently, there has been no neurological evidence to support or reject this hypothesis, as there has been no brain imaging studies of ToM development. The results of a few recent developmental brain imaging studies seem to support this hypothesis because these studies have found clear age-related differences in several brain regions involved in ToM and related socio-cognitive functions [Liu, 2005; Kobayashi et al. 2007a; Moriguchi et al., 2007; Wang et al., 2006a]. These results support the theory-theorists' main tenet: some major differences exist between adults' ToM (a.k.a., *folk psychology*) and children's ToM, which develops throughout life. These studies provide some initial evidence for significant changes in the neural basis of ToM and related social cognition between the first 10 years of childhood and adulthood [Liu, 2005; Kobayashi et al., 2007a; Moriguchi et al., 2007; Wang et al., 2006a]. Interestingly, the majority of these studies [Kobayashi et al., 2007a; Moriguchi et al., 2007; Wang et al., 2006a] did not find any behavioral differences between the age groups in the FB/irony task performance. This implies that the changes that may occur in the neural basis underlying ToM throughout development may not directly affect ToM performance but that children's way of understanding ToM may be different from adults'. In addition, Wang et al. (2006a) suggested that the developmental change reflects increasing automatization of ToM/irony understanding as people age.

One notable difference between adults and children in the ToM related brain activity found in our study is that even though both adults and children activated the mPFC, children activated more ventral mPFC areas than adults [Kobayashi et al., 2007b]. Similarly, an event related-potential (ERP) experiment found more activity in ventral prefrontal area in 6 years-old children during the animation-based FB than the control condition [Liu et al., 2005]. Moreover, in Moriguchi et al's (2007) study, a significant positive correlation between ToM related dorsal mPFC activity and age was found. In the vmPFC the relationship was reversed: the activity decreased as age progressed. It has been suggested that the dorsal cingulate area is primarily dedicated to cognitive aspects of behaviors while the ventral cingulate area is more dedicated to emotional aspects of behaviors [see Bush, Luu, & Postner, 2000, for a review]. In line with these results, an ERP study [Sabbagh, 2004] found vmPFC/orbito-frontal activity while their subjects encoded others' emotions from eye gazes, but dorsal mPFC activity when they engaged in the cognition-based standard ToM task. These results suggest that ToM may require more emotional processing for children but more cognitive processing for adults. These results also seem to fit well with the Theory-theorists' prediction that more emotion-laden 'desire'-based ToM understanding precedes more cognition-laden 'belief'-based ToM understanding in development [Bartsch & Wellman, 1995].

Simulation ToM

A third theory, 'simulation' ToM theory, posits that people do not use any naïve theories of psychology when predicting and explaining the behaviors of others [Goldman, 1989; Harris, 1992]. The Simulationists agree that ToM development depends upon conceptual development, but they argue that the concepts are derived from a child's own direct experience of such states, rather than through some abstract theorizing. When explaining others' mental states, the child uses his/her own mental states as a model, very much like putting his/her mind into others' shoes [Harris, 1991, 1992].

Simulation theory has recently been embraced with enthusiasm by neurologists and cognitive scientists following the discovery of the 'mirror neuron' system [Fogassi et al., 2005; Iacoboni, 2005]. Robust activity in the mirror regions has been found in several studies that tested imitation [Decety et al., 1997; Iacoboni, 2005], discrimination of 'self' from 'other' [Decety & Chaminade, 2004], and reading of others' intentions [Burgess, Quayle, & Frith, 2001; Iacoboni et al., 2005). For example, significant brain activity in these areas was found when monkeys engaged in a task in which they had to infer an experimenter's intentions [Fogassi et al., 2005). Several brain imaging studies on human adults also found significant activity in the inferior parietal regions (i.e., a part of the mirror neuron system) while their subjects engaged in imitation tasks [Decety et al., 1997; Chaminade & Decety, 2002; Nakamura et al., 2004]. It has been suggested that these lower-levels of ToM processing (e.g., understanding intentions of others and imitation) form bases for higher-order ToM (e.g., inferring from others' beliefs) [Meltzoff & Brooks, 2001].

However, whether or not the 'mirror neuron' system is involved in higher-order ToM such as FB reasoning is still controversial. The major reasons are that the mirror neuron regions (the inferior parietal lobule [IPL] and inferior frontal gyrus [IFG]) are not commonly implicated as ToM candidate areas, and that the FB task requires subjects to identify reasons for the behavior and to predict the next action. 'Reasoning' is more than just 'decoding' in that it involves prediction of behavior based on the person's past mental states in addition to the capacity to attribute current mental states to others [Nichols & Stich, 2003; Sabbagh,

2004]. This reasoning might require some abstract theorizing, not only the detection of intentions through the 'simulation'. Another criticism of the simulation theory is that simulation theory cannot account for errors that people often make about their own mental state judgment [see Saxe, 2005, for a review].

A recent neuroimaging study that tested social norm violation within the person's own culture or others' culture did not support this theory [Saxe & Wexler, 2005]. Subjects employed the right TPJ more when the stories were about norm-violation within their own cultures than when they were about the same norm-violation in other cultures. These results argue against the main prediction of 'simulation' theory: other minds are represented fundamentally in terms of their similarity to the person's own mind. Our study with adults and children, however, found some support for this theory by showing convergent activity in the IPL for both cartoon- and story-based ToM tasks [Kobayashi et al., 2007a]. Similarly, Wang et al. (2006a) found a greater activity in the IFG area in children than in adults. One explanation of these results may be that mirror neuron regions are important for children (more than for adults) because these regions are involved in lower and implicit level of ToM processing. Taken together, these results may indicate that the human mirror neuron system may be involved in lower-level ToM processing (e.g., detection of intentions) that does not require higher-level abstract theorizing or reasoning behind the action.

Another point of contention involves the definition of ToM and empathy. While simulation process is often thought of as synonymous with the empathy (which is defined as an ability to identify another person's emotions and thoughts, and to respond to these with an appropriate emotion [Baron-Cohen, 2003; Wheelwright et al., 2006]), ToM and empathy may be different functionally as well as neuro-psychologically [Singer, 2006]. ToM has been conceptualized as the cognitive component of an empathizing system, the residual component being affective empathy [Chakrabarti & Baron-Cohen, 2006; Davis, 1994]. It is clear that affective empathy is not required in the type of ToM tasks used in many neuroimaging studies of ToM. It has been suggested that affective empathy and ToM tasks, especially FB tasks, may tap different psychological capacities. Specifically, affective empathy may be more related to the ability to infer and react to the emotions of others whereas ToM may be more narrowly related to reading the intentions and beliefs of others [Singer, 2006]. However, neuroimaging research using paradigms that tapped empathy has found brain activity in the candidate ToM regions (i.e., mPFC and ACC) [Jackson et al., 2006; Jackson et al., 2005; Lamm et al., 2007; Völlm et al., 2006]. These results suggest that there may not be a clear psychological boundary between empathizing and ToM and that at least in some brain regions these two have functional overlaps [see Oberman & Ramachandran, 2007]. Future research will have to investigate further details of these different levels of processing and neural networks involved in each.

A final but important point is that there is no direct evidence of the human mirror neurons that are homologous to the machaque brain. While it is easy to assume that humans have the same mirror neurons as the monkeys, there is no direct evidence of human mirror neurons that respond to action [Agnew, Bhakoo, and Puri, 2007]. Thus, the association among human mirror neuron, simulation and ToM remains speculative until further anatomical as well as functional characterizations are done.

Linguistic Determinism of ToM

Despite the observation that the FB reasoning seems to rely upon some verbal ability, all of the above theories of ToM (except the 'theory-theory' to a limited extent) downplay the contribution of linguistic ability to ToM development. The last of the four main theories of ToM emphasizes this component of ToM and is called 'linguistic determinism' [de Villiers, 2000; de Villiers and de Villiers, 2000]. These theorists follow the Whorfian theory of language and cognition, positing that ToM develops as language develops in children. A strong form of this hypothesis proposes that linguistic (primarily syntactic and semantic) ability constrains ToM ability. Main advocates of this hypothesis, de Villiers and her colleagues maintain that a sophisticated command of syntax, or more precisely, complement, is necessary for FB task understanding [de Villiers, 2000]. They argue that 3-year-olds fail the FB task because their syntactic commands are not fully developed to handle the propositions embedded in the sentences of the FB task. De Villiers and her colleagues tested 3-4 years-old children for FB and syntactic ability, and found correlation between the two [de Villiers, 2000]. Moreover, a longitudinal study [Astington & Jenkins, 1999] has found that earlier language (syntax and semantics) ability predicts later ToM performance and not vice versa, indicating that language competence is a prerequisite for competitive ToM performance. In addition, Morgan and Kegl's (2006) study on Nicaraguan Sign Language (NSL) signers supported the linguistic determinism in that the early signers (who had been exposed to the NSL before the first 10 years of age) did better in the ToM task than late signers (who had been exposed to the NSL after the first 10 years of age). Another source of evidence for the linguistic determinism hypothesis comes from studies on children with Asperger syndrome (AS) and high-functioning autism (HFA). These children are known to have relatively intact language skills (despite being impaired in social skills as much as children with low-functioning autism) and they both pass the standard first-order FB task somewhat easily compared to children with low-functioning autism [Landa, 2000]. Others have found that the understanding of 'belief' terms predicts the performance level of FB tasks in children with autism [Ziatas, Durkin, & Pratt, 1998].

As described above, strong linguistic determinists emphasize the contribution of the command in syntax to ToM. However, there is another version of 'linguistic determinism' which emphasizes the contribution of communicative development and the role of socio-cultural experience for ToM. This alternative version stresses non-theoretical, direct interpersonal or social knowledge for ToM understanding [Hobson, 1991; Tomasello, 2003]. Although the proponents of this weaker version of 'linguistic determinism' are in agreement with the idea that language plays a major role in ToM, they argue that language does not constrain ToM development. Their focus is more on culture-specific socio-communicative aspects than constitutive aspects of language and therefore follows the Vygotskyan tradition more closely. A few studies have supported this second version by demonstrating that performance on a FB task is improved by discussing perspectives on the same objects or events with others without any use of the sentential complements [Lohman & Tomasello, 2003; Harris, 2005].

It has been found that children/adolescents with HFA and AS pass the FB task [Baron-Cohen, O'Riordan, et al., 1999], presumably being helped by their more advanced language skills than children/adolescents with low functioning autism [Tager-Flusberg, 2000]. But the fact that children/adolescents with HFA/AS show little understanding of Faux Pass sentences

[Baron-Cohen, O'Riordan, et al., 1999] and irony (Leekam & Prior, 1994] indicates that the help of syntax for ToM in HFA/AS population is limited to non-inferential reasoning. Given that understanding of ToM requires inferential skill to go beyond the literal meaning and to read communicative intent of others [Sperber & Wilson, 2002], the higher-order ToM task performance in children/adolescents with HFA/AS may be constrained by the pragmatic aspects (i.e., reading communicative intentions and inferential reasoning) of language. Taken together, these results seem to support the second version of linguistic determinism suggesting that language is important for ToM not because of the syntactic aspects but because of the inferential/pragmatic aspects.

Relationship Between Language and ToM Development: Evidence from Neurological Studies of ToM

Neurological studies that examined the relationship between neural correlates of ToM and those of language have obtained mixed results similar to what behavioral studies have found. On the one hand, a severe aphasic patient, who had a wide-range of left hemisphere damage, showed intact performance in some nonverbal ToM tasks, despite failing all other syntax-related tasks [Varley & Siegal, 2000]. On the other hand, evidence suggests that processing of pragmatically coherent sentences also recruits the mPFC area primarily [Fersl & von Cramon, 2002]. Ours is the first study to compare the effects of language/culture on ToM development, and our results are consistent with this hypothesis. We found clear cultural/linguistic effects on the neural bases of ToM [Kobayashi et al., 2006; 2007b], and at least the cultural effects had little to do with syntax (as both cultural groups saw exactly the same cartoons). Thus, both behavioral and brain imaging results seem to support the notion that language is important for ToM not because of its constitutive aspects (i.e. syntax and semantics) but because of its pragmatic aspects.

Do We Use "Language" Regions of the Brain for ToM?

Consistent with the second version of 'linguistic determinism' of ToM, in several recent developmental studies of ToM and related social/cognitive functions, children employed some of the "language" regions for processing the story-based [Kobayashi et al., 2007a; 2007b; Wang et al., 2006b] and/or the cartoon/animation-based tasks [Dapretto et al., 2006; Kobayashi et al., 2007a; 2007b; Moriguchi et al., 2007; Ohnishi et al., 2004; Wang et al., 2006a]. In addition, a study found some interference on the FB reasoning by verbal shadowing in adults [Newton & de Villiers, 2007]. These results suggest that adults process ToM more verbally than children and ToM develops as "language regions" develop.

The classical language regions encompass Broca's area or Brodmann area (BA) 44/45 in the IFG, Wernicke's area or BA 22 in the STG, and the angular gyrus and supramarginal gyrus (SMG) [Carter, 1998]. Thanks to new findings from brain imaging studies on various linguistic processing, there is now a broad consensus that syntactic processes are subserved by the left STG and the IFG (specifically, BA 44 and frontal operculum [FO]) in adults [Bornkessel et al., 2005; Friederici et al., 2003; Moro et al., 2001]. Semantic processes, in contrast, are supported by the left middle temporal gyrus (MTG), the SMG, and BA 45/47 in the IFG in adults [Kotz et al., 2002; Poldrack et al., 1999]. Brain imaging studies of language in children or on development are still too scarce to reach a broad agreement on the specialization of those linguistic processes in the different areas of the brain. But increasing evidence suggests that language is less lateralized and involves broader regions in children than in adults [Brauer & Friederici, 2007]. Thus, in this chapter, I consider right hemisphere homologues of the aforementioned brain regions as language regions (in addition to the left hemisphere language regions). In what follows, I will discuss some of the major functions of the language regions, and whether or not ToM studies indicate involvement of those language regions in ToM development.

Inferior Frontal Gyrus

Traditionally, IFG or the Broca's area (see **Figure 1**) has been thought to be specialized for syntactic processing and speech [see Price, 2000, for a review]. In neuroimaging studies, the anterior portion of the left IFG (BA 47 and FO) has been implicated in semantic processing [see Poldrack et al., 1999, for a review] and the posterior left IFG (BA 44/45) for syntactical processing [Bookheimer, 2002; Dapretto & Bookheimer, 1999] as well as phonological processing, such as phoneme monitoring or rhyme judgments [Poldrack et al., 1999; Roskies et al., 2001; Temple et al., 2003]. In addition, the bilateral IFG (BA 45/47) activity was found when children processed semantics [Brauer & Friederici, 2007; Chou et al., 2006] and syntax [Brauer & Friederici, 2007] in sentential level.

In terms of the involvement of the IFG area in the ToM development, several neuroimaging studies in children found activity in the IFG while the child participants engaged in facial imitation [Dapretto et al., 2006], story- and cartoon-based irony [Wang et al., 2006a; 2006b] and ToM [Kobayashi et al., 2007a; Moriguchi et al., 2007] tasks. We found a three-way interaction in the left IFG (BA 45) for children and adults [Kobayashi, Glover, & Temple, 2007a]. Children employed this area more for the cartoon ToM condition, yet the adults used this area more for the story ToM condition. Similarly, in Wang et al.'s (2006a) study on irony processing, children recruited the left IFG (BA 44 and 45) more than adults. Moriguchi et al. (2007) also found activity in the right IFG (BA 45) when children/adolescents processed animation-based ToM task. These results may suggest that the IFG is important for ToM processing especially during childhood because of its role as a language center.

However, the fact that some of the developmental ToM brain imaging studies found the IFG activity during the nonverbal tasks [Kobayashi, Glover, & Temple, 2007a; Moriguchi et al., 2007] may indicate that IFG is important for ToM development because of its involvement in inhibitory control. Increasing evidence suggests that bilateral IFG is selectively involved in working memory-related response inhibition [Bunge et al., 2002; Garavan et al., 1999; see also Aron, Robbins, & Poldrack, 2004, for a review]. The greater activity in this area may represent a greater effort to inhibit the immediate and more salient (but wrong) responses in the ToM/irony stories/cartoons in children than in adults.

Another alternative interpretation is that the IFG plays an important role in processing ToM during childhood because of the human mirror neurons that are localized in this area [Agnew, Bhakoo, & Puri, 2007; Oberman & Ramachandran, 2007; Saxe, 2005]. In line with this conjuncture, several adult brain imaging studies implicated this area in nonverbal imitation [Buccino et al., 2004; Grèzes, Frith, & Passingham, 2004; Heiser et al., 2003] and ToM [Brunet et al., 2000; German et al., 2004; Kobayashi et al., 2007a]. The IFG activity in children during the nonverbal ToM [Kobayashi et al., 2007a; Moriguchi et al., 2007] and related social cognitive tasks [Dapretto et al., 2006; Wang et al., 2006b] may support this hypothesis given that nonverbal tasks do not usually involve language processing. However, since adults especially seem to process nonverbal ToM tasks verbally [Kobayashi et al., 2007a; Newton & de Villiers, 2007] and since the mirror neuron system is closely associated with language system in humans [Gallese, 2007; Oberman & Ramachandran, 2007; Siegal & Varley, 2002], future studies need to examine precisely to how much extent the human mirror neuron system is involved in ToM and language development.

Middle Temporal Gyrus

The left MTG has been implicated in processing visually-processed semantic knowledge [Binder et al., 1997; Kotz et al., 2002; Vandenverghe et al., 1996; see also Price, 2000, for a review]. The right homologous area has also been implicated in semantic and lexical analyses [Newman et al., 2001; Sevostianov et al., 2002; Tracy et al., 2003]. Moreover, this region has been suggested to be involved in a process of converting pictures to words [Sevostianov et al., 2002]. In addition, a recent neuroimaging study in children implicated the left MTG in sentential semantic processing [Chou et al., 2006].

Several recent neuroimaging studies of ToM and related social cognition studies in children implicated this area [Kobayashi, 2007; Moriguchi et al., 2007; Onishi et al., 2004; Wang et al., 2006a]. A few studies found bilateral [Onishi et al., 2004] or left MTG activity [Moriguchi et al., 2007] during animation-based ToM conditions in children/adolescents relative to control conditions. In our study, Japanese children showed more activity in the left MTG during the cartoon ToM condition, yet Japanese adults showed more activity in the same area during the story ToM condition [Kobayashi, 2007]. Similarly, in Wang et al. (2006a), adults used this area more for processing the cartoon-based irony task than children. Thus, children may use the MTG area more for the visual-based ToM and other related social cognition tasks because they try harder to convert the meanings of the cartoons/animations into words and sentences.

Superior Temporal Gyrus

The STG at/around Wernicke's area (see **Figure 1**) has been originally associated with speech comprehension [Wernicke, 1874]. Sitting anterior to Wernicke's area, the primary auditory cortex (BA 22) processes various auditory input including music [Koelsch, 2005; Koelsch et al., 2005; Limb et al., 2006] and speech or heard word comprehension [Pekkola et al., 2006; Patel, Bowman, & Rilling, 2006; Rimol, Specht, & Hugdahl, 2006]. There is now a broad consensus that in the adult brain, the STG is primarily involved in syntactic processing [Bornkessel et al., 2005; Friederici et al., 2003; Moro et al., 2001]. In the child brain, however, the STG activity was found for both syntactic and semantic aspects of the language [Brauer & Friederici, 2007].

The STG is not among the ToM regions (see **Figure 1**; see also Frith and Frith [2003], and Saxe, Carey, and Kanwisher [2004] for reviews). However, a few recent imaging studies have implicated the right STG area for some functions that may be related to ToM: i.e., empathy mapping through facial and hand-gesture imitations [Leslie, Johnson-Frey, & Grafton, 2004] and reading eye-gaze directions [Akiyama et al., 2006]. Also, increasing evidence from neurobiological studies suggests that the STG has reciprocal connections with both the mPFC area and the parahippocampal gyrus [see Price, 2005 for a review]. Onishi et al. (2004) found activity in the bilateral STG area when 7-13 year-old children processed animation-based ToM tasks. In our study, we found story and cartoon task-specific interaction in the left STG between the American adult and child groups: adults used this area more for the cartoon ToM condition, while children used this area more for processing the story ToM condition [Kobayashi, 2007a]. Similarly, Wang et al. (2006a) found a greater activity in the right STG in children while they processed the cartoon-based irony task than in adults.

It has been shown that language processing tasks normally recruit the left hemisphere, but processing of pragmatics employs the right hemisphere [Paradis, 1998]. Also, results of a few studies have indicated that processing of story-based FB tasks is like processing pragmatically coherent sentences [Ferstl & von Carmon, 2002; Siegal, Carrington, & Radel, 1996]. Thus, our speculation is that children use this area more than adults for understanding pragmatics in the ToM (and related socio-cognitive) stories more than adults do.

Supramarginal Gyrus and Angular Gyrus

The SMG and angular gyrus are adjacent to each other (see **Figure 1**). Both of these regions have been implicated in some aspects of language processing. Although the 19th century language model has described these areas as being specialized for visual word form processing, they are now considered as a part of a more general semantic analysis network [see Price, 2000]. For instance, in some silent reading studies these areas became activated when the subjects read meaningful sentences [Bottini et al., 1994; Bavelier et al., 1997]. In children, however, activity in the SMG was found during the syntactic (rather than semantic) violation in the sentences [Brauer & Friederici, 2007].

The TPJ area that has been implicated in the more recent brain imaging studies of ToM (Saxe & Kanwisher, 2003; Saxe & Wexler, 2005; Kobayashi, Glover, & Temple, 2007a] may include these areas if we consider it as a region with 10 or more square-centimeter surface as suggested by Saxe (2006). Most of the ToM neuroimaging studies that have implicated the TPJ area have used story-based tasks [Gallagher et al., 2000; Kobayashi, Glover, & Temple, 2007a; Saxe & Kanwisher, 2003; Saxe & Wexler, 2005]. Therefore, it is possible that the TPJ-SMG/angular gyrus network is recruited for ToM processing especially when the task requires some sentential semantic/syntactic analyses.

Alternatively, as the TPJ, these areas may be involved in 'self' and 'other' distinction. The SMG area, especially the right SMG, has been implicated in anosognosia, asomatognosia, or somatoparaphrenia,that occur after the brain injury [Feinberg, 2000; Berlucchi & Aglioti, 1997]. A hallmark of these psychiatric conditions is the lack of self-awareness and body knowledge [see Decety & Grèzes, 2006, for a review]. Besides our study, Ohnishi et al. (2004) implicated this area in nonverbal ToM in children using a geometric figures task. Since, in their experiment children were asked to indicate what they thought the central figures (e.g., triangles) were doing, their task might have tapped the distinction between 'self' (i.e., the central figure) and 'other' (i.e., other figure) rather than ToM per se. Thus, the TPJ-SMG/angular gyrus network may also be recruited ToM for the 'self' and 'other' distinction.

DEVELOPMENT OF ToM NEURAL BASES

Several recent neuroimaging studies of ToM and related social and cognitive function suggested that children's neural bases of ToM are not entirely the same as adults' [Kobayashi et al., 2007a; 2007b; Liu, 2005; Moriguchi et al., 2007; Wang et al., 2006]. Moreover, results from several neuroimaging studies have suggested that maturation of the prefrontal cortex continues throughout childhood and late adolescence [Giedd et al., 1999; Gogtay et al., 2004; Sowell et al., 2003]. These results imply that development of ToM (and possibly other socio-cognitive functions) is a more gradual process than had been previously thought, and that it continues until even late adolescence.

In the remainder of the chapter, I present a developmental model of neural bases of ToM based, in part, on the evidence from those recent developmental ToM brain imaging studies. This model I present here describes a universal developmental trajectory of ToM neural bases.

LIMITATIONS OF FOUR THEORIES OF TOM DEVELOPMENT AND A NEW MODEL OF NEURAL BASES OF TOM DEVELOPMENT

As I have described above, several recent developmental neuroimaging studies of ToM suggest that children's neural bases of ToM are different from adults' [Kobayashi, Glover, & Temple, 2007a; 2007b; Liu, 2005; Moriguchi et al., 2007; Wang et al., 2006] universally [Kobayashi, 2007]. The modality-specific age-related interactions found in our study are especially interesting. Children activated ToM regions (i.e., bilateral TPJ) more during the cartoon ToM condition, yet adults activated the same regions more during the story ToM condition [Kobayashi et al., 2007a]. These results suggest children's ToM neural correlates are more tied to a visual modality while adults' ToM neural correlates are more tied to a verbal modality. These results further imply language may affect ToM throughout development.

As described earlier, there are four main hypotheses of ToM development; 'modular', 'linguistic determinism', 'simulation', and 'theory,-theory' hypotheses of ToM. Among these, the 'modular' and 'simulation' theories have been suggested to have support from neurological and neuroscience studies (see Frith and Frith [2003] for the 'modular' theory, and Saxe, Carey, and Kanwisher [2004] for the 'simulation' theory). The 'modular' theory predicts a highly circumscribed brain region that is specialized for ToM. A strong modular theory would predict that this region would not be involved in other tasks, that no other regions would be involved in ToM, there would be no change in this region across development, and that only this region would be damaged in autism. However, as described above, increasing evidence suggests that autism involves multiple and distributed brain regions [Müller, 2007]. In addition, also as described earlier, a few studies of ToM development found differences in ToM specific activity between adults and children, indicating that ToM module (if it exists) changes throughout development. The 'simulation' theory predicts that the mirror neuron system is the most important for ToM. The mirror neuron system, however, seems to play only a limited role for ToM (see above).

The proponents of the other two developmental theories of ToM have had no neurological evidence to support or refute their theories, primarily because of scarcity of neurological studies of ToM in children. A few neuroimaging studies of ToM and related social and cognitive functions in children begin to address some of the predictions these theories might make about the neural bases of ToM. Our [Kobayashi, Glover, & Temple, 2007a] and several others' [Liu et al., 2005; Moriguchi et al., 2007; Wang et al., 2006a] results support some aspects of the 'theory-theory' hypothesis. The 'theory-theory' (in opposition to the modular theory) would predict major differences between adults' *folk psychology* and children's ToM (Wellman, Cross, & Watson, 2001]. Consistent with that prediction, age-related differences in the neural bases of ToM and related social and cognitive functions have been found [Kobayashi, Glover, & Temple, 2007a; 2007b; Moriguchi et al., 2007; Wang et al., 2006a]. The 'theory-theory' would also predict that adults' ToM is based more on a cognition-laden 'belief' concept, whereas children's ToM is based more on an emotion-laden 'desire' concept [Bartch & Wellman, 1995]. Results from a few studies have also supported this notion, finding that children recruit the vmPFC more than the dorsal mPFC [Kobayashi, Glover, and Temple, 2007a; Liu et al., 2005; Moriguchi et al., 2007]. As described above, the ventral aspect of the ACC and mPFC has been hypothesized to be involved in emotional processing and the dorsal aspect in cognitive processing. As described above, recent findings from brain imaging studies in children have also supported aspects of the second version of the 'linguistic determinism' hypothesis of ToM, showing differential recruiting of language regions during ToM processing depending on age of the subjects and modality of the task (see **Table 1**). Thus, I have constructed a neural developmental model of ToM incorporating aspects of both of these hypotheses of ToM development. Although this model has limitations due to the limitations of our study (and of a few other developmental brain imaging studies on ToM and/or related social cognition) and scarcity of pediatric data in the ToM neuroimaging literature overall, it attempts to incorporate the findings that have been presented here.

I hypothesize that during childhood (before the age of 12), ToM understanding is more closely linked to understanding of emotions, and that young children employ the vmPFC or the ventral part of PFC to process the highly emotion-laden ToM (**Figure 2**). At this earlier stage, especially younger children may understand ToM more in terms of the 'desire' concept than through the 'belief' concept. During late childhood through adolescence, our linguistic ability continues to develop as various language brain regions (e.g., the IFG, MTG, STG, and angular gyrus) mature and language continues to influence ToM development during this time. Finally, in adulthood, ToM is understood in terms of the 'belief' concept, and the dorsal aspect of the mPFC is employed to understand the cognition-laden ToM. However, this model is subject to further empirical testing. It has been suggested that the dorsal mPFC activity is associated with various social-cognitions, while the ventral mPFC is associated with self-referential process [Mitchell, Banaji, & Macrae, 2005]. Thus, alternatively, the ventral-emotion versus dorsal-cognition dichotomy is a bi-product of socio-cognitive versus self-referential dichotomy. Future neuroimaging studies that will systematically test both children (especially children of ages between 3 and 5 during when ToM performance dramatically improves) and adults with either internally- or externally-directed 'desire'- and 'belief'-related tasks will be useful for examining how the activity in the different brain regions is associated with the development of different concepts related to ToM and the self-referential process. Further testing of children and adults with various language processing tasks in combination with those tasks will be helpful for examining precisely what aspects of language play the quintessential role for the conceptual development and ToM.

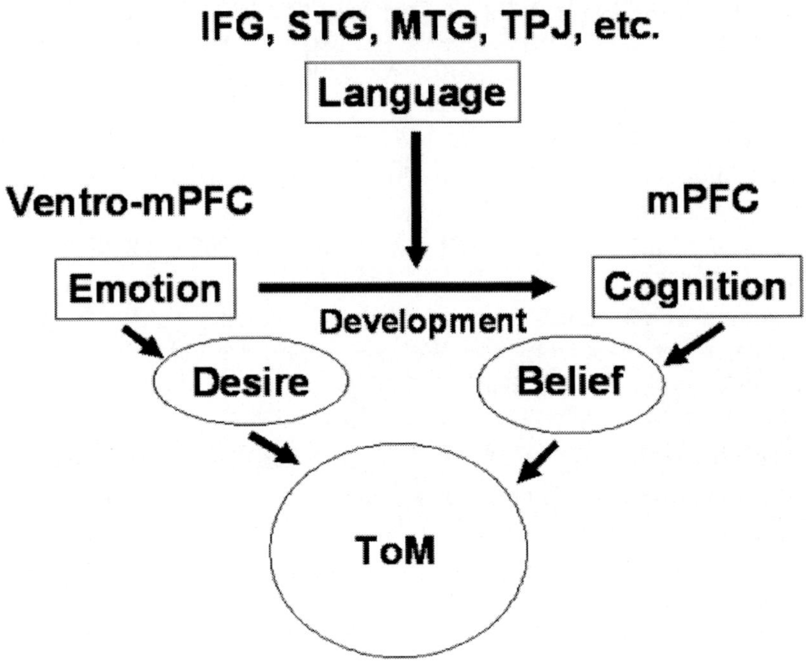

Figure 2.

Conclusion

To our knowledge, this is the first review to examine the neural correlates of ToM and other socio-cognitive functions in human development based on the most recent neuroimaging studies in children and adults for these functions. Increasing evidence suggests that neural correlates of ToM in children are different from those in adults and that ToM develops even throughout pre-pubertal childhood. These findings may also argue against 'modular' developmental hypothesis of ToM because this hypothesis predicts relatively unchanging innate ToM neural basis. 'Simulation' hypothesis of ToM has only a limited support from these recent results because of the limited involvement of the human mirror neuron regions (e.g., the IFG and IPL) in ToM processing. The new evidence also suggests that ToM development involves general (not only syntactic aspects of) language development. Thus, it supports the other two of the four major theories of ToM; 'theory-

theory' and the weaker version of 'linguistic determinism' of ToM. ToM development may be strongly associated with linguistic (especially pragmatics) and conceptual development.

These new findings may demand a rethink of 'modularity' in ToM (and other cognitive) development. This is not to say that specialized neural networks are not involved in the development of ToM, only that the neural correlates of ToM are neither innate nor informationally encapsulated, but subject to dramatic developmental changes based on the experience. Moreover, they indicate that the development of ToM may go hand-in-hand with language and other socio-cognitive development. These new findings support the Whorfian/Vygotskian hypothesis overall and imply that future neuro-psychological research will be benefited by emphasizing the socio-cultural influence on cognitive development more strongly.

ACKNOWLEDGMENTS

I thank Dr. Elise Temple, Dr. Barbara C. Lust, and Dr. Michael J. Spivey for discussion. I also thank Frank Randall for assistance.

REFERENCES

Agnew, Z. K., Bhakoo, K. K., & Puri, B. K. (2007). The human mirror system: A motor resonance theory of mind-reading. *Brain Research Reviews,* 54, 286-293.

Akiyama, T., Kato, M., Muramatsu, T., Saito, F., Nakachi, R., & Kashima, H. (2006). A deficit in discriminating gaze direction in a case with right superior temporal gyrus lesion. *Neuropsychologia*, 44(2),161-170.

Aron, A.R., Robbins, T.W., & Poldrack, R.A. (2004). Inhibition and the right inferior frontal cortex. *Trends in Cognitive Sciences,* 8(4), 170-177.

Astington, J.W., & Jenkins, J.M. (1999). A longitudinal study of the relation between language and theory-of-mind development. *Developmental Psychology,* 35(5), 1311-1320.

Baron-Cohen, S. (2000). Theory of mind and autism: A fifteen years. In S. Baron-Cohen, H. Tager-Flusberg, & D. Cohen (Eds.), *Understanding other minds: Perspective from autism* (2nd edition, pp. 3-20). Oxford: Oxford University Press.

Baron-Cohen, S., 2003. *The essential difference: men, women and the extreme male brain.* London: Penguin.

Baron-Cohen, S., Leslie, A.M., & Frith, U. (1985). Does the autistic child have a "theory of mind"? *Cognition,* 21, 37-46.

Baron-Cohen, S., Leslie, A.M., & Frith, U. (1986). Mechanical, behavioral and intentional understanding of picture stories in autistic children. British *Journal of Developmental Psychology,* 4, 113-125.

Baron-Cohen, S., O'Riordan, M., Stone, V., Jones, R., & Plaisted, K. (1999). Recognition of Faux Pas by normally developing children and children with Asperger syndrome or high-functioning autism. *Journal of Autism and Developmental Disorders,* 29, 407-418.

Baron-Cohen, S., Ring, H. A., Wheelwright, S., Bullmore, E. T., Brammer, M. J., Simmons, A., & Williams, S. C. (1999). Social intelligence in the normal and autistic brain: an fMRI study. *European Journal of Neuroscience,* 11, 1891-1898.

Bartsch, K., & Wellman, H. (1995). *Children talk about the mind.* New York: Oxford University Press.

Bavelier, D., Corina, D., Jessard, P., Padmanabhan, S., Prinster, A., Braun, A., et al. (1997). Sentence reading: A functional MRI study at 4 tesla. *Journal of Cognitive Neuroscience*, 9, 664-686.

Berlucci, A., & Aglioti, S. (1997). The body in the brain: Neural bases of corporeal awareness. *Trends in Neuroscience*, 20, 560-564.

Berthoz, S., Armony, J.L., Blair, R.J.R., & Dolan, R.J. (2002). An fMRI study of intentional and unintentional (embarrassing) violation of social norms. *Brain*, 125, 1696-1708.

Binder, J. R., Frost, J. A., Hammeke, T. A., Cox, R. W., Rao, S. M., & Prieto, T. (1997). Human brain language areas identified by functional magnetic resonance imaging. *Journal of Neuroscience*, 17, 353-362.

Bookheimer, S. (2002). Functional MRI of language: new approaches to understanding the cortical organization of semantic processing. *Annual Review of Neuroscience*, 25, 151-188.

Bornkessel, I., Zysset, S., Friederici, A. D., von Cramon, D. Y., & Schlesewsky, M. (2005). Who did what to whom? The neural basis of argument hierarchies during language comprehension. *Neuroimage,* 26, 221-233.

Boroditsky, L. (2001). Does language shape thought? Mandarin and English speakers' conception of time. *Cognitive Psychology,* 43, 1-22.

Bottini, G., Corcoran, R., Sterzi, R. Paulesu, E., Schenone, P., Scarpa, P., et al. (1994). The role of the right hemisphere in the interpretation of figurative aspects of language: A position emission tomography activation study. *Brain*, 117, 1241-1253.

Bowerman, M., & Choi, S. (2001). Shaping meanings for language: Universal and language-specific in the acquisition of spatial semantic categories. In M. Bowerman, & S. C. Levinson (Eds.), *Language acquisition and conceptual development* (pp. 475-511). Cambridge: Cambridge University Press.

Brambilla, P., Harden, A. Y., di Nemi, S. U., Caverzasi, E., Soares, J. C., Perez, J., & Barale, F. (2004). The functional neuroanatomy of autism. *Functional Neurology*, 19(1), 9-17.

Brauer, J., & Friederici, A. D. (2007). Functional neural networks of semantic and syntactic processes in the developing brain. *Journal of Cognitive Neuroscience,* 19(10), 1609-1623.

Brown, P., & Levinson, S. C. (1993). *Linguistic and nonlinguistic coding of spatial arrays: Exploration in Mayan cognition.* Working Paper 24. Nijmegen: Max Planck Institute for Psycholinguistics, Cognitive Anthropology Research Group.

Brunet, E., Sarfati, Y., Hardy-Bayle, M-C., & Decety, J. (2000). A PET investigation of the attribution of intentions with a nonverbal task. *Neuroimage,* 11, 157-166.

Buccino, G., Vogt, S., Ritzl, A., Fink, G. R., Zilles, K., Freund, H. J., & Rizzolatti, G. (2004). Neural circuits underlying imitation learning of hand actions: an event-related fMRI study. *Neuron*, 42(2), 323-334

Bunge, S. A., Dudukovic, N. M., Thomason, M. E., Vaidya, C. J., & Gabrieli, J. D. E. (2002). Immature frontal lobe contributions to cognitive control in children: evidence from fMRI. *Neuron,* 33, 301-311.

Burgess, P. W., Quayle, A., & Frith, C. D. (2001). Brain regions involved in prospective memory as determined by position emission tomography. *Neuropsychologia,* 39(6), 545-555.

Bush, G., Luu, P., & Postner, M. J. (2000). Cognitive and emotional influences in anterior cingulate cortex. *Trends in Cognitive Science*, 4(6), 215-222.

Carter, R. (1998). *Mapping the mind.* Berkeley: University of California Press.

Chakrabarti, B., & Baron-Cohen, S. (2006). Empathizing: neurocognitive developmental mechanisms and individual differences. *Progress in Brain Research,* 156, 403-417.

Chaminade, T., & Decety, J. (2002). Leader or follower? Involvement of the inferior parietal lobule in agency. *Neuroreport,* 13(15), 1975-1978.

Cheney, D.L., & Seyfarth, R.M. (1990). *How monkeys see the world: Inside the mind of another species*. Chicago: University of Chicago Press.

Choi, S., & Bowerman, M. (1991). Learning to express motion events in English and Korean: The influence of language-specific lexicalization patterns. *Cognition,* 41, 83-121.

Chomsky, N. (1980). *Rules and representations.* Oxford: Basil Blackwell.

Chou, T. L., Booth, J. R., Burman, D. D., Bitan, T., Bigio, J. D., Lu, D., et al. (2006). Developmental change in the neural correlates of semantic processing. *Neuroimage,* 29, 1141-1149.

Dapretto, M., & Bookheimer, S. (1999). Form and content: dissociating syntax and semantics in sentence comprehension. *Neuron*, 24, 427-432.

Dapretto, M., Davies, M. S., Pfeifer, J. H., Scott, A. A., Sigman, M., Bookheimer, S. Y., & Iacoboni, M. (2006). Understanding emotions in others: mirror neuron dysfunction in children with autism spectrun disorders. *Nature Neuroscience*, 9(1), 28-30.

Davis, M. H. (1994). *Empathy: a social psychological approach*. Boulder, CO: Westview Press.

Decety, J., & Chaminade, J. (2004). When self represents the other: A new cognitive neuroscience view of psychological intention. *Consciousness & Cognition,* 12, 577-596.

Decety, J., & Grézes, J. (2006). The power of simulation: imaging one's own and other's behavior. *Brain Research,* 1079(1), 4-14.

Decety, J., Grézes, J., Costes, N., Perani, D., Jeannerod, M., Procyk, E. et al., (1997). Brain activity during observation of actions. Influence of action content and subject's strategy. *Brain,* 120(10), 1763-1777.

Dehaene, S., Spelke, E., Pinel, P., Stanescu, R., & Tsivkin, S. (1999). Source of mathematical thinking: behavioral and brain-imaging evidence. *Science*, 284, 970-974.

De Villiers, J.G. (2000). Language and theory of mind: What are the developmental relationships? In S. Baron-Cohen, H. Tager-Flusberg, & D. Cohen (Eds.), *Understanding other minds* (2nd Edition, pp. 83-123). Oxford: Oxford University Press.

De Villiers, J.G., & de Villiers, P.A. (2000). Linguistic determinism and the understanding of false beliefs. In P. Mitchell, and K.J. Riggs (Eds.) *Children's reasoning and the mind* (pp. 191-228). East Sussex, UK: Psychology Press.

De Waal, F. (2001). *The ape and the sushi master: cultural reflections of a primatologist.* New York: Basic Books.

Feinberg, T. E. (2000). *Altered egos: How the brain creates the self.* New York: Oxford University Press.

Ferstl, E.C., & von Cramon, D.Y. (2002). What does the frontomedian cortex contribute to language processing: coherence or theory of mind? *Neuroimage,* 17, 1599-1612.

Fletcher, P.C., Happé, F., Frith, U., Baker, S. C., Dolan, R. J., Frackowiak, R. S. J., & Frith, C. D. (1995). Other minds in the brain: A functional imaging study of 'theory of mind' in story comprehension. *Cognition,* 57, 109-128.

Fodor, J. A. (1975). *The language of thought.* New York: Crowell.

Fodor, J. A. (1983). *The modularity of mind.* Cambridge, MA: MIT Press.

Fogassi, L., Ferrari, P. F., Gesierich, B., Rozzi, S., Chersi, F., & Rizzolatti, G. (2005). Parietal lobe: From action organization to intention understanding. *Science,* 308, 662-667.

Friederici, A. D., Rüschemeyer, S. A., Hahne, A., & Fiebach, C. J. (2003). The role of left inferior frontal and superior temporal cortex in sentence comprehension: Localizing syntactic and semantic process. *Cerebral Cortex,* 13, 170-177.

Frith, U. (2003). *Autism: Explaining the enigma.* Malden, MA: Blackwell Publishing.

Frith, U., & Frith, C. D. (2003). Development of neurophysiology of mentalizing. *Philosophical Transactions of the Royal Society of London, B, Biological Sciences,* 358(1431), 459-473.

Gallagher, H.L., & Frith, C.D. (2003). Functional imaging of 'theory of mind.' *Trends in Cognitive Sciences*, 7(2), 77-83.

Gallagher, H.L., Happé, F., Frunswick, N., Fletcher, P.C., Frith, U., & Frith, C.D. (2000). Reading the mind in cartoons and stories: an fMRI study of 'theory of mind' in verbal and nonverbal tasks. *Neuropsychologia*, 38, 11-21.

Gallagher, H.L., Jack, A.I., Roepstorff, A., & Frith, C.D. (2002). Imaging the intentional stance in a competitive game. *Neuroimage*, 16, 814-821.

Gallese, V. (2007). Before and below 'theory of mind': embodied simulation and the neural correlates of social cognition. *Philosophical Transactions of the Royal Society of London - Series B: Biological Sciences,* 362(1480), 659-669.

Garavan, H., Ross, T. J., Murphy, K., Roche, R. A. P., & Steln, E. A. (2002). Dissociable executive functions in the dynamic control of behavior: inhibition, error detection, and correction. *Neuroimage,* 17, 1820-1829.

German, T. P., Niehaus, J. L., Roarty, M. P., Giesbrecht, B., & Miller, M. B. (2004). Neural correlates of detecting pretense: Automatic engagement of the intentional stance under covert conditions. *Journal of Cognitive Neuroscience,* 16(10), 1805-1817.

Giedd, J. N., Blumenthal, J., Jeffries, N. O., Castellanos, F. X., Liu, H., Zijdenbos, A., et al. (1999). Brain development during childhood and adolescence: a longitudinal MRI study. *Nature Neuroscience,* 2, 861-863.

Goel, V., Grafman, J., Sadato, N., & Hallet, M. (1995). Modeling other minds. *Neuroreport,* 6(13), 1741-1746.

Gogtay, N., Giedd, J. N., Lusk, L., Hayashi, K. M., Greenstein, D., Vaituzis, A. C., et al. (2004). Dynamic mapping of human cortical development during childhood through early adulthood. *Proceedings of National Academy of Science, USA,* 101, 8174-8179.

Goldman, A. (1989). Interpretation psychologized. *Mind & Language*, 4, 161-185.

Gopnik, A., & Wellman, H.M. (1992). Why the child's theory of mind really is a theory. *Mind & Language,* 7(1-2), 145-171.

Grèzes, J., Frith, C. D., & Passingham, R. E. (2004). Inferring false beliefs from the actions of oneself and others: an fMRI study. *Neuroimage,* 21, 744-750.

Gusnard, D. A., Akbudak, E., Shulman, G. L., & Raichle, M. E. (2001). Medial prefrontal cortex and self-referential mental activity: relation to a default mode of brain function. *Proceedings of the National Academy of Sciences, U. S. A.* 98(7), 4259-4264.

Happé, F.G. (1993). Communicative competence and theory of mind in autism: a test of relevance theory. *Cognition,* 48, 101-119.

Happé, F., Ehler, S., Fletcher, P., Frith, U., Johansson, M., Gillberg, C., Dolan, R., Frackowiak, R., & Frith, C. (1996). 'Theory of mind' in the brain: evidence from a PET scan study of Asperger syndrome. *Neuroreport*, 8, 197-201.

Harris, P. L. (1991). The work of the imagination. In A. Whitman (Ed.), *Natural theories of mind: The evolution, development and simulation of everyday mindreading* (pp. 283-304). Oxford: Oxford University Press.

Harris, P. L. (1992). From simulation to folk psychology: The case for development. *Mind and Language,* 7, 120-144.

Harris, P. L. (2005). Conversation, pretense and theory of mind. In J. W. Astington, & J. A. Baird (Eds.), *Why language matters for theory of mind* (pp. 70-83). Oxford: Oxford University Press.

Hayes, C.M. (1998). Theory of mind in nonhuman primates. *Behavioral and Brain Sciences,* 21, 101-134.

Heiser, M., Iacoboni, M., Maeda, F., Marcus, J., & Mazziotta, J. C. (2003). The essential role of Broca's area in imitation. *European Journal of Neuroscience,* 17(5), 1123-1128

Hespos, S. J., & Spelke, E. S. (2004). Conceptual precursors to language. *Nature*, 430(6998), 453-456.

Hobson, R. (1991). Against the theory of "Theory of Mind." *British Journal of Developmental Psychology*, 9, 33-51.

Hresko, W. P., Reid, D. K., & Hammill, D. D. (1981). *The Test of Early Language Development.* Austin, TX: Pro-Ed.

Iacoboni, M. (2005). Neural mechanisms of imitation. *Current Opinion in Neurobiology,* 15, 632-637.

Jackson, P. L., Brunet, E., Meltzoff, A. N., & Decety, J. (2006). Empathy examined through the neural mechanisms involved in imagining how I feel versus how you feel pain. *Neuropsychologia* 44(5), 752-761.

Jackson, P. L., Meltzoff, A. N., & Decety, J. (2005). How do we perceive the pain of others? A window into the neural processes involved in empathy. *Neuroimage* 24(3), 771-779.

Kain, W., & Perner, J. (2005). What fMRI can tell us about the ToM-EF connection: false-beliefs, working memory, and inhibition. In W. Schneider, R. Schumann-Hengsteler, & B. Sodian (Eds.), *Young children's cognitive development* (pp. 189-217). Mahwah, NJ: Lawrence Erlbaum.

Kobayashi, C. (2007). *Language and thought: Cultural and linguistic influence on developmental neural bases of theory of mind.* Ph.D Thesis. Cornell University, NY.

Kobayashi, C., Glover, G. H., & Temple, E. (2006). Cultural and linguistic influence on neural bases of 'Theory of Mind': An fMRI study with Japanese bilinguals. *Bran and Language,* 98(2), 210-220.

Kobayashi, C., Glover, G. H., & Temple, E. (2007a). Children's and adults' neural bases of verbal and nonverbal 'Theory of Mind'. *Neuropsychologia,* 45, 1522-1532.

Kobayashi, C., Glover, G. H., & Temple, E. (2007b). Cultural and linguistic effects on neural bases of 'Theory of Mind' in American and Japanese children. *Brain Research,* 1164, 95-107.

Koelsch, S. (2005). Neural substrates of processing syntax and semantics in music. *Current Opinion in Neurobiology,* 15(2), 207-212.

Koelsch, S., Fritz, T., Schulze, K., Alsop, D., & Schlaug, G. (2005). Adults and children processing music: an fMRI study. *Neuroimage*, 25(4), 1068-1076.

Kotz, S. A., Cappa, S. F., von Cramon, D. Y., & Friederici, A. D. (2002). Modulation of the lexical-semantic network by auditory semantic priming: An event-related functional MRI study. *Neuroimage,* 17, 1761-1772.

Lamm, C., Batson, C. D., & Decety, J. (2007). The neural substrate of human empathy: effects of perspective-taking and cognitive appraisal. *Journal of Cognitive Neuroscience,* 19(1), 42-58.

Landa, R. (2000). Social language use in Asperger syndrome and high-functioning autism. In A. Klin, F.R. Volkmar, & S.S. Sparrow (Eds.), *Asperger syndrome* (pp. 125-155). New York: The Guilford Press, pp. 125-155.

Lane, R. D., Fink, G. R., Chau, R. M., & Dolan, R. J. (1997). Neural activation during selective attention to subjective emotion responses. *Neuroreport*, 8, 3969-3972.

Limb, C. J., Kemeny, S., Ortigoza, E. B., Rouhani, S., & Braun, A. R. (2006). Left hemispheric lateralization of brain activity during passive rhythm perception in musicians. *Anatomical Record. Part A, Discoveries in Molecular, Cellular, and Evolutionary Biology,* 288(4), 382-389.

Liu, D. (2005). *Neural correlates of children's theory of mind development.* Ph.D Thesis. University of Michigan, MI.

Liu, D., Sabbagh, M. A., Gehring, W. J., & Wellman, H. M. (2005, April). *An ERP study of 6-year-olds' theory of mind.* Poster presented at the 2005 annual meeting of the Cognitive Neuroscience Society, New York City, NY.

Lucy, J. A. (1992). *Grammatical categories and cognition: A case study of the linguistic relativity hypothesis.* Cambridge: Cambridge University Press.

Leekam, S. R., & Prior, M. (1994). Can autistic children distinguish lies from jokes? A second look at second-order belief attribution. *Journal of Child Psychology & Psychiatry,* 35: 901–15.

Leslie, A.M. (1992). Autism and the 'theory of mind' module. *Current Directions in Psychological Science*, 1, 18-21.

Leslie, A.M. (1994). Pretending and believing: issues in the theory of ToMM. *Cognition*, 50, 211-238.

Leslie, A. M., Friedman, O., & German, T. P. (2004). Core mechanisms in 'theory of mind'. *Trends in Cognitive Sciences*, 8(12), 529-533.

Leslie, K. R., Johnson-Frey, S. H., & Grafton, S. T. (2004). Functional imaging of face and hand imitation: Towards a motor theory of empathy. *Neuroimage*. 21(2), 601-607.

Liu, D., Sabbagh, M. A., Gehring, W. J., & Wellman, H. M. (2005, April). *An ERP study of 6-year-olds' theory of mind.* Poster presented at the 2005 annual meeting of the Cognitive Neuroscience Society, New York City, NY.

Lohman, H., & Tomasello, M. (2003). The role of language in the development of false belief understanding: A training study. *Child Development,* 74, 1130-1144.

Martin, R. C. (2003). Language processing: Functional organization and neuroanatomical basis. *Annual Review of Psychology,* 54, 55-89.

McDonough, L., Choi, S., & Mandler, J. M. (2003). Understanding spatial relations: Flexible infants, lexical adults. *Cognitive Psychology*, 46(3), 229-259.

Meltzoff, A. N., & Brooks, R. (2001). "Like Me" as a building block for understanding other minds: Bodily acts, attention, and intention. In B. F. Malle, L. J. Moses, & D. A. Baldwin (Eds.), *Intentions and intentionality* (pp. 171-191). Cambridge, MA: MIT Press.

Mitchell, J. P., Banaji, M. R., & Macrae, C. N. (2005). The link between social cognition and self-referential thought in the medial prefrontal cortex. Journal of Cognitive Neuroscience, 17, 1306-1315.

Morgan, G., & Kegl, J. (2006). Nicaraguan Sign Language and Theory of Mind: the issue of critical periods and abilities. *Journal of Child Psychology and Psychiatry,* 47(8), 811-819.

Moriguchi, Y., Ohnishi, T., Mori, T., Matsuda, H., & Komaki, G. (2007). Changes of brain activity in the neural substrates for theory of mind during childhood and adolescence. *Psychiatry & Clinical Neurosciences,* 61, 355-363.

Moro, A., Tettamanti, M., Perani, D., Donati, C., Cappa, S. F., & Fazio, F. (2001). Syntax and the brain: Disentangling grammar by selective anomalies. *Neuroimage*, 13, 110-118.

Müller, R. A. (2007). The study of autism as a distributed disorder. *Mental Retardation and Developmental Disabilities Research Reviews,* 13(1), 85-95.

Nakamura, A., Maess, B., Knösche, T. R., Gunter, T. C., Bach, P, & Friederici, A. D. (2004). Cooperation of different neuronal systems during hand sign recognition. *Neuoimage,* 23, 25-34.

Newman, A. J., Pancheva, R., Ozawa, K., Neville, H. J., & Ullman, M. T. (2001). An event-related fMRI study of syntactic and semantic violations. *Journal of Psycholinguistic Research,* 30(3), 339-364.

Newton, A. M., & de Villiers, J. G. (2007). Thinking while talking. *Psychological Science,* 18(7), 574-579.

Nichols, S., & Stich, S. P. (2003). *Mind reading: an integrated account of pretence, self-wareness, and understanding other minds.* Oxford: Oxford University Press.

Oberman, L. M., & Ramachandran, V. S. (2007). The simulating social mind: The role of the mirror neuron system and simulation in the social and communicative deficits of Autism Spectrum Disorders. *Psychological Bulletin,* 133, 310-327.

Ohnish, T., Moriguchi, Y., Matsuda, H., Mori, T., Hirakata, M., Imabayashi, E., Hirao, K., Nemoto, K., Kaga, M., Inagaki, M., Yamada, M., & Uno, A. (2004). The neural network for the mirror system and mentalizing in normally developed children: an fMRI study. *Neuroreport,* 15(9), 1483-1487.

Onishi, K. H., & Baillargeon, R. (2005). Do 15-month-old infants understand false beliefs? *Science,* 308, 255-258.

Paradis, M. (1998). The other side of language: Pragmatic competence. *Journal of Neurolinguistics*, 11, 1-10.

Patel, R. S., Bowman, F. D., & Rilling, J. K. (2006). Determining hierarchical functional networks from auditory stimuli fMRI. *Human Brain Mapping*, 27(5), 462-470.

Pekkola, J., Ojanen, V., Autti, T., Jaaskelainen, I. P., Mottonen, R., & Sams, M. (2006). Attention to visual speech gestures enhances hemodynamic activity in the left planum temporale. *Human Brain Mapping*, 27(6), 471-477.

Perner, J., & Ruffman, T. (2005). Infants' insight into the mind: How deep? *Science,* 308, 214-216.

Piaget, J. (1962). *Play, dreams, and imitation in childhood.* New York: Norton.

Poldrack, R. A., Wagner, A. D., Prull, M. W. Desmond, J. E., Glover, G. H., & Gabrieli, J. D. (1999). Functional specialization for semantic and phonological processing in the left inferior frontal cortex. *Neuroimage,* 10, 15-35.

Premack, D., & Woodruff, G. (1978). Does the chimpanzee have a theory of mind? *Behavioral and Brain Sciences,* 1, 515-526.

Price, C. J. (2000). The anatomy of language: contribution from functional neuroimaging. *Journal of Anatomy*, 197, 335-359.

Price, J. L. (2005). Free will versus survival: Brain systems that underlie intrinsic constrains on behavior. *Journal of comparative neurology*, 493, 132-139.

Rimol, L. M., Specht, K., & Hugdahl, K. (2006). Controlling for individual differences in fMRI brain activation to tones, syllables, and words. *Neuroimage*, 30(2), 554-562.

Roskies, A. L., Fiez, J. A., Balota, D. A., Raichle, M. E., & Peterson, S. E. (2001). Task-dependent modulation of regions in the left inferior frontal cortex during semantic processing. *Journal of Cognitive Neuroscience*, 13, 829-843.

Roth, D., & Leslie, A. M. (1998). Solving belief problems: towards a task analysis. *Cognition*, 66, 1-31.

Sabbagh, M. A. (2004). Understanding orbitofrontal contributions to theory-of-mind reasoning: Implications for autism. *Brain and Cognition*, 55, 209-219.

Sabbagh, M.A., & Taylor, M. (2000). Neural correlates of theory-of-mind reasoning: an event-related potential study. *Psychological Sciences*, 11(1), 46-50.

Sanfey, A. G., Rilling, J. K., Aronson, J. A., Nystrom, L. E., & Cohen, J. D. (2003). The neural basis of economic decision-making in the ultimatum game. *Science*, 300, 1755-1758.

Saxe, R. (2005). Against simulation: the argument from error. *Trends in Cognitive Science*, 9(4), 174-179.

Saxe, R., Carey, S., & Kanwisher, N. (2004). Understanding other minds: linking developmental psychology and functional neuroimaging. *Annual Review of Psychology,* 55, 87-124.

Saxe, R., and Kanwisher, N. (2003). People thinking about thinking people: the role of the temporo-parietal junction in "theory of mind." *Neuroimage*, 19, 1835-1842.

Saxe, R., & Wexler, A. (2005). Making sense of another mind: the role of the right temporo-parietal junction. *Neuropsychologia,* 43, 1391-1399.

Scholl, B. J., & Leslie, A. M. (1999). Modularity, development and 'theory of mind.' *Mind & Language,* 14(1), 131-153.

Schultz, R.T., Romanski, L.M., & Tsatsanis, K.D. (2000). Neurofunctional models of autistic disorder and Asperger syndrome: Clues from neuroimaing. In A. Klin, F.R. Volkmar, & S.S. Sparrow. (Eds.), *Asperger syndrome* (pp. 172-209). New York: Guilford Press.

Sevostianov, A., Horwitz, B., Nechaev, V., Williams, R., Fromm S., & Braun A. R. (2002). fMRI study comparing names versus pictures of objects. *Human Brain Mapping,* 16(3), 168-175.

Siegal, M., Carrington, J., & Radel, M. (1996). Theory of mind and pragmatic understanding following right hemisphere damage. *Brain and Language*, 53, 40-50.

Siegal, M., & Varley, R. (2002). Neural systems involved in 'theory of mind'. *Nature Reviews,* 3, 463-471.

Sinclair, M. (1970). The transition from sensory-motor behavior to symbolic activity. *Interchange*, 1, 119-126.

Singer, T. (2006). The neuronal basis and ontogeny of empathy and mind reading: Review of literature and implications for future research. *Neuroscience and Behavioral Reviews,* 30, 855-863.

Southgate, V., Senju, A., & Csibra, G. (2007). Action anticipation through attribution of false belief by 2-year-olds. *Psychological Science,* 18(7), 587-592.

Sowell, E. R., Peterson, B. S., Thompson, P. M., Welcome, S. E., Henkenius, A. L., & Toga, A. W. (2003). Mapping cortical change across the human life span. Nature Neuroscience, 6: 309–315.

Sperber, D., & Wilson, D. (2002). Pragmatics, modularity, and mind-reading. *Mind & Language,* 17(1-2), 3-23.

Surian, L., Caldi, S, & Sperber, D. (2007). Attribution of beliefs by 13-month-old infants. *Psychological Science,* 18(7), 580-586.

Tager-Flusberg, H. (2000). Language and understanding minds: Connection in autism. In S. Baron-Cohen, H. Tager-Flusberg, & D. Cohen (Eds.), *Understanding other minds: Perspective from autism* (2nd Edition, pp. 124-149). Oxford: Oxford University Press.

Temple, E., Deutsch, G. K., Poldrack, R. A., Miller, S. L., Tallal, P., Merzenich, M. M., & Gabrieli, J. D. (2003). Neural deficits in children with dyslexia ameliorated by behavioral remediation: evidence from functional MRI. *Proceedings of the National Academy of Sciences, USA,* 100(5), 2860-2865.

Tomasello, M. (2001). Perceiving intentions and learning words in the second year of life. In M. Bowerman, & S. C. Levinson (Eds.), *Language acquisition and conceptual development* (pp. 132-158). Cambridge, UK: Cambridge University Press.

Tomasello, M. (2003). The key is social cognition. In D. Gentner, & S. Goldin-Meadow (Eds.), *Language in mind: Advances in the study of language and thought* (pp. 48-57). Cambridge, MA: MIT Press.

Tracy, J., Flanders, A., Madi, S., Natale, P., Delvecchio, N., Pyrros, A., & Laskas, J. (2003). The brain's response to incidental intruded words during focal text processing. *Neuroimage,* 18(1), 117-126.

Valsiner, J. (1989). *Human development and culture: The social nature of personality and its study.* Lexington, MA: Lexington Books.

Vandenberghe, R., Nobre, A. C., & Price, C. J. (2002). The response of left temporal cortex to sentences. *Journal of Cognitive Neuroscience,* 14, 500-560.

Varley, R., & Siegal, M. (2000). Evidence for cognition without grammar from causal reasoning and 'theory of mind' in an agrammatic aphasic patient. *Current Biology,* 10, 723-726.

Venkatraman, V., Siong, S. C., Chee, M. W., & Ansari, D. (2006) Effect of language switching on arithmetic: a bilingual FMRI study. *Journal of Cognitive Neuroscience,* 18(1), 64-74.

Völlm, B. A., Taylor, A. N. W., Richardson, P., Corcoran, R., Stirling, J., McKie, S., Deakin, J. F. W., & Elliot, R. (2006). Neural correlates of theory of mind and empathy: a functional magnetic resonance imaging study in a nonverbal task. *Neuroimage,* 29(1), 90-98.

Vogeley, K., Bussfeld, P., Newen, A., Herrmann, S., Happé, F., Falkai, P., Maier, W., Shah, N.J., Fink, G.R., & Zilles, K. (2001). Mind reading: Neural mechanisms of theory of mind and self-perspective. *Neuroimage*, 14, 170-181.

Vygotsky, L. S. (1967). *Thought and language.* In E. Hanfmann, & G. Vakar (Eds. and Trans.). Cambridge, MA: MIT Press.

Wang, A. T., Lee, S. S., Sigman, M., & Dapretto, M. (2006a). Developmental changes in the neural basis of interpreting communicative intent. *Social, Cognitive and Affective Neuroscience,* 1, 107-121.

Wang, A. T., Lee, S. S., Sigman, M., & Dapretto, M. (2006b). Neural basis of irony comprehension in hcildren with autism: the role of prosody and context. *Brain*, 129(4), 932-943.

Wellman, H.M., Cross, D.C., & J. Watson. (2001). Meta-analysis of theory of mind development: The truth about false belief. *Child Development,* 72(3), 655-684.

Wernicke, C. (1874). *Der aphasiche Symptomenkomplex.* Bresiau, Poland: Cohen and Weigert.

Wheelwright, S., Baron-Cohen, S., Goldenfeld, N., Delaney, J., Fine, D., Smith, R., Weil, L., & Wakabayashi, A. (2006). Predicting autism spectrum quotient (AQ) from the systemizing quotient-revised (SQ-R) and empathy quotient (EQ). *Brain Reseach,* 1079, 47-56.

Whorf, B.L. (1956). *Language, thought, and reality: Selected writing of Benjamin Lee Whorf.* (J.B. Carroll, ed.). Cambridge, MA: MIT Press.

Wimmer, H., & Perner, J. (1983). Belief about belief: representation and constraining function of wrong beliefs in young children's understanding of deception. *Cognition,* 13, 103-128.

Ziatas, K., Durkin, K., & Pratt, C. (1998). Belief term development in children with autism, Asperger syndrome, specific language impairment, and normal development: Links to theory of mind development. *Journal of Child Psychology and Psychiatry,* 39(5), 755-763.

In: Children and Language: Development, Impairment … ISBN 978-1-60692-395-5
Editor: Michael A. Reed

Chapter 2

IS A STORY THE SAME AS THE SUM OF ITS PARTS? THE DEFERENTIAL EFFECTS OF CONTEXT AND ISOLATED WORD TRAINING ON READING FLUENCY

Sandra Lyn Martin-Chang[1]
Concordia University Montreal, Quebec, Canada

ABSTRACT

The first priority for novice readers is to understand that the letters they see in written language correspond to the sounds they hear in speech. Once children grasp the letter-to-sound pairings afforded to them by the alphabetic principle, they can begin to identify some of the written words that are contained in their spoken vocabularies. At this point, the question becomes whether reading practice should take place in stories (context) or in lists (isolation). Two camps have emerged with opposing views on this topic. On the one hand, investigators have shown increased long-term word recognition when children practice reading words in isolation.

In contrast, it has also been suggested that reading words in context can act as a secondary self-teaching mechanism. Proponents of this view argue that the added value of context increases reading ability beyond that achieved by other methods of training. At present, then, the evidence on best training practices (context vs. isolation) is mixed. The studies discussed here begin to unify these two differing perspectives by elucidating the circumstances that mediate the utility of each type of training. In brief, during the five training studies reviewed, context training dominated isolated word training with regards to word acquisition. However, after words were learned, retention over an eight-day interval approached ceiling under both conditions. Finally, fluency transfer (reading words quickly and accurately in new texts or new lists) was maximized when the congruency between training and testing was high; words trained in isolation were read more fluently in novel lists, whereas words trained in context were read more fluently in novel stories. To conclude, the decision of which training method to use cannot be made independently from the task to be done after training has ceased. However, if the goal of

[1] Author Note: Correspondence should be addressed to Sandra Martin-Chang who is now at, 1455 De Maisonneuve Boulevard West, Montreal, Quebec, Canada, H3G 1M8. Tel: (514) 848-2424 x 8932, fax: (514) 848-4520, email: smartinc@education.concordia.ca

instruction is to have students who excel during training, remember what they have learned, and who use their learning to read new texts fluently, the research plainly suggests that training in context is a more fruitful method of instruction than isolated word training.

INTRODUCTION

The sight of an infant taking his or her first steps sends parents scrambling for video cameras – and with good reason. Those steps, however unsteady and tenuous, open up avenues for exploration beyond anything the infant could previously imagine. Along a similar vein, hearing a child read his or her first few words is an exciting and awe-inspiring event; although they may be cautious and tentative, those words mark the entrance into literacy. However, unlike motor development, which follows a natural progression from stepping to walking to running, without the aid of formal training reading often fails to progress from word-by-word decoding to fluent reading. Research has shown that even when interventions successfully improve reading accuracy, it is inordinately difficult to "close the fluency gap" once children have fallen behind their peers (Torgesen, Rashotte, & Alexander, 2001). Torgesen et al. attributed this difficulty to the loss of reading experience in the slow and plodding reader. When reading is fluent, it frees children to think about *what* they are reading without allotting finite resources attending to *how* they are reading it. Until skill development has reached this level, the benefits associated with reading are often too minimal for children to justify the effort it requires. It is for this reason that non-fluent readers tend to participate in other activities rather than spending their time engaging with print (Stanovich, 1986). It would seem that fluency is a natural precursor of reading enjoyment.

As educators and parents, then, our goal is clear: to make the transition from non-reader to fluent reader as seamless as possible. But obvious questions remain: What methods of training increase the chances of achieving fluency? Should words be read in games, grocery lists, recipes, and flashcards (isolation)? Or should every effort be made to get children reading meaningful passages (context) right from the start? This chapter addresses these issues by describing a series of experiments illuminating the role of context in the development of reading fluency.

The Struggle for Fluency

On June 22, 2004, the headline of the Toronto Star entitled, "New Help For Reading", described a plan to quadruple the number of reading specialists in the public school system by 2006 (Boyle, 2004). Education Minister Kennedy explained: "If we don't get basic literacy by 8 years old and advanced [fluent] literacy by 12, there will be immense struggle ahead for that particular student".

The $150 million-budget increase came in response to the finding that half of Ontario students were failing to meet provincial reading standards (Boyle, 2004). This is not a phenomenon unique to Canada – in 2000, it was reported that a similar number of children were failing to meet grade level standards in the United States (Smith, Borkowski, & Whitman, 2008). The long-term educational prognoses for children who are meeting reading standards are very different from those who are not. The "Matthew Effect" (Stanovich, 1986) plots two learning trajectories resulting from high and low levels of reading proficiency. On the one hand, children who easily grasp the correspondence between print and sound upon entering school are clearly advantaged. They are able to use these skills to set up early sight vocabularies (Ehri, 1999; Share, 1995), which encourage extra-curricular reading activities (Stanovich, 1986). Reading for enjoyment acts to further strengthen core phonological abilities, which in turn, expand sight word vocabularies (Perfetti, 1992). As reading becomes ever more facile, a greater allotment of cognitive resources can be dedicated to text integration and comprehension (laberge & Samuels, 1974; Perfetti & Roth, 1981; Stanovich, 1980). At this point, reading is said to be 'fluent.' The culmination of these events results in increasingly skillful readers, reading more advanced material, for greater lengths of time (Stanovich, 1986). This description does not, however, adequately summarize the experience for most poor readers.

Children who struggle in the beginning stages of reading often become disenchanted with print, and as a result, receive substantially fewer self-initiated reading experiences than their skilled peers. This carries a double impact for poor readers; it denies them much needed reading practice and excludes them from a rich source of knowledge and vocabulary (Stanovich, 1986). While the discrepancies between good and poor readers at the initial stages of instruction may seem transient, empirical evidence suggests otherwise. As shown by a 10-year longitudinal study, the ease of acquiring reading skills in Grade 1 accounted for a significant amount of variance in reading ability in Grade 11. Moreover, the children who learned to read more easily in Grade 1 continued to find greater enjoyment in reading a decade later (Cunningham & Stanovich, 1997). A recent study also found a positive relationship between print exposure and reading rate in adults (Martin-Chang & Gould, in press). University students who read more for pleasure also read faster and had higher comprehension scores than students who read less (as measured by an updated Author Recognition Test and an Activity Preference Questionnaire).

One of the consequences of the effortful, halted reading, characteristic of poor readers is that meaningful phrases in texts are processed exceedingly slowly. It is estimated that skilled readers in Grade 4 process as many as 24 idea units per minute; this is contrasted with poor readers who average only eight (Jenkins, Fuchs, van den Broek, Espin, & Deno, 2003). It is perhaps for this reason that reading fluency (the number of words read correctly per minute) serves as a better predictor of reading comprehension than more standard measures, such as question answering skills, recall ability, or performance on cloze tasks (Fuchs, Fuchs, Hosp, & Jenkins, 2001; Jenkins et al., 2003). For instance, Spear-Swerling (2006) found that the best marker of fourth grade comprehension was a measure of oral reading fluency taken in third grade. Accordingly, fluency is recognized as one of the primary goals of reading instruction (Kuhn et al., 2006; Kuhn & Stahl, 2003).

The Ontario government, then, is correct in allotting more funds to early reading instruction. However, there is a longstanding debate over which method of instruction carries the most benefit for the beginning reader. For example, researchers who encourage the direct instruction of phonics credit phonological decoding as being the single most influential skill in successful reading (for review see Mody, 2003; Shankweiler et al., 1999; Shankweiler & Fowler, 2004). They argue that children learning an alphabetic language, such as English, do not need to waste resources memorizing word forms or predicting words from context. Children who grasp the alphabetic principle can capitalize on the systematic relations from letters to sounds in order to "see" the way words are pronounced (Ehri, 1992, 1993, 1999, 2004). Moreover, as language continues to shift and develop, children can use letter-sound conversion skills in order to read words that are newly invented (e.g., names for children's toys such as "Webkinz" or "Bakugan"), or words given new, unusual, spellings (e.g., slang terms such as "phat").

However, for the last several decades the instructional approach endorsed in Canada has focused on contextual reading, pushing the role of phonological skills to the periphery. In fact, according to Goodman (1992), it was Canadians who popularized the term "whole language" in reference to text-based reading programs. Text-based reading strategies orient children toward using cues from pictures, semantics and syntax to aid in word identification. As exemplified by the following statement from a language arts textbook, text-based reading programs are still highly regarded by some Canadian educators.

Often it is assumed that phonemic awareness instruction is the most important component of the reading program for young children, put phonology is only one of the four language systems [...] while it is important to help children understand how language works, such instruction should not lead to isolated skill instruction, separate from meaningful reading and writing experiences (Tompkins, Bright, Pollard, & Winsor, 2005, p. 93).

Indeed, a brief survey of the materials used within the realm of education shows that the definition of 'reading' often entirely fails to include word reading accuracy as part of it's description. In these documents the role of word reading is down played and the focus is placed instead on the "interactive process between the reader and the text" (Progress in International Reading Literacy Study, 2006). For example the International Association for the Evaluation of Educational Achievement (2004) described 'reading' as "the ability to [...] construct meaning from a variety of texts" (International Association for the Evaluation of Educational Achievement, 2004). Many researchers would agree with this statement, however they would posit that accurate word reading is a fundamental component passage comprehension.

For example, Compton, Appleton, and Hosp (2004) explored the text characteristics associated with fluent reading in second grade children. They measured texts in terms of passage readability (i.e., using the Flesch-Kincaid and Spache measures), decodability, high frequency words, multisyllabic words and average sentence length. In contrast to the view that word reading accuracy plays an inferior role in passage reading, Compton et al. Found that reading fluency increased as the number of highly frequent and easily decodable words increased; no such relationship was found with passage readability.

Research examining the development of prosodic reading (fluent reading with appropriate intonation and timing) has also highlighted the importance of word reading accuracy. Schwanenflugel et al. (2004) found that the children who read with most advanced prosody while reading passages also had the fastest word decoding skills. They stated that "as children became skilled word decoders, reading prosody took on a culturally normative character" (p. 127). Importantly, these authors also concluded that prosody was less related to comprehension than to word decoding. Based on these findings, it seems misguided for educators to concentrate exclusively on the role of "meaning making" in reading, without acknowledging the important role of word decoding skills.

Outside of the Education field, there has been mounting concern over the effectiveness of whole language instruction. Investigators who argue that the main focus of reading instruction should be letter names and sounds disagree with the premise that children should rely on non-alphabetic cues as a primary form of word identification (Ehri, 1992, 1993, 1999; Gough & Wren, 1999; Johnston, 2000; Perfetti, 1992, 1999; Share, 1995; Stanovich & Stanovich, 1999). Code-based strategies of reading encourage the use of letter-sound conversion rules to decode unknown words (Ehri, 1999; Perfetti, 1999; Share, 1995). The conflict over the direct instruction of decoding skills has become one of the main points of contention between proponents of whole language and supporters of a code-based approach to reading instruction. As indicated by its name, the whole language philosophy posits that language learning should not be broken down into smaller component skills. Instead, children should learn how to read in a similar fashion as they learn how to speak, via exposure. It is argued by Goodman (1973) that showing children the systematic correspondences between letters and sounds by using worksheets or by other direct approaches, focuses the child on the print and inadvertently detracts from the meaningfulness of the text as a whole. A second tenet of the whole language tradition is that reading lessons must involve "real" texts. Proponents of whole language propose that learning to read using children's stories highlight the similarities between the written word and speech (Dalh, 1979; Goodman, 1965, 1967, 1992) which ultimately improves both the motivation and the ability to read.

Reading in Context

The idea of learning to read words within connected text has gained some favor, even among investigators who have rejected all other aspects of whole language. For although there is now an impressive database underscoring the importance of phonological skills to reading development, it is still unclear whether contextual reading offers opportunities for learning beyond those experienced from reading words out of context (Nation & Snowling, 1998; Tunmer & Chapman, 1995, 2002). If contextual reading functions as a secondary self-teaching mechanism, it follows that children should be more successful learning to read words in stories compared to in isolation. Dahl (1979) asked a group of children to read passages to a criterion of 100 words per minute, at which point training on a new story began. A second group of children were trained to read 800 words presented individually to a criterion of 60 words per minute. A third group acted as controls and received only classroom instruction over the lengthy training interval. Despite of the extensive amount of single word exposure in Dahl's study, she reported the greatest gains in accuracy, speed, and comprehension, for children who practiced reading in context. Reading words in isolation accrued no more benefits than regular classroom instruction. Dahl concluded that practicing words in passages was necessary to integrate the skills required for proficient reading.

In a more recent investigation, Archer and Bryant (2001) compared learning words in isolation and in sentence contexts. They asked 6 and 7-year-old average readers to read from the Schonell reading list until 8 items were missed. The 8 unknown words for each participant were then divided into 2 groups of 4, half of which were taught within the context of meaningful sentences, while the others were taught via flash cards. Each target word was presented 3 times during training. Archer and Bryant found that children required fewer trials to learn the target words during context training compared to isolated word training.

Nation and Snowling (1998) have also reported that reading in context may benefit children who experience atypical difficulty learning to read. For example, many dyslexics, despite having persisting phonological difficulties, achieve levels of functional literacy that approximate those of average readers. Nation and Snowling credit this achievement to the ability to draw from context to facilitate learning. They observed that children with dyslexia gained the most from reading in context compared to both average readers, and readers with specific comprehension problems. Based on this finding they concluded that dyslexics might be using context as a secondary self-teaching mechanism to enhance overall reading ability.

Strengthening the view that context facilitates learning in children with reading disabilities, Jenkins et al. (2003) compared children's word reading accuracy while reading meaningful passages versus reading randomized word lists. Jenkins et al. reported that "about a third [of reading disabled students] demonstrated impairment in list reading but not in context reading. Apparently, some students with reading disability derived enough facilitation from context to escape the impairment classification for reading accuracy" (Jenkins et al., 2003, p.243). Further, Stanovich has demonstrated that the long-term effects of text reading are not limited to poor readers. Print exposure has been credited with improving several reading related skills in children of all ability, including vocabulary, reading speed, decoding ability, reading comprehension, and general world knowledge (Cunningham & Stanovich, 1997; Martin-Chang & Gould, in press; Stanovich, 1986; Stanovich, West, Cunningham, Cipielewski, & Siddiqui, 1996). This has led some investigators to ask whether the ability to use context could be a source of individual differences in the development of reading skill.

Context Use as a Source of Individual Differences

Tunmer and Chapman (1995) examined the relationship between language prediction skill (as measured by performance on a cloze task) and reading ability in approximately 300 children. They found that language prediction skill made an independent contribution to reading ability even when phonological recoding skills were taken into consideration. Yet, Tunmer and Chapman continued to stress the importance of letter-to-sound correspondences, noting that children with *emerging* phonological skills showed the largest improvements from reading in context. In contrast, children who lacked a basic understanding of the alphabetic principle were unable to combine the graphophonemic cues from the print and the contextual cues from the text. The unique variance in reading ability accounted for by prediction skill led Tunmer and Chapman to conclude that the ability to use context is a source of individual differences in reading.

Nation and Snowling (1998) came to a similar conclusion when examining the word reading skills of children with comprehension difficulties. These children have a range of deficits in drawing inferences, integrating sentences, and monitoring metacognitive aspects of comprehension. Children with comprehension difficulties tend to be quick and accurate readers, therefore these comprehension problems are observed in spite of adequate phonological skill. However, when Nation and Snowling divided a group of children matched on phonological skill into those with and without comprehension difficulties, they found differences in word reading ability despite both groups having similar levels of phonological awareness. Poor comprehenders had difficulty reading words that could not be sounded out by regular grapheme-phoneme conversion rules. Nation and Snowling proposed that children with comprehension difficulties are unable to capitalize on the contextual support offered from text. Consequently they show deficits reading words that benefit from being learned in context – such as those that are irregular or infrequent. Like Tunmer and Chapman (1995),

Nation and Snowling concluded that the ability to benefit from semantic support is a source of individual differences in reading skill.

Context versus Lists

While the concept of learning to read within connected text has gained popularity, very few empirical studies have been dedicated to examining the outcomes associated with contextual training. Before the results from our series of experiments are discussed, however, some important terms must first be defined.

There is no question, of course, that context is crucial to many aspects of reading advancement. For example, context is necessary for both learning new word meanings (e.g., discovering that a "hansom" refers to a horse and buggy in the Narnia series), and for deciphering which word meaning (e.g., pig *pen* vs. writing *pen*) or pronunciation (e.g., *read* this, vs. she *read*) to use in a given sentence. However, there is far less consensus over whether context helps children reliably translate letter strings into spoken words. It is this specific facet of context that remains to be clarified, and thus forms the basis of the experiments described below.

Even within this fairly narrow definition of reading, context training could benefit children in three different ways; context could enable children to read more words accurately at the time of reading (acquisition), to remember more words learned during training (retention), or to read those words more fluently when they are encountered in novel situations (transfer).

Experimental Overview

The current chapter reviews the results of five training experiments that shared a common research design. When discussing the work below I purposely focus on the commonalities among the five experiments (i.e., the results observed during acquisition, retention, and transfer), rather than on the properties unique to each (i.e., number of participants, number of items in material sets, etc.) in order to highlight the consistent pattern of findings that emerge when the body of work is considered as a whole (more detailed descriptions can be found in Martin-Chang & Levy, 2005, 2006; and in Martin-Chang et al., 2007).

The experiments reported here consisted of two phases: a training phase, and a test phase. During the training phase, each child was taught to read different sets of target words under experimentally distinctive conditions. Although the number of actual target words varied between experiments (ranging from a minimum of 10 to a maximum of 85 target words per condition) the number of training trials was held constant so that each target word was viewed 12 times throughout training. Each word appeared twice in the training materials, therefore accuracy was measured throughout phase 1 to gauge the amount of learning taking place over the 6 learning trials (2 words per story x 6 trials = 12 word repetitions in total).

In phase 2, the children were tested to determine how many words from each condition could be read in different situations. Depending on the experiment, retention was tested by giving children the same materials used during training (e.g., stories or lists), or the amount of fluency transfer was tested by providing the children with novel materials containing trained words (e.g., new stories or lists). The findings for accuracy, retention and transfer are discussed below.

Acquisition

Traditionally, investigations into the role of context have focused on the number of additional items that are read when children are presented with stories compared to scrambled word lists. Although the exact values vary, it is now generally agreed upon that if word identification is difficult because of characteristics surrounding the reader (e.g., low ability, inexperience, second language learner, etc.), or the text (e.g., too advanced, visually degraded, etc.) performance improves when words are presented in context (e.g., Archer & Bryant, 2001; Biemiller, 1970; Landi, Perfetti, Bolger, Dunlap, & Foorman, 2006; Nicholson, 1991). My colleagues and I were interested in an issue related to this finding, namely we wondered if we could capitalize on the added value of context observed during single reading trials to create optimal situations for word acquisition during training.

This question has been addressed by a series of experiments working with good, poor and average readers in Grades 2, 3, and 4 (Martin-Chang & Levy, 2005, 2006; Martin-Chang et al., 2007). As described above, a within-subjects design was employed in each of the experiments so that every child was taught to read two sets of different words; one set was taught in context, the second set was taught in isolation. In the context condition words were incorporated into meaningful stories. The stories we used were not predictable (i.e., Pilot studies using our materials have shown that when cloze procedures were employed, undergraduate students were not able to guess the identity of the target words), therefore children needed to attend to the print in order to arrive at correct word pronunciations. In the isolated word conditions, words were presented individually. In some cases, they were shown on a computer screen, in others they were presented on individual flashcards, but in both cases items in the isolated word condition were presented out of context.

One of the methodological considerations involved when comparing context and isolated word training, is that the children who have the most to gain by reading words in context (less skilled readers), generally come across the most difficulty when faced with reading a whole passage. Levy (2001) encountered this problem during an experiment where she trained good and poor readers to read two sets of words, one set was incorporated into a story and the second set was shown within a computer game. Although Levy reported no differential effects of context training for fluency gains (accuracy, reading rate, and comprehension) in novel passages containing trained words, a limitation of the study was that the number of word exposures was not held constant between the two training conditions. Due to the fact that the children could only read a passage once or twice during the same amount of time in which they could read several lists, the items in the isolated word conditions received, on average, double the number of repetitions during training compared to those in the context condition.

Building on the findings reported from Levy and her colleagues (Faulkner & Levy, 1999; Levy et al., 1997), Ring, Brown and Black (2008) compared reading improvements resulting from context and isolated word training in a group of 9-year-old students at risk for reading failure. Using a between-subjects design, Black et al. had children read either passages or lists containing target words adhering to specific vowel-consonant patterns (information regarding the target words can be obtained from the Texas Scottish Rite Hospital for Sick Children). Training occurred in small groups (app. 5 students), 3 to 4 days a week for 15-20 minutes a session. At the completion of training, greater gains on standardized tests of reading rate, reading accuracy, and word attack skills were reported in the children who received the isolated word training. These findings fit nicely with the corpus of work showing that training words in isolation improves subsequent reading of passages containing those same words. However, two key methodological points of this study bear consideration. First, in isolated word training the target words were presented to the children in a meaningful passage before they were pulled out of context and trained in isolation. It is possible that reading the words in a story at the onset of training set up a conceptual framework that influenced how the words were interpreted when they were later read in isolation. Second, because the experimenters controlled for training time (15-20 minutes) rather than word repetition, it is possible that the words read in isolation received more training trials than the words presented in context.

In order to avoid similar complications in the series of experiments reported here, we controlled for word repetition between the two experimental training conditions rather than reading time. We also equated task difficulty by ensuring that children were reading single words in both conditions. In order to do this, we employed a shared reading paradigm in the context condition where the participants read the target words and the experimenter read the remainder of the story. Word acquisition was measured as the number of target words read correctly during each training trial.

As depicted in Figure 1, the first trial of training replicated the well-established contextual facilitation effect in all five experiments (Alexander, 1998; Archer & Bryant, 2001; Kim & Goetz, 1994; Landi et al., 2006, Nation & Snowling, 1998; Nicholson, 1991; Nicholson,Bailey, & McArthur, 1991). Poor readers in third and fourth grade (Experiments 1 and 3) and average readers in second grade (Experiments 2, 4, and 5) were able to read substantially more items when the words were first encountered in context.

But would the initial boost in word reading accuracy be carried over the remaining learning trials? Based on our data, the answer seems to be 'yes'. The initial benefits of reading in context were maintained throughout an extended training program; at the end of 12 word repetitions, children with poor and average abilities were reading reliably more words in context compared to in isolation. This was a very robust finding, as evidenced by the consistent pattern of results observed across all five experiments. It is also especially noteworthy because every child received both methods of training. Regardless of how well the students were reading at the end of isolated word training they were reading statistically more accurately after context training. In sum, the data presented in this chapter suggest that the benefits provided by context – specifically, enabling children to repeatedly pair written words with correct pronunciations, accumulate over time to result in measurable increases in word reading accuracy.

In addition to word reading accuracy, reading rate was measured throughout training in 3 of the 5 experiments. As would be expected, children of all ability (good, average, poor) became faster at reading the materials as training progressed. Because the units of measurement varied between the two conditions (individual words were measured in milliseconds in the isolated word condition, story readings were measured in minutes in the context condition), we were not able to comment on whether words were read faster in context or in isolation during training.

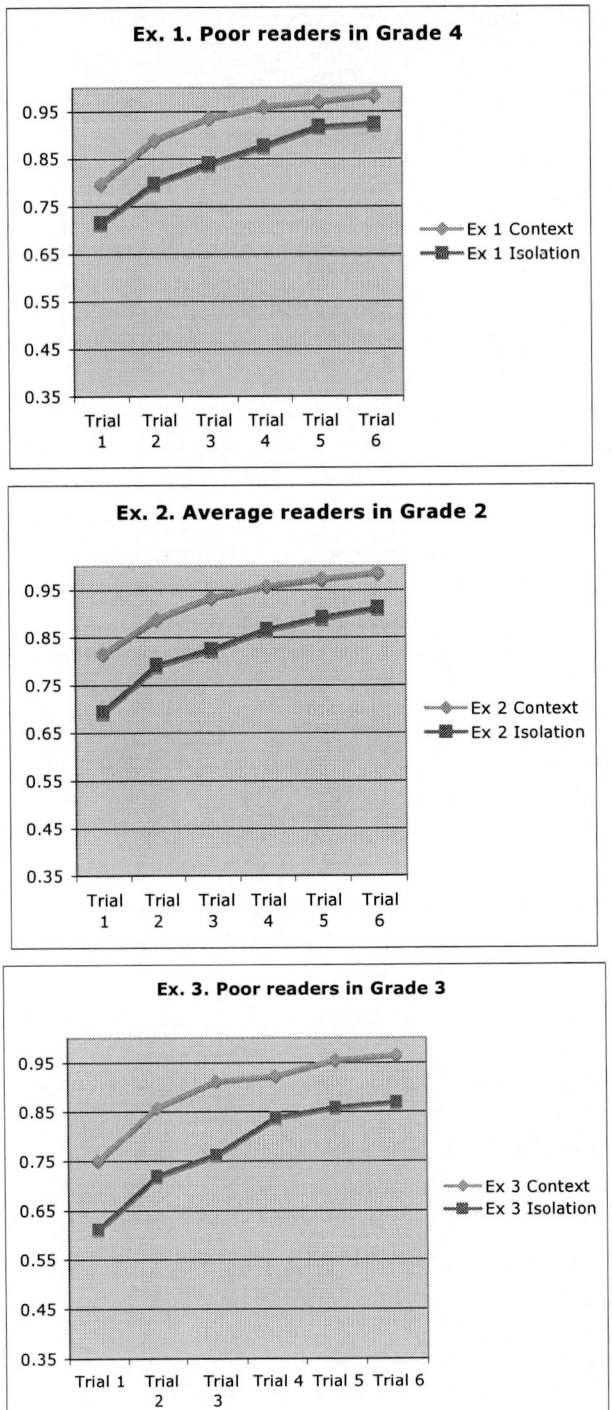

Figure 1. (Continued)

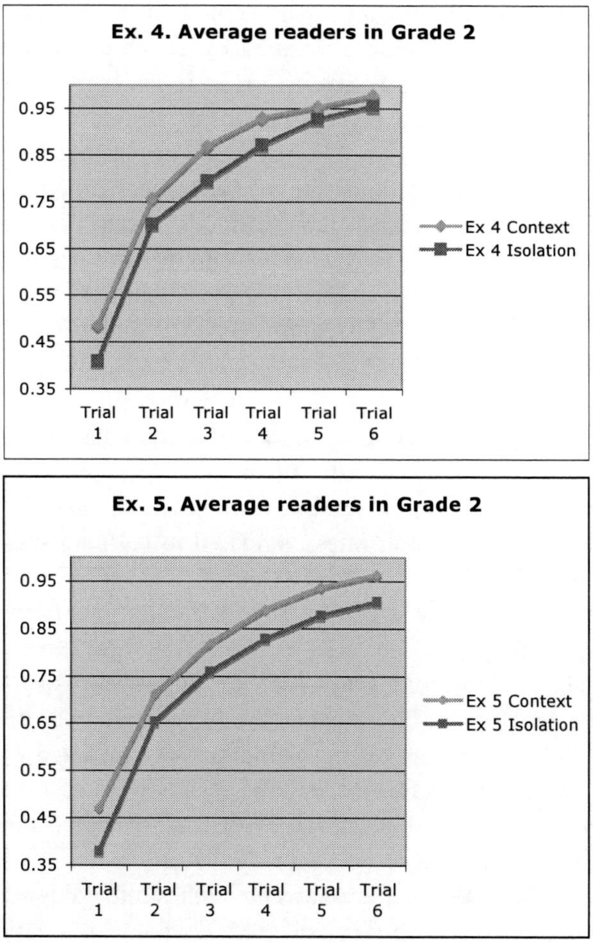

Figure 1. Ratio of words acquired as a function of training condition and trial

Retention

Torgesen et al. (2001) outlined five major factors that have the potential to disrupt reading fluency: 1) how well context is used to aid in word identification, 2) how many words in the passage are recognized by sight, 3) how quickly those sight words are read, 4) how quickly unknown words are read, and 5) how quickly word meanings are identified. With regards to using context to aid in word identification, the findings reviewed above have shown that reading words in context increases the number of successful learning trials that occur during training. Poor and average readers in Grades 2, 3, and 4 could name more words presented in context at every trial during training compared to words presented in isolation. Nonetheless, as Torgesen identifies in his second point, the paramount goal of training is to *permanently* increase the number of words children can recognize by sight. This begs the question of whether words learned in context are remembered as well as words learned in isolation.

One of the first studies to address this issue compared the effects of teaching words in isolation to teaching words that were accompanied by a picture. Samuels (1967) found that children entering first grade were more likely to read items correctly during training if the words were illustrated. However, the inverse pattern of results was reported at test; fewer words from the picture conditions were accurately read once stripped of contextual cues. In a second experiment, Samuels tracked the rate of word acquisition during the reading of illustrated and unillustrated storybooks. Again he observed that poor readers in the isolated word (no-picture) condition were able to read significantly more words on a subsequent word identification task compared to children in the illustrated condition.

Singer, Samuels and Spiroff (1973) examined the cumulative effects of pictures and sentences on the word acquisition of children in Grades 1 and 2. Words could be presented in one of four conditions: a) alone, b) in a sentence, c) with a picture, or d) in a sentence that was also accompanied by a picture. As the number of extraneous cues associated with target words increased (pictures and context) so did the number of repetitions required to reach the criterion of two successive error free readings. Once more, learning words in isolation resulted in the best long-term retention rates compared to learning words in the presence of sentences or illustrations.

Nemko (1984) also examined whether reading instruction was more profitable in context or in isolation. Using a fully crossed, within subject design, Nemko trained and tested children in isolation and in context. During each condition the words were presented once with feedback (in either isolation or context) and then immediately again without feedback (in isolation or in context). This training/testing paradigm was repeated 6 times. Only 4 words were taught in each condition, therefore no training results were reported. The 6 testing trials were combined to result in a total accuracy score out of 24. Nemko reported the best performance when target words were presented in isolation during both training and test (isolation-isolation = 19.39). Words were learned with similar degrees of accuracy in the remaining three conditions (isolation-context = 15.22, context-isolation = 14.35, context-context = 14.75). Thus, once again, learning was maximized in isolation.

Additional support comes from Johnston (2000) who trained children in Grade 1 to read words using 3 training methods: a) rereading, b) sentence context, and c) word banks. The amount of contextual support available to the reader systematically declined over the three training conditions. The rereading technique focused solely on the text as a whole and provided the greatest source of contextual constraint. In contrast, moderate contextual support was available in the sentence context treatment. Finally, the word bank technique used personalized sets of flashcards and consequently focused the children at the level of individual words. Johnston reported that all children, regardless of skill level, read more words correctly in the word bank condition, whereas the least amount of learning was recorded in the rereading condition. Thus, it seems that as reading becomes facilitated by context, the amount of attention allotted to the print decreases, resulting in compromised word learning.

Consistent with these accounts, Landi and colleagues (Landi et al., 2006) identified a number of words that second graders were unable to read in isolation. The children then read half of the words once in isolation, and the other half once as the final word in a predicable sentence. During the single training trial, Landi et al. noted that children had higher accuracy rates for words presented in context. Yet, when the words were presented in isolation after a 7-day retention period, all of the items were read with similar accuracy. Perhaps more telling, when Landi et al. considered only those words that were read correctly during the practice trial, they found that the retention rates were superior for words that were initially read in isolation. These findings lend support to Samuels (1967) argument, suggesting that while context may result in more accurate on-line recognition, it might also *reduce* the need to attend to the print which inadvertently results in corresponding reductions in long-term word acquisition.

The notion that words learned in context might be more easily forgotten was investigated in Experiments 4 and 5 reported in the present chapter (see Martin-Chang et al., 2007 for more details). During this set of experiments average readers in Grade 2 were first screened to identify two sets of words that could not be read in context. Once again, a within-subjects design was used so that each child learned half of the unknown words within a story while the remaining words were learned via flashcard training. The acquisition curves for these experiments are depicted in Figure 1 (Experiments 4 and 5). Eight days after training finished, the children were presented with the same materials used during training. The retention rates were highly encouraging. We found that once children learned a set of words, either in context or in isolation, very little forgetting took place over the 8-day interval. For example, in Experiments 4 and 5 participants learned to read 97% and 96% of the words presented during context training. After a week delay, they were able to read 98% and 97% of the words respectively. The non-significant increase from phase 1 to phase 2 seemed to suggest that the children were treating the retention task as an additional learning trial. The results were similar for words learned in isolation. At the end of isolated word training children were reading approximately 94% and 91% of the words correctly; once more, retention fell by only 1% and 3% after the 8-day delay (93% and 88% accuracy, respectively). There was no significant change in accuracy over the retention period for words trained in context or isolation in either Experiment 4 or 5. So why then, have others reported a drop in retention following context training and why we were unable to replicate it?

Transfer

Fluency affords children the ability to read never-before-seen text in a fashion that is easy, automatic and effortless (Meyer & Felton, 1999). Therefore, it is not enough that children can read words in the same materials used during training, they must also be able to easily access word representations from memory so that unfamiliar texts containing familiar words can be read fluently. In addition to word acquisition and retention, our group has also explored how memorial representations formed under one set of circumstances (i.e., in context or in isolation), are transferred to aid in the reading of novel texts. Specifically, several of our studies have been aimed at determining whether one method of training (either context or isolation) offers advantages for optimal fluency transfer.

Some pertinent work in this area has come from the work of Levy and her colleagues (Bourassa, Levy, Dowin, & Casey, 1998; Faulkner & Levy, 1994, 1999; Levy, Abello, & Lysynchuk, 1997; Levy, 2001). For instance, Bourassa et al. (1998) asked poor readers in fourth grade to read a training story 4 times in succession on day 1 of their experiment. On day 2, the training story was read one additional time after which the children were asked to read a transfer story and a control story. Both passages were novel, however the transfer story contained many of the words that had been practiced in the initial training passage, whereas the control story contained very few trained words. Bourassa et al. reported faster and more accurate reading of the transfer passages compared to the control passages. Importantly, they also found comprehension improvements in the transfer stories, suggesting that training words in one context can lead to heightened understanding of those same words when they are encountered in a new context at a later time.

Bourassa et al. (1998) also examined whether training words in context would transfer into the more fluent reading words presented isolation. Similar to the first experiment, poor readers in fourth grade read a training story 4 times in succession on the first day of the investigation. On the second day, the training story was read one additional time, however, at this point the children were asked to read two lists: one list containing trained words, and the second list containing untrained words. Bourassa et al. reported improvements in both reading rate and accuracy when words that were initially trained in context were later read in isolation.

The work of Bourassa et al. (1998) substantiated the claim that learning to read words at one level (text or word) transfers to several other levels. However, Bourassa et al. did not directly compare the efficacy of two methods of training. Therefore, they were unable to comment about whether one method of training (either context or isolation) resulted in enhanced fluency transfer. Our work was aimed at addressing this interesting gap in the literature.

Our basic research question, then, focused on how well children could read trained words when faced with new materials. As such, the transfer tasks were presented to the participants as new activities. No mention was made of the fact that the new stories or lists contained the same words that had been practiced during training. A methodological challenge associated with measuring fluency transfer in this way is creating materials that contain a high degree of word overlap between the training and testing passages that do not overlap in content. In the context condition, this was achieved by employing a shared reading paradigm during training that required the participants to read only individual target words. The remaining words, which were read by the experimenter, were used to create a semantic framework that was distinct from the transfer passage. For example, one of the training stories revolved around a Halloween party occurring in a third grade classroom. In this story, words such as **only, branch,** and **breeze** could be meaningfully incorporated into the story as finishing details describing the atmosphere of the classroom (e.g. "The **only** sound the kids heard was a **branch** in the **breeze** tapping on the window."). In contrast, the transfer passages were much shorter because they contained only words that had been trained in phase 1 (during transfer the children read the entire story, therefore the passages did not contain any extraneous words read by the experimenter). For example, the transfer passage accompanying *The Halloween Story* was about two young boys who make discovery in the woods. In *The Owl's Nest* the words **only, branch** and **breeze** were used to setup the main scene that takes place in the forest. In the isolated word condition, the transfer lists were made "novel" by adding a large number of untrained words at test. In both conditions, fluency transfer was monitored by tracking how accurately and quickly the trained words were read in the novel materials (passages and lists). Furthermore, reading comprehension was also measured in two of the experiments to ensure that the increase in reading speed did not come at the expense of reading for meaning.

We found that when children were required to read passages at phase 2, fluency transfer was the highest when training occurred in context at phase 1 (Martin-Chang & Levy, 2005;

Martin-Chang et al., 2007). We noted that children read new passages containing trained words more accurately after context training compared to isolated word training. This finding held after a 1-day delay (Martin-Chang & Levy, 2005) and an 8-day delay (Martin-Chang et al., 2007). In addition, both good and poor readers in fourth grade and average readers in second grade read the novel transfer passages faster following context training compared to isolated word training (Martin-Chang & Levy, 2005).

Interestingly, we observed the exact opposite findings when participants were asked to read novel lists during phase 2. Namely, good and poor readers in Grade 3 (Martin-Chang & Levy, 2006) and average readers in Grade 2 (Martin-Chang et al., 2007) read more accurately and quickly in isolation, when they had first received training in isolation.

Taking the transfer results from all five experiments into consideration, we are left to conclude that our original research question, asking "which method of training leads to universally better fluency transfer", was overly simplistic. Instead, a more profitable question asks "what are the circumstances that mediate the best method of training for fluency transfer". It would appear that the most advantageous method of training for optimal fluency transfer is directly dependent on the task employed at test.

Retention or Transfer?

It will be recalled that: a) several researchers have reported that words learned in context are more susceptible to being forgotten than words learned in isolation, and that b) the data reported from Experiment 3 failed to replicate this finding. However, even a brief examination of the literature shows that many investigators have failed to differentiate between retention and transfer. For example, the 'retention tasks' reported in numerous studies involve reading words in lists at test (c.f. Archer & Bryant, 2001; Johnston, 2000; Landi et al., 2006; Samuels, 1967; Singer et al., 1973). Under these circumstances *retention* was measured when words had been both practiced and tested in isolation, whereas accuracy *transfer* was measured for words that had been practiced in context but tested in isolation. This may account for the retention advantage for words both learned and tested in isolation in the studies discussed above.

Our findings fit nicely with this interpretation. In our experiments, retention was highest when the tasks presented during training and test were identical. Although retention was somewhat lower when learning had to be transferred to a novel task, advantages remained when the tasks during training and testing were congruent (both in context or both in isolation). In contrast, sharp decreases in retention were noted when the tasks presented during training and testing were incongruent (context to isolation, or isolation to context). Given this finding, it is interesting to note that many standardized reading tests involve reading words in isolation, even though it is widely acknowledged that children are rarely required to read words in isolation in day-to-day life.

CONCLUSION

The importance of instilling young children with early reading success cannot be overestimated. The goal for educators is to make early reading instruction as valuable and rewarding as possible for all children, and to quickly minimize the gap between good and poor readers when difficulties arise (Cunningham & Stanovich, 1997; Stanovich, 1980, 1986; Stanovich et al., 1996). Research has clearly documented the effects of contextual facilitation during on-line word recognition in poor and inexperienced readers (Nation & Snowling, 1998; Nicholson, 1991; Perfetti & Roth, 1981; Stanovich, 1980). Consistent with these reports, all five experiments reviewed here found that poor and average readers were able to name substantially more words on trial 1 in context compared to in isolation. The self-teaching hypothesis (De Jong & Share, 2007; Share, 2004) argues that every time a word is read correctly the child gains the opportunity to acquire word specific orthographic information about that individual word. If words have a greater likelihood of being read correctly in context, it follows that contextual reading should result in greater word learning than isolated word training. Our data support this hypothesis. The benefits associated with contextual reading on trial 1 were maintained over training. Poor and average readers were naming reliably more words at the completion of context training compared to isolated word training in all five experiments. We went on to demonstrate that the benefits of learning words in context does not come at the cost of poor retention; words learned in context were retained just as accurately as words learned in isolation. These results are consistent with the premise that contextual reading offers opportunities for word acquisition beyond those experienced from reading words out of context (Nation & Snowling, 1998; Tunmer & Chapman, 1995, 2002).

An examination of the transfer phases reveals a second general trend in the data. Namely, fluency transfer (as defined by reading speed and accuracy) is maximal when there is a high degree of congruency between the tasks employed at training and at test. For example, when the transfer task involves reading words *in context*, good and poor readers showed equivalent benefits in reading speed when practice takes place *in context*. In addition, these increases in speed occurred with no loss in reading comprehension. On the other hand, when the transfer task involves reading words *in isolation*, good and poor readers showed equivalent gains in reading speed after practicing words in *isolation*. Similarly, words are read more accurately in an unfamiliar passage when they were first trained in context, whereas words are read more accurately in isolation when they are first trained out of context.

Summary of Findings

This chapter opened by suggesting that context training could affect the development of reading fluency in three distinct ways. Taken together the results reviewed here show that for acquisition, children reliably experience more success when learning words in context. Both children of poor and average reading skill learned more items, in fewer trials, when the words were incorporated into meaningful passages. With respect to retention, words learned in context and in isolation are remembered equally well after a week long delay, as long as the children were given the same materials at test as they were given during training. The situation becomes slightly more complicated when measuring the transfer of fluency; here, either form of training can offer measurable benefits above the other, depending on the kinds of materials the children will need to read after training has finished.

Educational Implications

Reading, like walking, has the ability to grant access to new and unseen places – but only to those who posses adequate skill. Torgesen et al. (2001) suggested that fluency deficits remain resistant to remediation due to the lack of print exposure in the non-fluent reader. When reading is effortful and slow children simply choose to do other things. This notion finds support from the results reported by Martin-Chang and Gould (in press) showing that the slowest readers in university were also the least likely to read for enjoyment.

In spite of the heated and discrepant views that are often brought to the table with regard to reading pedagogy, most researchers would agree that the goal of instruction is to provide children with the ability to read stories quickly, accurately, and with comprehension. Training is not an end unto itself; the ultimate goal is to give children the skills and motivation to be able to read for enjoyment. With this in mind, the data presented here suggest that, after children are well versed in the alphabetic principal, training words in context offers benefits over and above teaching words in isolation (Martin-Chang & Levy, 2005, 2006; Martin-Chang et al., 2007). However, the fact that isolated word training can sometimes result in superior performance (i.e, when children are asked to read out of context at test) serves as an important reminder that there is nothing magical about learning to read words in stories 'per se'. Instead, it is simply the high degree of congruency between training (school) and test (extracurricular reading) that is expected to improve fluency transfer.

Acknowledgments

I wish to thank Megan Ladd and Christopher Martin-Chang for their careful reading this chapter. I would also like to gratefully acknowledge financial support SSHRC for the experiments summarized herein.

References

Alexander, J. C. (1998). Reading skill and context facilitation: A classic study revisited. *The Journal of Educational Research, 9,* 314-318.

Archer, N., & Bryant, P. (2001). Investigating the role of content in learning to read: A direct test of Goodman's model. *British Journal of Psychology, 92,* 579-591.

Biemiller, A. (1970). The development of the use of graphic and contextual information as children learn to read. *Reading Research Quarterly, 11,* 75-96.

Bourassa, D., Levy, B. A., Dowin, S., & Casey A. (1998). Transfer effects across contextual and linguistic boundaries: Evidence from poor readers. *Journal of Experimental Child Psychology, 71,* 45-61.

Boyle, T. (2004, June 22). New help for reading. *Toronto Star,* pp. A1, A19.

Compton, D., Appleton, A., Hosp, M. (2004). Exploring the relationship between text-leveling systems and reading accuracy and fluency in second-grade students who are average and poor decoders. *Learning Disabilities Research, 19,* 176-184.

Cunningham, A. E., & Stanovich, K. E. (1997). Early reading acquisition and its relation to reading experience and ability 10 years later. *Developmental Psychology, 33,* 934-945.

Dahl, P. R. (1979). An experimental program for teaching high speed word recognition and comprehension skills. In J.E. Button, T.C. Lovitt, & T. D. Rowland (Eds.), *Communications research in learning disabilities and mental retardation* (pp. 33-65). Baltimore, MD: University Park Press.

De Jong, P., Share, D. (2007). Orthographic learning during oral and silent reading. *Scientific Studies of Reading, 11,* 55-71.

Ehri, L. (1992). Reconceptualizing the development of sight word reading and its relationship to recoding. In P. Gough, L. Ehri, & R. Traiman (Eds.), *Reading acquisition* (pp. 107-143). Hillsdale, NJ: Lawrence Erlbaum Association.

Ehri, L. (1993). How English orthography influences phonological knowledge as children learn to read and spell. In R.J. Scholes (Ed.), *Literacy and language analysis* (pp. 21-43). Hillsdale, NJ: Lawrence Erlbaum Association.

Ehri, L. (1999). Phases of development in learning to read words. In J. Oakhill & R. Beard (Eds.). *Reading development and the teaching of reading* (pp. 97-108). Oxford, England: Blackwell.

Ehri, L. (2004, June). *Learning to read words: Theory, findings and issues.* Paper presented at the 11th Annual meeting for the Society of Scientific Study of Reading, Amsterdam, Netherlands.

Faulkner, H. J., & Levy, B.A. (1994). How text difficulty and reader skill interact to produce differential reliance on word and content overlap in reading transfer. *Journal of Experimental Child Psychology, 58,* 1-24.

Faulkner, H. J. & Levy, B.A. (1999). Fluent and nonfluent forms of transfer in reading: Words and their message. *Psychonomic Bulletin and Review, 6,* 111-116.

Fuchs, L. S., Fuchs, D., Hosp, M. K., & Jenkins, J. R. (2001). Oral reading fluency as an indicator of reading competence: A theoretical, empirical, and historical analysis. *Scientific Studies of Reading, 5,* 239-256.

Goodman, K. S. (1965). A linguistic study of cues and miscues in reading. *Elementary English*, *42*, 639-643.

Goodman, K. S. (1967). Reading: A psychological guessing game. *Journal of the Reading Specialist, 6,* 126-135.

Goodman, K. S. (1973). The 13th easy way to make learning to read difficult: A reaction to Gleitman and Rozin. *Reading Research Quarterly, 8,* 484-493.

Goodman, K.S. (1992). I didn't found whole language. *The Reading Teacher, 46,* 188-199.

Gough, P. B., & Wren, S. (1999). Constructing meaning: The role of decoding. In J. Oakhill & R. Beard (Eds.), *Reading development and the teaching of reading* (pp. 59-78). Oxford, England: Blackwell.

International Association for the Evaluation of Educational Achievement. (2004). Retrieved June 16, 2008, from http://www.iea.nl/.

Jenkins, J. R., Fuchs, L. S., van den Broek, P., Espin, C., & Deno, S.L. (2003). Sources of individual differences in reading comprehension and reading fluency. *Journal of Educational Psychology, 95,* 719-729.

Johnston, F. R. (2000). Word learning in predictable text. *Journal of Educational Psychology, 92,* 248-255.

Kim, Y.H., & Goetz, E.T. (1994). Context effects on word recognition and reading comprehension of poor and good readers: A test of the interaction-compensatory hypothesis. *Reading Research Quarterly, 29,* 178-188.

Kuhn, M.R., & Stahl, S. A. (2003). Fluency: A review of developmental and remedial practices. *Journal of Educational Psychology, 95,* 3-21.

Kuhn, M.R., Schwanenflugel, P.J., Morris, R.D., Mandel Morrow, L., Gee Woo, D., Meisinger, E.B., Sevcik, R.A., Bradley, B., Stahl, S.A. (2006). Teaching children to become fluent and automatic readers. *Journal of Literacy Research, 38,* 357-387.

LaBerge, D., & Samuels, S. J. (1974). Toward a theory of automatic information processing in reading. *Cognitive Psychology, 6,* 293-323.

Landi, N., Perfetti, C.A., Bolger, D., Dunlap, S., & Foorman, B. (2006). The role of discourse context in developing word form representations: A paradoxical relation between reading and learning. *Journal of Experimental Child Psychology, 94,* 114-133.

Levy, B.A. (2001). Moving the Bottom. In M. Wolf (Ed.), *Dyslexia, fluency, and the brain* (pp. 357-379). Timonium, MD: York Press.

Levy, B.A., Abello, B., & Lysynchuk, L. (1997). Transfer from word training to reading in context: Gains in reading fluency and comprehension. *Learning Disability Quarterly, 20,* 173–188.

Martin-Chang, S. L., & Levy, B.A. (2005). Fluency transfer: Differential gains in reading speed and accuracy following isolated word and context training. *Reading and Writing, 18,* 343-376.

Martin-Chang, S. L., & Levy, B.A. (2006). Word reading fluency: A transfer appropriate processing account of fluency transfer. *Reading and Writing, 19,* 517-542.

Martin-Chang, S. L., Levy, B. A., & O'Neil, S. (2007) Word acquisition, retention, and transfer: Findings from contextual and isolated word training. *Journal of Experimental Child Psychology, 96,* 37-56.

Martin-Chang, S. L., & Gould, O. N. (in press). Revisiting print exposure: Exploring differential links to vocabulary, comprehension and reading rate. *Journal of Research in Reading.*

Meyer, M. S., & Felton, R. H. (1999). Repeated reading to enhance fluency: Old approaches and new directions. *Annals of Dyslexia, 49,* 283-306.

Mody, M. (2003). Phonological basis in reading disability: A review and analysis of the evidence. *Reading and Writing: An Interdisciplinary Journal, 16,* 21-39.

Nation, K., & Snowling, M. J. (1998). Individual differences in contextual facilitation: Evidence from dyslexia and poor reading comprehension. *Child Development, 69,* 996-1101.

Nemko, B. (1984). Context versus isolation: Another look at beginning readers. *Reading Research Quarterly, 19,* 461-467.

Nicholson, T. (1991). Do children read words better in context or lists? A classic study revisited. *Journal of Educational Psychology, 83,* 444-450.

Nicholson, T., Bailey, J., & McArthur, J. (1991). Context cues in reading: The gap between research and popular opinion. *Reading, Writing, and Learning Disabilities, 7,* 33-41.

Perfetti, C.A. (1992). The representation problem in reading acquisition. In P. Gough, L. Ehri, & R. Trieman (Eds.), *Reading acquisition* (pp. 147-174). Hillsdale, NJ: Lawrence Erlbaum Associates.

Perfetti, C.A. (1999). Cognitive research and the misconceptions of reading education. In J. Oakhill & R. Beard (Eds.), *Reading development and the teaching of reading* (pp. 42-58). Oxford, England: Blackwell.

Perfetti, C.A., & Roth, S. F. (1981). Some of the interactive processes in reading and their role in reading skill. In A.M. Lesgold, & C.A. Perfetti (Eds.), *Interactive processing in reading* (pp. 269-297). Hillsdale, NJ: Lawrence Erlbaum Associates.

Progress in International Reading Literacy Study. (2006). *An international perspective on fostering reading development.* Retrieved June 16, 2008, from http://timss.bc.edu/ pirls2006/index.html.

Ring, J., Brown, S., Black, J. (2008). Reading fluency instruction for students at risk for reading failure: Effects of two approaches to improving reading rate. Presentation at the Society for the Scientific Study of Reading, Asheville, NC.

Samuels, S. J. (1967). Attentional progress in reading: The effect of pictures on the acquisition of reading responses. *Journal of Educational Psychology, 58,* 337-342.

Schwanenflugel, P. J., Hamilton, A. M., Kuhn, M. R., Wisenbaker, J. & Stahl, S. A. (2004). Becoming a fluent reader: Reading skill and prosodic features in the oral reading of young readers. *Journal of Educational Psychology, 96*, 119-129.

Shankweiler, D., & Fowler, A. (2004). Questions people ask about the role of phonological processing in learning to read. *Reading and Writing: An Interdisciplinary Journal, 17*, 483-515.

Shankweiler, D., Lundquist, E., Katz, L., Stuebing, K. K., Fletcher, J. M., Brady, S., et al. (1999). Comprehension and decoding: Patterns of association in children with reading difficulties. *Scientific Studies of Reading, 3,* 69-94.

Share, D. (1995). Phonological recoding and self-teaching: Sine qua non of reading acquisition. *Cognition, 55*,151-218.

Share, D. (2004). Orthographic learning at a glance: On the time course and developmental onset of self-teaching. *Journal of Experimental Child Psychology, 87,* 267-298.

Singer, H., Samuels, S. J., & Spiroff, J. (1973). The effect of pictures and contextual conditions on learning responses to printed words. *Reading Research Quarterly, 9,* 555-567.

Smith, L.E., Borkowski, J.G., Whitman, T.L. (2008). From Reading Readiness to Reading Competence: The Role of Self-Regulation in At-Risk Children. *Scientific Studies of Reading, 12*, 131 – 152.

Spear-Swerling, L. (2006). Children's reading comprehension and oral reading fluency in easy text. *Reading and Writing, 19,* 199-220.

Stanovich, K. E. (1980). Toward an interactive-compensatory model of individual differences in the development of reading fluency. *Reading Research Quarterly, 16,* 32-71.

Stanovich, K. E. (1986). Matthew effects in reading: Some consequences of individual differences in the acquisition of literacy. *Reading Research Quarterly, 21,* 360-407.

Stanovich, K. E., & Stanovich, P. J. (1999). How research might inform the debate about early reading acquisition. In J. Oakhill & R. Beard (Eds.), *Reading development and the teaching of reading* (pp. 12-41). Oxford, England: Blackwell.

Stanovich, K.,E., West, R.F., Cunningham, A.E., Cipielewski, J., & Siddiqui, S. (1996). The role of inadequate print exposure as a determinant of reading comprehension problems. In C. Cornoldi & J. Oakhill (Eds.), *Reading comprehension difficulties* (pp.15-32). Lawrence Erlbaum Associates: New Jersey.

Tomkins, G. E., Bright, R. M., Pollard, M. J., & Winsor, P. J. T. (2005). *Language arts: Content and teaching strategies.* Toronto, ON: Pearson Education Canada.

Torgesen, J. K., Rashotte, C. A., & Alexander, A.W. (2001). Principles of fluency instruction in reading: Relationships with established empirical outcomes. In M. Wolf (Ed.), *Dyslexia, fluency, and the brain* (pp. 357-379). Timonium, MD: York Press.

Tunmer, W.E., & Chapman, J.W. (1995). Context use in early reading development: Premature exclusion of a source of individual differences? *Issues in Education, 1,* 97-100.

Tunmer, W.E., & Chapman, J.W. (2002). The relation of beginning readers' reported word identification strategies to reading achievement, reading-related skills, and academic self-perceptions. *Reading and Writing: An Interdisciplinary Journal, 15,* 341-358.

In: Children and Language: Development, Impairment … ISBN 978-1-60692-395-5
Editor: Michael A. Reed

Chapter 3

CHILDREN'S LANGUAGE AND LITERACY LEARNING DURING A SCIENCE CONCEPT INQUIRY

Ni Chang
Indiana University, South Bend, Indiana, USA

INTRODUCTION

Using children's literature to assist in science inquiry and in knowledge building in other subject areas has been on the rise due to the benefits of supporting children's language and literacy learning. However, published research has reported a substantial variation in the methods of utilizing children's literature to support learning and language development. A deficiency in the association between reading and writing, and in the amount of time children are given to write has also been reported. "Writing was not linked to reading, and students seemed to spend relatively little time composing" (Allington, Guice, Li, Michelson, & Baker, 1995). In some classrooms in the United States, science is separately taught and given relatively less time in comparison with English/Language Arts (Royce & Wiley, 2005). In the real world, however, when it comes to learning science concepts, children do not often separate science from other subject areas that assist them in the inquiry, because the human brain naturally makes meaningful connections when new information is presented (Bredekamp & Copple, 1997). "One of the most important constants throughout human development is that all domains of development are interrelated. Development in one dimension influences and is influenced by development in other realms" (Bredekam & Copple, 1997, p. 144). Furthermore, Allington, et al also found ". . . hardly any art or drama activities linked to the reading children were doing in any of the classrooms" (p. 10). Therefore, the purpose of this study was to examine what might provide a scaffolding to a child's language and literacy competencies when reading was closely connected to writing and when art was linked to reading in the process of acquiring a science concept. The underlying research question is "What does an integrated curriculum provide to facilitate and how does an integrated curricular approach mediate children's language and literacy competencies when they are engaged in acquiring a science concept?"

Theoretical Framework

Science Inquiry through Integrated Curriculum

Children advance science understanding through various means, such as exploration, discovery, cooperation, collaboration, experimentation, and reading. Literature affords children ample opportunity not only to become familiar with science concepts, but also to gain language and literacy competencies if books are meticulously and thoughtfully selected and if adult-child reading interactions are appropriately designed (Chang, 2007). Curricular integration is at the heart of linking science with children's literature, which allows children to focus on scientific and literary elements at the same time (Cho & Kim, 1998). "Literature is not only an area of language development, but the center of integration for the entire curriculum through a whole language approach" (Cho & Kim, 1998, p. 3).

Literature-Based Science

This literature-based science approach to teaching signifies an integrated curriculum that falls into what Huck (1992) classified a comprehensive literature program. In comprehensive literature program, books permeate every area of the curriculum. Teachers read aloud to children and encourage them to respond to books through discussion, drama, art, and writing (Machado, 2007). As children learn science, they use the language arts skills, such as listening, speaking, reading, writing, and viewing to comprehend science concepts under discussion. Gambrell and Mazzoni (1999) reasoned that this comprehensive approach enables teachers to interlock various activities in a logical fashion, making activities meaningful to young children. These activities provide children not only with book skills, but also with a sense of lifelong literacy learning.

Literature-based science may help generate meaningful language learning activities that enable children not only to learn science through language, but also to learn language and to learn about language, which is supported by Halliday (1989 in the International Reading Association (IRA) & National Council of Teachers of English (NCTE), 2006-2007). Learning through language refers to the fact that children's learning takes place through the use of language. Learning language occurs through listening, speaking, reading, writing, and viewing. Learning about language implies that children develop an understanding of how language works. When children are situated in a learning environment in which these three aspects operate together, the learning context is meaningful and supportive for literacy development and learning makes sense to young children.

Sense-making learning also comes from children's books. Children's picture books afford children plenty of exciting and rich scientific experiences and encourage inquisitive minds. It is believed that linking science with children's books helps improve children's attitudes toward science, increase their interest in science, and promote their confidence in scientific abilities. In addition, "Connecting science with children's books has a potential to provide children with a richer, more realistic, and broader view of the nature and scope of science" (Cho & Kim, 1998, p. 5). In such a meaningful context for learning science, children are able to identify science with their life experience in a familiar setting (Cho & Kim, 1998).

Learning becomes easy to children as book content is related and interesting to them and allows them to describe what they know orally and visually/pictorially.

Reggio Emilia Approach to Science Inquiry

Art, such as visual/pictorial representations or symbolic expression in Reggio schools, is not at all a separate entity of curriculum, but an integrated part of the learning process, through which children are able to freely and comfortably express themselves. The Reggio Emilia approach to early childhood education advocates a curriculum that brings unity and continuity to teaching and learning. An analysis of science education research literature from an early childhood perspective enables Stegelin (2003) to conclude that the Reggio Emilia Approach can exceptionally and uniquely promote conceptual change within the constructivist paradigm. Reggio educators provide a scaffold for children's learning of concepts by engaging them in meaningful dialogues and by offering them with occasions for discovery. Learning, from Reggio educators' point of view, is a complex and upward spiral rather than a linear learning process (Malaguzzi, 1993). Children govern their own rate of learning as they develop a high level of curiosity with which they are likely to develop an ability to ask questions and a willingness to discover on their own. Learning moves back and forth, but in an advanced fashion. This notion is also construed through an understanding that children are intelligent, powerful, competent, capable, creative, curious, and elastic (Rinaldi, 1998). These attributes of young children are sufficient enough to make a persuasive conclusion: children are natural science researchers (Stegeline, 2003).

The U.S. science education goal is to promote self-directed thinkers and to challenge students to master science concepts necessary for helping them to build a solid knowledge base so they can understand the world around them (Stegelin, 2003). Additionally, the National Science Education Standards (1996) specified what science concepts that students, at varying developmental and grade levels, should know and understand (National Research Council, 1996). Since the Reggio Emilia Approach is intended to encourage young children to explore, discuss, and reflect upon key concepts, the inclusion of Reggio Emilia into early childhood science education is likely to make learning science concepts a much more stimulating, encouraging, and unforgettable experience (Stegelin, 2003).

Reggio educators affirm that visual documentation is critical to the learning and assessing processes (Gandini, 2002) and, hence, visually documenting children's learning process and its outcomes in various formats is essential to teaching and learning (Edwards, Gandini, & Forman, 1998; Stegelin, 2003). Reggio educators place more emphasis on a learning process rather than on a product. Children's learning processes can supply teachers with information about "how children arrive at specific conclusions, how they scaffold from one level of understanding to the next and how similar or different children's cognitive processes are at different levels of development (Fu, Stremmel, & Hill, 2003 in Stegelin, 2003, p. 165). Documentation thus should focus more on children, on actual ongoing learning experiences, and on children's thoughts, perceptions, and ideas (Katz & Chard, 1996) to reveal varying levels of children's understanding of certain concepts (Chang, 2007). This practice also works as a qualitative tool for assessment (Chang, 2007), because it assists teachers in planning for "how to provoke and encourage children's learning to the next and more complex level of understanding" (Stegelin, 2003, p. 165).

Since its beginning, curriculum is designed based on children's interests, prior knowledge, and/or life experiences, which work as a guiding torch throughout children's learning experiences. Curriculum is not designed in advance, but emergent based on children's interests and needs. Emergent curriculum usually is reflected through inquiry-based projects, from which general educational goals are set forth. During the process of its implementation, possible outcomes as a result of pedagogical decisions may occur consistent with perceived needs and young children's levels of learning, which result from their oral expressions as well as from expressions by the use of visual/pictorial language (Chang, 2007; Edwards, Gandini, & Forman, 1998).

From Pictorial Representation to Visual Literacy

Drawing is something that naturally attracts most young children. According to Sulzby (1996), most kindergarteners draw and scribble as they write to express themselves (in Machado, 2007). Given paper and drawing tools, children leave marks to create symbols, representing their observations, perceptions, wishes, ideas, understandings, knowledge, impressions, and feelings (Chang, 1996; Machado, 2007).

Durkin (1966) found that scribbling and drawing played a major role in forming a starting point of children's curiosity about written language. The development of literacy should begin prior to children's formal schooling, which can be partially achieved through activities that allow children to gain awareness of "associating spoken words with their graphic representations" (International Reading Association (IRA) & National Council of Teachers of English (NCTE), 2006-2007, n.d.).

One such activity is talking about drawings. Some of the symbols created by young children may be readily recognizable to adults while some others require a young author's interpretation or explanation to unveil the represented meaning (Chang, 2007), as these symbols are "unique and represent the word in the child's own way" (Machado, 2007, p. 491). Therefore, talking about drawing is essential and important (Chang, 2007). When an adult pays attention to children's graphic language and accept children's comments and ideas, children learn their thoughts are valued (McCormick, 1988), which may propel youngsters' continued effort to share their inner world (Machado, 2007). Dialogical interactions are also opportunities for children to recognize that created symbols can be read, spoken, or talked about and, at the same time, to see their thoughts can be written for expression and communication (Machado, 2007; McCormick, 1988).

Young children's creative writing ability has been strongly encouraged by many educators and researchers, such as Stauffer (1970), because it is basic to reading and a precursor to writing (Oken-Wright, 1998). Standards set forth by the IRA and NCTE (2006-2007) expect teachers to develop "curriculum and instruction that make productive use of the emerging literacy abilities." Viewing or visual representations integrated into curriculum or inquiry-based projects can be powerful in assisting children in acquiring a science concept, as all these multi-faceted means, including reading aloud, speaking, thinking, and writing/drawing simultaneously come into play, aiding the inquiry. It is a meaningful learning process, providing ample room for children to "adjust their use of spoken, written, and visual language to communicate effectively with a variety of audiences and for different purposes"

(IRA & NCTE standard #4) and ". . .to accomplish their own purposes (e.g., for learning, . . . and the exchange of information" (IRA & NCTE standard #12).

Visual literacy or viewing has been commonly recognized by the IRA as well as many researchers and experts in the early childhood literacy field. Through visual images, considered as a language, a child's perception of the world is made known (Weismann, 1970). Visual literacy represents one's ability to perceive, produce visual messages, and to think visually about images (Machado, 2007). Since "the primary literacy of the twenty-first century will be visual" (Machado, 2007, p. 165), children should have experiences that allow them to shift from word to illustration and vise versa. Visual literacy is a critical skill that can assist children in their learning across different educational disciplines, such as math, science, art, and language. It improves children's cognitive, reading, writing, and creative skills. The needed skills also include attending behaviors, discrimination, identification, and analysis (Machado, 2007). Visual thinking, visual arts, visual intelligence, and visual awareness all depend on one's ability to note various characteristics, including line, shape, color, texture, number, and various dimensions (Machado, 2007).

Stieglitz (1972) believed that the sense of sight played a crucial role as a basic source of information about one's immediate environment, because it not only involves the eye, but also the brain. When encountering something visual that either is of one's own interest or relates to one's past experiences, one has to make a note of it based on previous knowledge and ideas and to link it with feelings and emotions. Eye receptors note the perceived object or event with its unique characteristics relating to an individual's purpose in noting this particularity. If children are encouraged to note down their learning through graphic representations, this act functions as recording and demonstrating their understandings. When communicating with others about what has been seen, they not only have a chance to use language and to advance its growth, but also are able to trace and revisit their discoveries and actions. "The exercise is an instrument for reflection . . . Reflection can lead to a refinement of ideas and further search and discovery" (Machado, 2007, p. 165).

Morrow and Asbury (2003) highly recommended that visual literacy be integrated with speaking, listening, reading, and writing. It thus requires instruction to be explicit and well orchestrated, because when discussing children's creative art, the discussion gives teachers insights into what children are thinking through their reading and talking about visual cues and symbols (Machado, 2007). In this process, the adult and child are deliberately seeking meaning from children's expressed views and experiences (Barry, 1999 in Machado, 2007). Visual images and conversations about visual representations are conducive to advancing children's understanding of abstract concepts (Burmark, 2002) and concurrently promote language competencies.

Reading Aloud

The benefits of reading aloud have long been acknowledged by teachers and researchers alike in the early childhood field. Reading aloud enables children to hear and see picture books, which is advantageous to an increased interest of children in print. Reading aloud promotes children's concentration, develops their auditory perception, builds vocabulary, enlarges grammar, enhances thinking, and develops brain power. In addition, it widens the imagination, which, in turn, advances the creativity that is conducive to problem solving.

Reading aloud teaches children skills necessary to "differentiate the significant ideas in the content from the less important and to place the important ideas in a logical sequence" (Homeschool-curriculum-for-life.com, n.d.). According to Strickland (1990), reading-aloud activities are positive and beneficial to children's development because interactive behaviors exhibited by an adult and a child include "questioning, scaffolding (modeling dialogue and responses), praising, offering information, directing discussion, sharing personal reactions, and relating concepts to life experiences" (in Machado, 2007, p. 591). These practices are fundamental to conceptual development and the advancement of the language arts skills, including listening, speaking, reading, writing, and visual literacy. In addition, children's oral vocabulary increases as a result of active and oral participation in these activities. Oral vocabulary refers to words that are spoken and that are heard (Machado, 2007). Children's vocabulary, in turn, plays a crucial role in their comprehension and ease of learning to read (the National Reading Panel, 2000) just as "Oral vocabulary is a key in making the transition from oral to written forms" (Machado, 2007, p. 543). Therefore, teachers are expected to involve children in discussions about books to arrive at these recognized and worthwhile ends.

When talking about what has been read, children develop the ability to think and express their ideas (Homeschool-curriculum-for-life.com, n.d.). To acquire language, children need not only to engage with language for a certain purpose, but also to be situated in a social context. Two people interact with each other, in part, through the medium of language. While using language to communicate, a dyad of two individuals pays attention to one another, constructing meanings and influencing thoughts as well (Fries, n.d.). Discussions guided by sensitive adults help construct meanings and clarify comprehension that otherwise would distance children from the learning process. In dialogical communication, children's responses can offer teachers valuable clues, allowing them to know how to effectively work out the next step of instruction to further promote learning (Chang, 1996; Chang, 2007). Effective ways, aiming to encourage children to use language authentically, apparently need to be seriously sought out by concerned teachers in an effort to enhance children's learning and their language competencies (Machado, 2007).

Purposeful teacher dialogues with children, working as a stimulant, are intended to promote the mental and language growth of young children. In these intellect-building encounters, teachers explain and talk with children about objects and interesting concepts in order to "advance further discovery or to help put the discovery or experience into words" (Machado, 2007, p. 113). Dialogues enable teachers to be exposed to aspects of children's inner world, their concept learning, and feelings, which are deemed valuable in a continuum of teaching and dyadic interactions (Chang, 2007).

METHODOLOGY

Subjects and Site

The participants of the study included 71 children, ages 4-8, and 71 pre-service teachers across four semesters (spring and fall, 2005, spring, 06, and spring 07) from a Midwest comprehensive university. Most of the children (38%) were five years old, who were either in preschool or kindergarten (see Table 1).

Table 1. Demographics of Young Participants Ages 4-8

Age	Gender		Total
	Boy	Girl	*n*
4	3	8	11 (15%)
5	14	13	27 (38%)
6	8	11	19 (27%)
7	4	5	9 (13%)
8	2	3	5 (7%)
Total	31 (44%)	40 (56%)	71 (100%)

The majority of adult and young participants were Caucasians.

The adult participants in this institution were all Block One students (most were juniors). Block One is the first block for which the students must enroll after entering into a teacher education program to gain their baccalaureate degree and teaching licensure. These participants were identified through an early childhood course, "Inquiry in Math and Science." The college students were intentionally sampled because they had received rigorous training prior to actually working with young children on a one-on-one basis either in a school setting or in an alternative setting comfortable for both the adult and the child. The intentional sampling was also employed due to the participants' first-hand experiences of working with a child on a science concept.

Data Collection

Under the guidance of the researcher/ trainer (hereafter referring to as the researcher), each adult participant must exert an effort to tap into the interests of a child who would be the interactive partner of the adult. A child might be a cousin, a relative's child, or a child from a school where the participant was engaged in field experience. With an established intimate knowledge of the child, a science concept was determined. The participant planned and refined an integrated curriculum, consisting of English/Language Arts (book sharing and conversations), Science (a scientific concept) and Art (children's drawings). What an adult participant was required to do included (1) searching for a children's picture book conveying an accurate science concept and (2) designing a hands-on-activity that was plainly and simply related to the chosen concept. Based on the lesson plan that had been approved by the researcher, the interaction was implemented and was either tape recorded or videotaped before being transcribed. Each pre-service teacher must submit a written report, documenting his or her learning reflection besides the transcription of the conversation. The information provided by these students allowed the researcher to explore what opportunities an integrated curriculum provided to facilitate and how an integrated curricular approach mediated children's language and literacy competencies when they were engaged in acquiring a science concept.

Data Analysis

The data were analyzed qualitatively and quantitatively. The analysis of the conversation on the transcripts were based on the following: A) Halliday's Model of Language Functions (1973) was used to examine young children's utterances (see Table 2) and B) the language and literacy development information provided by Otto (2006) (see Table 3) coupled with Halliday's Language Functions was adopted to explore adult utterances in terms of opportunities provided to young children for oral language and literacy acquisition. The data were coded in line with Halliday's Model of Language Functions as well as the language and literacy development information provided by Otto. The coded data then were tallied and their individual frequencies were calculated to partially answer the research question concerning opportunities that the children had in the development of language and literacy competencies when interacting with adults in the process of learning science.

Table 2. Halliday's theory transformed for the purpose of data analysis

Code	Meaning	Example
Personal (P)	to express opinions or emotions	-I'll make something that you really like. - Doesn't make any.
Regulatory (R)	to influence the behaviors of others	-You do that other thing. - Mommy, smell this one.
Informative/ Representational (I)	to give information facts and information	-I made a Daddy snowman. -They help him, they help him walk like this.
Instrumental (IS)	to express their needs	-I need help making a robot.
Interactional (IN)	to form relationships	Mommy.
Imaginative (IM)	to express creative language	-Why do you have all those ears?
Heuristic (H)	to seek information and ask questions	-How do you make purple?
Yes or no answer		-Yeah. -No.

Even though the codes were predetermined in light of Halliday's theory and information congregated by Otto, the researcher also employed the constant comparative method suggested by Creswell (2002) and Lincoln & Guba (1985). This analysis was employed to examine the data to identify significant and meaningful patterns in relation to the research question, focusing on opportunities for offering scaffolding for young children's language and literacy uses. This exercise was undertaken continuously throughout the analysis process for data refinement.

Table 3. Codes of the language and literacy development information provided by otto

Code	Name	Meaning	Example
LL	Low level questions	Requiring a little thinking or a listener having an answer already	What color is this marker? Why did you draw this picture?
HL	High-level question	Stimulating a listener's thinking	Why is not a caterpillar's color the same as a butterfly's? How is rain formed?
CQ	Clarification question	Intending to understand better the message of what was just said.	Child: They are fireworks. Adult: You drew fireworks?
RQ	Recitation question	Knowing the answer, but intending to check for understanding	Adult: What is the first letter of your name? Child: My name starts with J.
IQ	Information questioning	Intending to know information	Adult: What are those giggly lines on your pictures?
TATQ	There-and-then question	Focusing on things or events not presented in the immediate context	Adult: We went to that apple orchard last year. Did you remember? Child: I do not remember. But I like apples.
*LES	Expansion or recasting	Completing what a child was just said into a full sentence to demonstrate more complex syntax, morphology, semantics, and phonology.	Child: A bird. Adult: Yes. I see the bird is flying to the South because Fall is approaching.
*LER	Repetition	Repeating what was just said	Child: This is a dinosaur. Adult:

*Linguistic scaffolding (LS)

Knowing the data thoroughly, the researcher coded and interpreted the data with different symbols and words representing language and literacy development. For example, READ/BO-IM denotes the impact that a book had on a child. LIT/VO-WR refers to a child's initial desire to write (see Table 4). The purpose of coding was to form categories emerging from the data that had the same content based on the researcher's carefully considered judgments. In the constant comparative method process, the data were constantly compared internally within a context and externally across categories. That is, the analysis was done by comparing incidents applicable to each category and then by classifying the coded data based on their individual categories. Even though the data were categorized according to their individual characteristics, the information within each category was further compared, being focused on similarities and differences.

Table 4. Codes used for categorizing language development

Code	Interpretation	Example
LIS/FO-DI	Listening through following direction	S: Now, you are going to get to do an activity to help you remember what the order of the colors in the rainbow look like. S: These are arches that are representing each of the colors in the rainbow. S: I would like you to try and order them in the order they go in according to what you have learned. S: Do you think you can do that for me? G: Yeah. Y
LIS/MA-DE	Listening through mathematical concept development	H: Can you count out the eight legs for me? K: One, two, three, four, five, six, seven, eight. [pointing to picture as he counts]
SP/BO-WA	Speaking through book walk	S: In this picture what colors do you see in the rainbow? G: [Points at the colors] Red, orange, yellow, green, blue, and purple.
SP/WO-RE	Speaking through word recognition	N: Do you remember what they are called? A: Um…. N: (Made the sound of the letter "t.") A: Tadpole. (She smiles)
SP/TU-TA	Speaking through turn taking and vocabulary learning	M: . . . The pumpkin seed grew into a pumpkin . . . T.J.: Ummm, that thing (pointing to the sequence card with a sprout on it). M: That's right, it's a sprout. T.J.: Sprout
SP/IN-IN	Through an investigating process of a child's interest	T: What are you interested in nature? T: And what do you know about [it]? K: Frogs—some are poisonous and some are not. K: They are different colors green, blue. K: Green are not poisonous. . . .

Table 4. (Continued)

Code	Interpretation	Example
READ/THINK	Ability to think while being read	Child: "I made sure to get the tongue right this time. I saw in the book that I didn't draw it right the first time. Child: "Do snakes really do that, or do snakes really need that?" while listening to a book.
READ/THINK	Ability to connect with one's own prior knowledge	While talking about the book content to enhance the child's understanding of the physical characteristics of an ant, MyKaila commented, "Don't touch the eyes" when the location of the ant's eyes were being discussed.
READ/VO-RE	Repeating what was being read voluntarily	An adult sounded out each word carefully while pointing at each of the words. Adult: One….Tiny….T..u..r..t..l..e. T-U-R-T-L-E. Child: Oh! Turtle! T-u-r-t-l-e. Turtle, that sounds like purple to me. P-u-r-p-l-e! Expect instead of p's there are t's!
READ/REPE	Adult's requesting a child to repeat words	Adult: Can you repeat those words after me? … Adult: Thorax (pointing to the thorax). Child: Thorax. Adult: Abdomen. Child: Abdomen.
READ/BO-IM	Empowerment of the book on a child's learning	Adult: So the egg turns into a tadpole? Child: Yeah, didn't you read the story?
READ/LIBRARY	Building a concept of a library's functionality	Child: Can I take the book too? Adult: How about I write down the title and who wrote it, then she can get it at your school library? Child: Yeah and I am going to check the book out when we go to the library
LIT/PH-EN	Phonological enhancement	R: Alright, I'll write and you tell me what to say. A: (points to the largest elephant) R: You want to tell me about this elephant first? A: Happy. Happy Elephant. Happy Elephant R: You want it to say Happy…

Table 4. (Continued)

Code	Interpretation	Example
LIT/LA-PI	Asked to label pictures	M: If you could please label what you are drawing, that would be of great help. A: Okay, here is the picture, and it is labeled too.
LIT/VO-WR	Voluntary labeling and writing	E: But let me write something down here (opens the book that Shannon just has read to him to a page with the names of different butterflies and starts to write down a specific type).
LIT/EN-WR	Encouraged to write	A: This is a baby frog. (She pointed to the smallest frog) J: Do you think that you could write "baby frog?" A: Yep (She writes 'baby.')
LIT/AS-WR	Asked to write a name	J: Can you put your name on it? A Is that a good N?
LIT/VO-RE	New vocabulary development	A child was exposed to and learned three new big words when acquiring a science concept of the water cycle:, evaporation, condensation, and precipitation
VIS/DRA	Mental ability to recognize differences visually and symbolically	Tyler quickly pulled his drawing close to him and attempted to modify it soon after viewing the picture of a spider on the book cover.
VIS/TA-DR	Talking about drawing	H: Can you tell me . . . about what you have drawn this time? K: Sure! I drew the sun in the corner, because snakes need heat. Then, I drew some rain, lots and lots of rain, because snakes need a lot of water. . . .

Categories that were, in some way, connected with one another and that were needlessly overlapping were combined together. For example, some questions that were categorized as low-level questions (LLQ) according to language and literacy information by Otto (2006). Examples are "Do you know what I want you to do for me now?" "Do you think you can do that for me?", "Can you tell me about your drawing?" "What is the first stage of a butterfly's life cycle?" A continuous comparison within the category show that although these questions all fell into the category of LLQ (low-level questions), the last two questions also were labeled as IQ adult. IQ denotes information questions according to Halliday's Language Function Model (1973).

Collected drawings and the researcher's notes were referenced to verify and refine the data, as were the communicative notes between the researcher and the participants. Reliability was sustained by the researcher's effort to code and re-code the data and to classify categories consistently across the four semesters.

RESULTS AND DISCUSSION

The study was intended to explore what opportunities an integrated curriculum provided to facilitate and how an integrated curricular approach mediated children's language and literacy competencies when they were engaged in acquiring a science concept. While a child was acquiring a science concept, several different subject areas, such as language arts, math, and arts were involved and assisted the learning process.

During the dialogical interaction, adult participants mostly asked the children low-level questions (LLQ) (34.45%) or shared ideas with the children (P adult) (34.08%). Young participants, in contrast, primarily offered information (I child) (60.23%) or stated their own ideas and thoughts (P child) (26.55%) (see Table 5).

The following will first present the analysis of questioning that occurred throughout a lesson in order to demonstrate what opportunities an integrated curriculum provided to facilitate and how an integrated curriculum mediated children's language and literacy acquisition in the process of learning a science concept. To further respond to the research question, the findings will also be presented specifically related to five areas of language arts development, namely, listening, speaking, reading, writing, and visual literacy/viewing.

QUESTIONING

Questioning technique was vastly utilized throughout a lesson to maintain the verbal interactions. The analysis shows that most of the low-level questions asked by the adults served either to seek information (RQ adult) (32.69%) or to solicit answers that they already knew (recitation questions--IQ adult) (31.26%). In interacting with the children, the adults infrequently utilized clarification questions and closed-ended questions that elicited either yes or no answers (see Table 6). The finding is consistent with the Otto's (2006) notion that questioning is essential to interactions, as it is one of the principal strategies to elicit responses from listeners.

Table 5. Children's Utterances In Light of Halliday's Model of Language Functions

Semester	LLQ	HLQ	IQ	CQ	P	I	R	H	IS	IN	Total	Y/N
Spring 05	57	1	3	6	110	200	15	6	4	0	402	74
Fall 05	29	2	0	0	161	351	1	6	2	0	552	67
Spring 06	22	3	0	0	87	246	13	10	0	0	381	103
Spring 07	19	4	0	0	105	253	3	17	5	2	408	82
Total	127	10	3	6	463	1050	32	39	11	2	1743	326
	7.28%	.56%	.17%	.34%	26.55%	60.23%	1.83%	2.31%	.62%	.11%	100%	

Table 6. Adults' utterances in light of both the language and literacy development information provided by Otto (2006) and Halliday's language functions

Semester	LLQ	HLQ	RQ	CQ	IQ	TATQ	P adult	I adult	R adult	LSE	LSR	Total	Y/N
Spring 05	229	8	53	2	63	1	271	67	83	1	0	659	4
Fall 05	307	2	73	3	97	0	276	105	58	2	2	752	5
Spring 06	318	15	109	4	124	0	282	164	100	3	2	884	18
Spring 07	283	28	154	13	88	2	234	160	78	31	10	824	6
Total	1137	53	389	22	372	3	1063	496	319	37	14	3119	33
	34.45%	1.70%	32.69%	1.85%	31.26%	.25%	34.08%	15.90%	10.23%	1.19%	.45%	100%	

There were various purposes for an adult to ask questions in the learning of a science concept. Questions, according to Machado (2007), encouraged the children to ponder and to express their thoughts verbally, which allow the adults to check children's understanding of concepts. During the interactive process, the adult participants modified questions to fit specific language levels of the children in order for them to respond with ease. In this process, the adults helped the children experience "turn-taking" (Otto, 2006; Pine, 1994), active listening, speaking, thinking, and following directions to further his or her language development (Otto, 2006). Exposing children to questioning also impacts their five aspects of language knowledge, including phonetics, semantics, syntax, morpheme, and pragmatics (Otto, 2006).

According to Otto (2006), phonetic knowledge involves children's receptive awareness and production of language-related sounds (phonemes). Semantic knowledge refers to children's receptive and expressive vocabulary. Syntactic knowledge means children's ability to use utterances comprised of more than three words. Morphemic knowledge indicates young children's linguistic competencies in communicating intended meaning more precisely with an ability to change word structures. Pragmatic knowledge is about children's ability to use language for a wider range of purposes, such as requesting permission, expressing emotions, or making judgments.

Attracting the attention

Seianna utilized questioning at the very beginning of a lesson to attract the attention of Gabby, a five-year-old child (see below). To respond to the question, Gabby had a chance to listen and to be exposed to the structure of a complete sentence as the adult expanded the words she just had said.

S: What do you think this is a picture of? [RQ adult, LLQ adult]
G: [*Smiles and her eyes get really big*] A rainbow! [I child]
S: You are right! [P adult]
S: It is a rainbow. [P adult] [LSE adult]

The structure of the question is short and well formed with no false start. The question asked is contextual, which was closely associated with the immediate context (the picture held in the teacher, Seianna's hand). It promotes the act of communication to enhance the child's language acquisition (Otto, 2006). The excitement observed in the child's eyes served as a vehicle to prepare the child for the subsequent dialogue.

A conversational interchange between a five-year-old boy, Josiah, and an adult, Sarah, in this same fashion can also be illustrated as below:

S: What do you think these are [in my hand]? [RQ adult LLQ adult]
J: [giggling] Seeds. [I child]
S: Yes, they are seeds. [LSE adult]

The first recitation question asked by both of the adults served the purpose of attracting the child's attention to a lesson that was about to start. The adults utilized a linguistic scaffolding technique to fill in words to make complete sentences out of the children's utterances: from "A rainbow" to "It is a rainbow" or from "Seeds" to "[T]hey are seeds." This behavior of expanding or filling in words to a child's verbal expression provides a means to enhance the child's acquisition of language competencies and is widely recognized by researchers (Machado, 2007, Otto, 2006). In addition, the adult's repetition of these key words, such as "rainbow" and "seeds" is intended to "reinforce pronunciation and to confirm the meaning of what the child said" (Otto, 2006, p. 51). Scaffolding technique is characterized by Bruner (1978) and Wells (1986) as a supportive teaching strategy with challenge, constituting responsive communication, open-ended questioning technique, and the facilitation of the child's initiatives (Machado, 2007).

Setting the stage

The questioning technique continued as an adult made an effort to prepare a child for the participation in the lesson. Seianna posed the following questions in order for Gabby, five years old, to concentrate on the scope of this lesson.

S: Have you ever seen an actual rainbow? [IQ adult, LLQ adult]
G: [*Smiles*] Yeah, it's in the sky and on the road like water. [I child]
S: What did the rainbow look like? [RQ adult, LLQ adult]
G: Like colors. [I child]
S: What colors did you see? [IQ adult, LLQ adult]
G: Green, red, yellow, blue, and uh [rolls her eyes up to think] pink. [I child]

The information question, "Have you eve seen an actual rainbow?" (IQ) led the child to share with the adult what she knew about a rainbow. With the adult's continual inquiry: "What colors did you see [on the rainbow]?" the child verbally described her prior knowledge of the science topic of the sequential colors of a rainbow, which, from the child's point of view, was comprised of five different colors. Not only did the adult get to know the child's knowledge level of the colors of the rainbow, but also encouraged the child to use her language skills to describe her mental picture about a rainbow (productive-expressive speech). In the second short episode, the adult asked two information questions with one recitation question, and the child was able to understand them all (receptive speech). The number of words constituting the questions yielded about the same number of words from the two responses from the child (I child) with 18 words each. The questions were well formed and fairly simple in their structure. Following the adult's questions did not seem to be difficult for Gabby. This conversational interaction with accurately modeled utterances allowed the child to think in order to provide information and impacted on the child's comprehension and language growth (Otto, 2006).

In a similar way, Sarah also captivated Josiah's attention (a five-year-old child) with a number of questions:

S: Do you know where they [seeds] are from? [RQ adult LLQ adult]
J: Maybe an apple. [I child]

S: You are right. [P adult]
S: These are apple seeds that will eventually turn into apples. [LES adult]
[Sarah brings out a whole apple to show.]
S: . . . Do you know how an apple grows? [RQ adult LLQ adult]
J: Uh-huh. [Y child]

In the dialogic interaction between Sarah and Josiah, with the concrete materials, seeds, displayed in front of the child, the child's attention was quickly captured. This paved the way for the child's concentration on the recitation question (RQ) posed by the adult. The child's comprehension of the question elicited a short response (I child). This, in turn, allowed Sarah to employ a linguistic scaffolding strategy (Otto, 2006) as she extended the child's short responses, "Maybe an apple" by saying, "These are apple seeds that will eventually turn into apples." It is a way to fill out what a child has said (Otto, 2006; Reich, 1986; Wells, 1986). Expansion or recasting (Camarata, 1995) used as a linguistic scaffolding strategy helps advance the child's acquisition of language skills (Machado, 2007; Otto, 2006). Expansion models more complex syntax, morphology, semantics, and correct pronunciation (phonology) (Machado, 2007; Otto, 2006). It is contingent on the experience of a child encountered at the very moment. The responsive communication of the adult expands the syntactic composition of the child's utterance (Machado, 2007).

In addition, Sarah's verbal statement helped facilitate Josiah's language skills because they are closely tied to the jointly focused objects (seeds and an apple). "Referents of utterances found in the immediate context give the young child a visible connection between the oral symbol and its actual referent" (Otto, 2006, p. 48).

Requesting a Drawing

After the expansion of the child's utterance, Sarah brought out a real apple. This additional concrete material further excited Josiah, age 6, and helped activate his prior knowledge. At this moment, Sarah requested a drawing from Josiah in order to receive detailed information of what a child knew about the growth cycle of an apple:

S: Can you show me with a picture how an apple grows? [LLQ adult]
[Josiah picks up the red crayon. He draws a tree with apples on it. He also adds his name to the picture.] (see Figure 1)

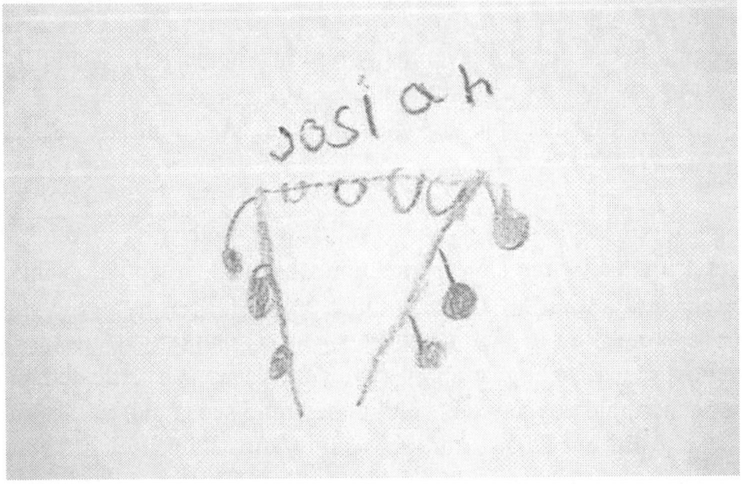

Figure 1. Josiah's first attempt to describe the growth cycle of an apple

A similar situation took place in the interaction between Seianna and Gabby, age 5:

S: Can you draw me a picture of how the colors appear in a rainbow? LLQ adult]
G: [Giggles] Yeah.

[Gabby picks up the green crayon first and draws the top of the rainbow. She then grabs the purple crayon and draws the next arch in the rainbow. She then continues with the red crayon, followed by the yellow crayon, the orange crayon, and finally ending the rainbow with the blue crayon.]. (see Figure 2)

The verbal exchange between the adult and child enabled the child to focus on the science concept. The children's active listening seemed to allow them to understand the requests. While the questions facilitated the children's listening, the children had an opportunity to learn that a mental image can be expressed through a graphic representation (Paquette, Fello, & Jalongo, 2007).

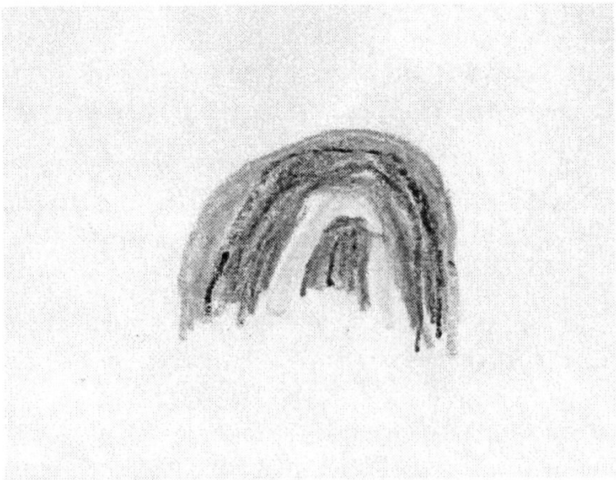

Figure 2. Gabby's prior understanding of the rainbow colors

Sometimes, when a request is made, the child's action does not directly reflect what had been requested. An adult then flexibly takes advantage of this opportunity to engage the child in a scaffolded conversation to enhance his or her acquisition of language competencies (Otto, 2006). In addition, the adult's intimate listening facilitated the child's language skills (Machado, 2007). The following segment of conversation illustrates the supportive scaffolding that the adult provided to the child's listening, speaking, turn-taking, and direction following skills.

J: Yeah, can you draw that [tornado] for me? [IQ adult LLQ adult]
G: I like this new crayon. It's pointy. [P child]
J: I like new crayons too. [LSR adult]
J: This box has lots of new crayons if you want to use those. [LSR adult LSE adult]
G: This looks like my tornado friend. [P child]
J: Your mom told me you have a tornado friend. [LSR adult]
She says it makes big messes just like a tornado. [P adult]
Is that what you're drawing? [IQ adult LLQ adult]
G: Yeah. [Y child]

This conversation, unlike the two that were presented earlier, did not take in the pattern of the child's quick compliance with the adult's request. Unexpectedly, the conversation focus shifted from tornados to crayons. Yet, Jenni let six-year-old Gena assume control over the conversation by consciously following the lead of the child. After her information question (IQ adult), Jenni realized that the child's focus at that time was on the new crayons provided. With the understanding that a young child usually is fascinated by new writing tools, Jenni patiently waited for the child's enthusiastic exploration of the drawing tool. Yet, to facilitate the child's linguistic skills, Jenni followed suit by repeating the child's utterance about the new crayons: "I like new crayons too." The repetition changed the sentence as structured by the child to show her more complex sentence structure achieved by switching from the singular (this new crayon) to the plural (new crayons). In the meantime, she extended the sentence to make it more complex in its structure: "This box has lots of new crayons if you want to use those." The child then quickly changed a topic from new crayons to that of tornados: "This looks like my tornado friend." By this lead, Jenni made an attempt to shift the child's focus to the science topic by emphasizing the key words, "a tornado friend," in the sentence, "Your mom told me you have a tornado friend." The repetition serves to confirm the child's utterance. The next sentence was further intended to arouse the child's interest in the topic. The question that Jenni asked afterwards purposefully lured the child back to the topic of the tornado formation. In this process, Jenni facilitated the child's turn-taking, listening, speaking, and direction following, because the child had to listen to Jenni carefully in the entire interchanging communication in order to follow and respond to the questions. This finding is consistent with the notion made by Otto (2006). Jenni was able to maintain the conversation even though the topic appeared to be derailed at a time, because she employed contingent questioning to pose a series of questions that were built on Gena's response to engage the child's thinking and oral responses (Otto, 2006; Trousdale, 1990). Moreover Jenni's ability to verbally map (Otto, 2006) what Gena said shows that she was able to take into account the developmental level of the child's receptive language skills. The action of the child's drawing of tornados and the science topic itself promote the child's conceptual development. "Verbal mapping is not just idle chatter on the part of an adult. Instead, it involves a conscious focus by the adult on the concepts and vocabulary relevant to the ongoing learning activity" (Otto, 2006, p. 49). In a communication loop, a child does initiate a change of a topic. An adult sensitive to the changed topic quickly becomes responsive by providing supportive scaffolding to sustain the communicational flow. As the topic of tornados was being discussed, the child was exposed to syntactic, morphemic, and phonemic knowledge related to the concept, extending and expanding the child's receptive and expressive language (Otto, 2006).

Eliciting Prior Knowledge

In soliciting the content of a drawing, an adult's information question was an opportunity for a child to use language to describe what appeared on a piece of paper (see the dialogue below-S denotes Sarah and J represents Josiah, age 6):

S: Okay, can you tell me what is happening in your picture? [IQ adult LLQ adult]
J: They are growing, a tree and the apples are growing. [I child]

The child described his picture in roughly two complete sentences: "They are growing" and "the apples are growing." The child was able to comprehend the adult's complex question that is composed of a compound structure with one main clause and one subordinate clause. In addition, it also involves the aspects of semantics, syntax, and morpheme. It is apparent that the child had no difficulty understanding the question and responded with correct morphology: "They are growing. . . the apples are growing" besides selecting an appropriate verb and forming grammatically correct sentences. The information also enabled Sarah to gain some insight about Josiah's understanding of the growth cycle of an apple.

The verbal exchanges taking place between Seianna and Gabby, a five-year-old child, further show language enhancement as a result of the information question posed by the adult:

S: . . . Can you describe your picture to me? [LLQ adult]
G: It's a pretty rainbow with lots of colors. [I child]
G: It has purple in it. [I child]
G: That's my favorite color! [*Smiles*] [P child]
S: It is a pretty rainbow. [P adult]
S: You did a very good job drawing the arches and filling them each in with different colors. [P adult]

The adult's low-level question (LLQ) elicited three complete sentences with the first sentence structure being more complex than the other two: "It's a pretty rainbow with lots of colors." Not only did the child describe the drawing, but also expressed her own feeling about a certain color (P child). The pictorial explanation by the child was then acknowledged by the adult. The acknowledgement made the child see that her utterances were understood by the adult and that the rainbow was shaped in arches and did have different colors: "It is a pretty rainbow. You did a very good job drawing the arches and filling them each in with different colors." All the utterances about the picture that Gabby produced coupled with the verbal expression about the colors of a rainbow prior to the drawing fairly well informed Seianna of how much the child knew about the rainbow colors (see Figure 2).

Gauging the Comprehension

After book reading and follow-up discussions, communication continued with questions and answers. Seianna utilized a series of questions to gauge where four-year-old Gabby was conceptually. Concurrently, the child was assisted in solidifying or constructing the science concept by speaking and thinking.

S: Okay, now I am going to ask you some questions that relate to what we have just read from the book and we will not use the book to find the answers this time. [R adult]
G: Uh…okay. [Y child]
S: What colors are in the rainbow? [RQ adult LLQ adult]
G: [Takes her time recalling the colors and thinks carefully to herself] Red, orange, mmm… yellow, uh….green, uh…blue, and purple! [I child]
S: Great job! [P adult]
S: You named all of them and in the correct order too. [P adult]
S: I am so proud of you. [P adult]
S: What color is always on top? [RQ adult LLQ adult]
G: Red. [I child]
S: Good job. [P adult]
S: What color is always on the bottom? [RQ adult LLQ adult]
G: Purple! [I child]
G: That's my favorite color! [Smiles]. [P child]

The initial directional statement was relatively long for a young child. However, the child seemed to be able to follow it: "Uh . . . okay." The recitation question made the child think hard before sharing the answer verbally. The targeted and purposeful praise further inspired the child to cooperate with the adult. Soon after the adult posed another recitation question (RQ adult LLQ adult), the child's quick response consistently showed her close attention to the adult's question: "Red." The next response given by the child clearly demonstrated her listening comprehension, because instead of asking the second color of the rainbow, the adult gave an unexpected twist to solicit the answer of the last color of the rainbow. Accurately, the child was able to answer: "Purple." Not only did she answer the question, but also expressed her comment on the color: "That is my favorite color." This interactive segment strengthened the child's listening ability, but offered the opportunity for the child to communicate orally with the adult. Literal or low-level questions (Genishi & Dyson, 1984; Otto, 2006) serve to have children recall facts or learned concepts and help establish a basic level of comprehension and understanding. In the meantime, questions like these enable adults to perceive whether children are on the right track in the learning process (Otto, 2006).

Jaime engaged McKenzie (a five-year-old child) with questions and answers in order to informally gauge the child's level of understanding of the growth cycle of a pumpkin. This interactive process not only was an opportunity to reinforce the child's acquisition of the science concept, but also exposed the child to more formal language structure.

J: How does a pumpkin start out? [RQ adult LLQ adult]
M: By seed. [I child]
J: Good! A pumpkin starts out as a seed. [I adult] [LSE adult]
J: Then what does that seed grow into? [RQ adult LLQ adult]
M: Um……..a stem and leaf. [I child]
J: Right! The seed grows from the ground into a little green stem you can see above the ground. [I adult] [LSE adult]
J: In the book they call that little stem a sprout. [I adult]
M: Oh yeah. I forgot. [P child]

Jaime's two recitation questions resulted in three utterances from the child. The incomplete sentences by the child as the information, e.g., "By seed" and "a stem and leaf," then were expanded by the adult: "A pumpkin starts out as a seed" and " . . the seed grows from the ground into a little green stem you can see above the ground." In this verbal interaction, the adult was modeling for the child by expanding the sentences to show the child how to structure a formal sentence with the correct tense (starts), a correct corresponding verb phrase (starts out) and a correct use of a preposition (as). This effort can further promote the child's understanding of semantics, syntax, morpheme, and phonetics (Otto, 2006). Otto recognizes the expansion of a child's utterance as linguistic scaffolding; it is the adult's attempt to use language in a supportive manner for children to communicate and to express their insights.

The second sentence is more complex than the first one, because it has a main clause, "The seed grows from the ground into a little green stem" with an adjective sub-clause, "you can see above the ground" to modify "a little green stem." Exposed to this sentence, the child again was reinforced with the correct selection of a verb and a correct verb tense use. This learning opportunity provided the child with more to know, including how to use spatial words, such as "above," another verb phrase, "grow into," a prepositional phrase, "from the ground," an adverb phrase, "above the ground." Also in this learning process, the child was further informed of the usefulness of the book and learned a new vocabulary word, "sprout."

Hands-on Activity

To help Kevin (a five-year-old child) further construct a concept of physical characteristics of a spider, Hannah provided him with Styrofoam balls, pipe cleaners, glue, black buttons, etc to create a spider. The questions that Hannah asked passed the dialogical turn to the child in order to bring out Kevin's understanding of the physical characteristics of a spider:

H: Which part of your spider is the front? [RQ adult LLQ adult]
[Kevin points to the front of his spider.]
H: How do you know? [RQ adult LLQ adult]
K: It has legs. [I child]
H: So, you remembered that the legs are on the front body part? [CQ adult LLQ adult LSE adult]
K: Yes. [Y child]

H: Good job! [P adult]
H: That is an awesome spider! [P adult]
K: I put two eyes on the top of the head so that it can see if someone is trying to kill it. [I child]
H: Wow, the book did say that some spiders have eyes on the top of their head. [LSE adult]

Questioning in this discourse consists of one clarification and two recitation questions. These two types of questions informed the adult about Kevin's level of understanding of the science concept. Linguistically, Kevin had several attempts to use language to communicate while solidifying his newly acquired knowledge by Hannah's repetition of "legs" in the sentence: " . . you remembered that the legs are on the front body part?" (CQ adult LLQ adult LSE adult) following the child's utterance of "It has legs" (I child). Because of the appropriate questions raised by Hannah, even the adult's personal expression: "This is an awesome spider!" could inspire Kevin to add more information by speaking a complex sentence: "I put two eyes on the top of the head so that it can see if someone is trying to kill it" (I child). This oral expression, on the other hand, reflected the focused attention that the child had on the book content while it was being read to him. The adult then provided linguistic scaffolding by adding plural nouns to the sentence and by changing the sentence structure. Her response was, "Wow, the book did say that some spiders have eyes on the top of their head." Such a response facilitated the child's language acquisition (Otto, 2006).

Gauging the Learning Outcome

In the end of the learning process, another drawing was solicited in order for an adult to "assess" a learning outcome. This was an opportunity for Josiah, six years old, to use language to share what had been learned with Sarah.

S: Can you tell me about your picture? [IQ adult LLQ adult]
J: First the seed came, then the tree, then the bud, then the flower, and then the apple. [I child]

This information-seeking provided the child with an opportunity to express what he confidently knew about the life cycle of an apple. Although the question only had 7 words, the child responded with 17 words.

In a similar case, Gabby also acquired not only the new science concept, but also new vocabulary. Moreover, she was able to freely express herself.

S: . . can you tell me about your picture? [IQ adult LLQ adult]
G: Yes, I colored a rainbow with colors in order. [I child]
S: What is the order of the colors you drew? [RQ adult LLQ adult]
G: Red, orange, yellow, green, blue, and purple. [I child]

The child demonstrated to the adult, as a result of the question, that she learned new vocabulary, "in order." It also shows her capability to make a relatively more complex sentence with two prepositional phrases: "with colors" and "in order." The second recitation question posed by Seianna was a complex sentence with a main clause and a subordinate clause. However, the child was able to follow with a response that was conceptually correct even though Gabby had just acquired it (see Figure 3). Otto (2006) theorized that the way a question is worded by an adult would influence how a child would structure his or her response.

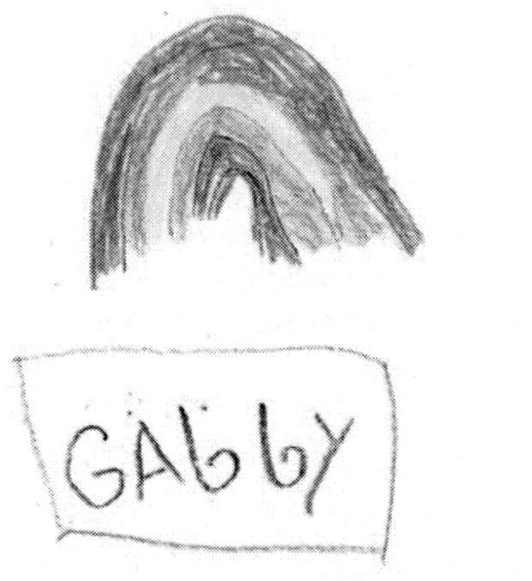

Figure 3. Gabby's post-learning drawing

The general finding shown above was also in line with another notion made by Otto, (2006) and by Trousdale (1990). The sustainability of the conversations demonstrates the adults' uses of contingent questioning, which composes a series of questions building on each other to engage children's thinking and elicit oral responses. Taking into consideration the child's responses, follow-up questions were thereby formulated (Otto, 2006; Trousdale, 1990).

FIVE LANGUAGES ARTS AREAS

To further respond to the research question, the following text will set forth opportunities the young participants had specifically related to five areas of language arts development, namely, listening, speaking, reading, writing, and visual literacy/viewing in the process of learning a science concept through an integrated curriculum.

Listening

While engaging the children in the learning of a science concept, the adults facilitated the children's listening acquisition through questioning. Yet, the study also found that a child's listening skills were facilitated through the following:

Following directions

For the child to construct a learned science concept, a hands-on activity was provided after book reading and follow-up discussion. Although ittle verbal exchange happened during this interaction, prior to a child's engagement in the activity, he or she had to listen in order to know how this activity worked (see the example given below). S denotes Seianna, an adult, while G denotes Gabby, a five-year-old child:

S: Now, you are going to get to do an activity to help you remember what the order of the colors in the rainbow look like. [R adult]
[Seianna shows her the colored arch pieces.]
S: These are arches that are representing each of the colors in the rainbow. [P adult]
S: I would like you to try and order them in the order they go in according to what you have learned. [R adult]
S: Do you think you can do that for me? [LLQ adult]
G: Yeah. [Y child]
[The child grabs the pieces and begins to lay them out on the table.]
G: [Talks out loud as she places each piece in its order] Red, orange, yellow, blue, green, purple. [P child]

Seianna's instruction was quite long. It consists of two regulatory speeches and one personal speech. Although the adult's comment in between those two long regulatory speeches was relatively short, it was a complex sentence with a main clause and an adjective sub-clause, describing the arches. To this five-year-old child, Gabby, it provided a change in following the direction. While Gabby was listening to the instruction, she had to actively process the adult's utterance in order to understand what she was hearing. The child's response, in return, shows to the adult that Gabby was successful in receiving the information. Machado (2007) supported the practice as she believed that listening required practice since it is a learned behavior. Sometimes, children hear, but may not understand what they have heard. "Language development depends on the auditory process" by sustaining attention span and following directions (Machado, 2007, p. 244).

Learning Mathematics

Listening took place through the child's engagement in mathematics learning. After reading aloud, Hannah and her five-year-old child, Kevin, were engaged in a book walk about "the physical characteristics of a spider." The book walk not only granted the child an enhanced understanding of the number of legs that a spider has, but also reviewed and practiced counting, solidified cardinal number (four), and reinforced his spatial sense (on this side) (see the conversation below):

H: Now, let's look at this book again. [R adult]
H: And we are going to point to the parts as we read them. [R adult] Okay?
H: Can we point to the parts of the spider as we read them? [LLQ adult]
K: Uh-huh. [Y child]

H: Can you count out the eight legs for me? [LLQ adult]
K: One, two, three, four, five, six, seven, eight. [pointing to picture as he counts] [I child]
H: How many legs are on this side? [pointing at book] [RQ adult LLQ adult]
K: Four. [I child]
H: How many legs are on this side? [pointing at book] [RQ adult LLQ adult]
K: Four. [I child]
H: Yes. [Y adult]

This episode of book walk promoted the child's listening by having the child's attention drawn on the adult's utterances. In this practice, the child's attentive listening made him respond to every step that the adult expected him to do. His answers confirmed that the child was able to decipher the adult's spoken language as he understood what a cardinal number is. Learning the physical characteristics of a spider involved learning or reviewing the mathematical concept. At the same time, it encouraged the child's careful listening. Discussion following a read-aloud helps develop young children's language skills (Short, Kauffman, & Kahn, 2000; Soundy, Guha, & Qin, 2007). The adult's affirmative answer "Yes" to the child's responses became a rewarding experience that continued to sustain the child's attention to learning (Machado, 2007).

Recognizing Words

N: Okay, now we'll go back through the book. [R adult]
N: You were right that in the first stage of a frog's life cycle they are eggs. [I adult]
N: They are wrapped in jelly. [I adult]
N: The second stage they have gills. [I adult]
N: Do you remember what they are called? [LLQ adult]
A: Um....
N: (Made the sound of the letter "t.")
A: Tadpole. (She smiles) [I child]

Although the child did not say a lot, the combination of the regulatory speech (R adult) and information speech to provide information, either to verify what a child knew or to reinforce the new concept (I adult), encouraged the child to listen. Because of her attentive and active listening, the child knew when it was time for her to respond: "Um . . ." Quickly reacting on the child's cue, the adult retaught the child with an elicitation method. This episode shows that interaction between an adult and a child works as an opportunity for promoting a letter sound (phoneme) and vocabulary construction (Otto, 20006).

Reading Aloud

Reading aloud evoked a child's thinking when a child had a great interest in the topic covered by the book. This is consistent with Machado's (2007) notion that listening is a learned behavior. Although it seemingly appears to be passive and receptive, listening promotes a child's thinking and encourages the child to interpret what has been read to him or her, which, in turn, draws more attention from the child to the book being read. After Kevin, a five years old child, drew his first picture of the physical characteristics of a spider, Hannah read a children's book, Spiders by Monica Hughes. Kevin was looking intently at the pictures while the book was being read aloud. His apparent active thinking about the book content led him to make a heuristic speech to query the picture in the book: "What are these sticking out?" [pointing to the hairs on the spiders legs]. The answer given by the adult encouraged his further thinking by closely listening to the book: "Let's keep reading the book and see if it tells us." This encouragement, in turn, piqued the child's interest in the book. His desire to seek the answer from the book grew. Duke and Pearson (2002) and Johnson (2009) supported the use of authentic books that may be enjoyable to children and that may increase the children's desire to read. Johnson further posited, "A child who is engaged in reading employs both his mind and his heart. . ." (p. 48). Kevin's displayed behavior completely demonstrates this notion. It was because of careful listening and his deep engagement of his heart and mind that he asked a higher-level question.

Table 7. Adult and child utterances across the four semesters

	Spring 05		Fall 05		Spring 06		Spring 07	
	Adult	Child	Adult	Child	Adult	Child	Adult	Child
1	43	28	20	13	93	28	56	22
2	36	18	25	9	39	12	74	37
3	28	6	33	23	46	22	73	36
4	36	30	33	22	83	23	60	36
5	27	26	39	27	32	18	51	13
6	31	30	18	8	68	25	96	34
7	70	61	22	25	44	20	46	12
8	31	15	60	45	46	33	72	40
9	21	8	37	18	40	26	24	30
10	36	26	41	20	82	28	54	19
11	33	12	46	60	42	17	64	25
12	29	21	70	48	56	19	30	37
13	46	15	60	46	27	27	72	25
14	34	28	23	14	120	59	25	21
15	52	37	64	31	66	24	33	21
16	46	7	16	16				
17	26	17	25	30				
18	34	17	35	23				
19			60	35				
20			25	39				
Total	659	402	752	552	884	381	830	408
Average	36.6	22.3	37.6	27.6	58.9	25.4	55.3	27.2

Speaking

Through the science concept learning experiences, the total utterances of the adults were 3125. The average utterances for each adult were 45.96 either in the form of a statement or that of a question. In contrast, the young participants spoke 1743 times with 25.63 times as the average. The results excluded utterances made by adults during reading aloud (see Table 7). Oral language is a key area of literacy development in the early childhood field (Strasser & Seplocha, 2008).

Discussing Book Content (Book Walk)

After reading a carefully selected book, an adult often would engage a child in an activity to discuss the book content. Machado (2007) posited that dynamic classroom discussion lent itself to the development of literacy competency. Discussion of the book by means of a book walk not only develops the child's oral language acquisition, but also is conducive to the child's listening comprehension as reading a book once may not effectively help young children construct the meaning of a story (Machado, 2007). The discussion in the form of book walk, if enjoyed by both adult and child, may further the child's listening, thinking, and speaking. In this process, the child has to pay attention to what is being said, use language to think, and then verbalize his or her thoughts. The acquisition of language competency is promoted when a reciprocal interaction between an adult and a child is built on a communication that is authentic and substantive (Machado, 2007). The following dialogue taking place between Seianna and Gabby (a five-year-old child) about "the sequential colors of a rainbow" illustrates these aspects.

S: In this picture what colors do you see in the rainbow? [RQ adult LLQ adult]
G: [*Points at the colors*] Red, orange, yellow, green, blue, and purple. [I child]
S: What color appears on top in the picture? [RQ adult LLQ adult]
G: Red! [I child]
S: Do you think it is always on top? [IQ adult LLQ adult]
G: Mmm…yes! [Y child]
S: Let's check it by re-reading the page that describes the order. [R adult]

The book walk specifically highlighted this particular science concept. Centering on it, both of the parties' attention was focused on the page under discussion. As the adult raised the question: "In this picture what colors do you see in the rainbow?" the child's thinking was evoked, "Yes, what exactly am I seeing in this picture?" The child must take a quick action to examine the page in order to find proper words to answer this question. The answer to this recitation question (RQ adult LLQ adult) represented the child's undivided attention to the page: "Red, orange, yellow, green, blue, and purple" (I child). Although there was no apparent confirmation from the adult to the child's answer, the adult's continual questioning, "What color appears on top in the picture?" signaled to the child that the naming of each color was correct. In the meantime, the question elicited one-word response from the child, based on which the adult framed another question, "Do you think it is always on top?" In this question-and-answer process, these two recitation questions (RQ adult LLQ adult) exposed the child to syntactic, pragmatic, morphemic, and semantic knowledge about the science concept. The first question was a question with "what" as a starting word, which was followed by a noun, a verb, an adverb phrase, and a prepositional phrase. Whereas the second question was structured with a main clause "Do you think" and an objective sub-clause: "it is always on top." The child was able to hear the pronunciation of each word spoken by the adult and to process the way these questions were formed. The hesitated response from the child: "Mmm . . . yes" quickly allowed the adult to determine the next-step action: "Let's check it by re-reading the page that describes the order"(R adult). The verbal interaction during the book walk inspired the child to want to know about colors of a rainbow. Apparently, the child gained the understanding of the concept by the adult's discussing and analyzing the text.

In learning a science concept of the life cycle of a flower, Sara, a five-year-old child, demonstrated her increased capability in speaking (see the episode below). L denotes Lena and S denotes Sara.

L: How many stages did this seed go through before it was an adult flower? [IQ adult LLQ adult]
S: Um?
L: Let's go through them together and we'll count using our fingers, ok? [R adult]
S: Yeah. [Y child]
L: First is the…? [RQ adult LLQ adult]
S: Seeds! [I child]
L: Yes, then the root grows…? [RQ adult LLQ adult]
S: Down to the ground. *(Sarah is pointing her finger down toward the floor).* [I child]
L: Wow, you are doing great. Next the…? [RQ adult LLQ adult]
S: Green thing grows up to the sky. *(Sarah is using her finger to indicate the growth of the shoot).* [I child]
L: The green thing is called a shoot and it grows up to the sky just like you said. [I adult]
L: What is the last stage in the flower's lifecycle? [RQ adult LLQ adult]
S: The flower and the leaves come. [I child]
L: How many stages are there? [RQ adult LLQ adult]
S: One, two, three, four. [I child]
L: Yes. There are four stages. [I adult]

The child's brain was moving as she was listening to the questions posed by the adult. She had to pay very close attention in order to fill in the blanks that the adult deliberately made. In this verbal interaction, while sharing what she knew about each stage of the life cycle of a flower, the child was able to use the adverb phrase "down to the ground" to describe the second stage after the seeds are planted in dirt. The next sentence shows the child's ability to describe the third stage. Instead of using one word to represent it, the child used several words to express her knowledge in this regard: "Green thing grows up to the sky." This expression also reflected her awareness of morpheme (grows up) and her ability to use the preposition phrase: "to the sky." The adult, who was sensitive and responsive to the child's reply, provided linguistic scaffolding (Machado, 2007; Otto, 2006), expansion or recasting (Camarata, 1995) for the child's utterance with the presentation of a new vocabulary word, “shoot.” The adult’s scaffolding had an effect on the child’s thinking and speech; the language scaffolding helped the child use inner speech to clarify her thinking. “Interactive teachers provide verbal assistance and nudge discovery based on their individual child’s degree of sophistication” (Machado, 2007, p. 222). The child’s four responses as information giving (I child) presented her evolved language abilities from one word, “seeds” to one whole sentence: “The flower and the leaves come.” It is consistent with the report by Snow and Tabors (1993) that a discussion led by an adult following book reading is powerful in developing a child’s complex oral language, vocabulary, and story understanding via the child’s use of language. These are critically essential in young children’s later literacy tasks (Machado, 2007).

Additionally, Lena was assisted in acquiring a concept of cardinal number when she was asked to sum up the stages that she and the adult were just jointly counted together. Instead of reporting “four” as a cardinal number, indicating a number of stages in this set, the child counted it again. Lena’s sensitivity, based on Sara’s utterances, quickly intervened the process by directing the child’s attention to the cardinal numeral “four:” “. . .There are four stages.” This short learning experience enabled Sara not only to learn a new word, “shoot,” but also had a chance to solidify counting and a cardinal number that further enhanced the understanding of the science concept being studied. The learning experienced by Sara is also consistent with the notion by Otto (2006) and Tizard (1981). Both the adult and the child were situated in a context that both adult and child were cognizant of, forming an immediate learning context, which is advantageous of learning. Furthermore, Sara, due to the one-on-one interaction with the adult, obtained more opportunities to respond and to speak than children in a group setting (Otto, 2006).

Turn-Taking and Vocabulary Learning

T.J. (a four-year-old child) had fun learning a concept of the pumpkin’s growth cycle. The child’s interest and enjoyment propelled his thinking of and active participation in the activity. Interacting with the adult afforded this child an opportunity not only to enhance listening, speaking, thinking, and following directions, but also to enlarge his vocabulary. M denotes Michelle, an adult while T.J. denotes a four-year-old boy.

M: Okay, let’s read these and fill in the missing words. [R adult]
M: T.J. planted a pumpkin . . . [P adult]
T.J.: SEED! [I child]
M: Good job! The pumpkin seed grew into a pumpkin . . . [P adult]
T.J.: Ummm, that thing (pointing to the sequence card with a sprout on it). [I child]
M: That’s right, it’s a sprout. [P adult]
T.J.: Sprout [P child]
M: The pumpkin sprout grew into a pumpkin . . . [P adult]
T.J.: A plant. [I child]
M: You are just so smart! [P adult]
M: The pumpkin plant grew into a pumpkin . . . [IQ adult]
T.J.: Ummm, a flower? [I child]
M: Good! The pumpkin flower grew into a . . . [P adult]

T.J.: PUMPKIN! [I child]
M: The pumpkin (grew) and (grew) and (grew) until… [P adult]
T.J.: grew and grew and grew until I TOOK IT HOME! [P child]

The turn-taking exercise drew the child's close attention to the activity. He had to listen well in order to partake in the activity. The child's verbal expression demonstrates that this four-year-old had fun interacting with the adult by filling in the blank left by Michelle. He started to become more and more comfortable while this exercise was unfolding. Toward the end, the child spoke more than one word: "grew and grew and grew until I TOOK IT HOME!" In this interaction, T.J. had to comprehend words spoken by Michelle, to comply with the rule of turn-taking, and to search for proper words deriving from his understanding of a science concept. This illustrated dialogue is in line with the perspectives of Machado (2007) and Otto (2006) that a child is able to acquire an understanding of changing roles in a dialogic conversation. A speaker can become listener and vice versa. Completing simple sentences or filling in missing words is a teaching technique promoting language skills (Machado, 2007; Otto, 2006).

Investigating the Child's Interests: A Process

Prior to teaching six-year-old Kolton, Trista was in search for an appropriate topic. In this interview process, the child was given an opportunity to share enthusiastically and impressively with Trista what he knew. The respect shown by the adult's attentive listening to Kolton encouraged him to develop more linguistically (Machado, 2007) by unveiling his knowledge:

T: What interests you in nature? [IQ adult LLQ adult]
T: And what do you know about [it]? [IQ adult LLQ adult]
K: Frogs—some are poisonous and some are not. [I child]
K: They are different colors green, blue. [I child]
K: Green are not poisonous. [I child]
K: All frogs croak at dark. [I child]
K: They eat flies and dragon flies. [I child]
K: Butterflies—caterpillars turn into butterflies. [I child]
K: Their colors are white, orange, and black. [I child]
K: Crickets—Austin chases crickets, croak out in the dark, hide in dark places. [I child]
K: Snakes—there are different kinds rattle snakes, king snake, some are poisonous. [I child]
K: Uncle Andrew has snakes. [I child]
K: Big, big enough to eat people, but maybe not eat mice, and different creatures. [I child]
K: Spiders—hairy spiders, little spiders, daddy long legs protect people, stick to stuff, bite people, big hairy ones bite also. [I child]

With "What interests you in nature?" as a starting question, the child seemed to receive a signal that the adult was here with great intention to listen to what he knew about nature. The right question elicited the flood of answers from the child, which consisted of 12 sentences (I child). Some of them have more than two verb phrases, e.g. "Austin chases crickets, croak out in the dark, hide in dark places," "Big, big enough to eat people, but maybe not eat mice, and different creatures." These 12 sentences also demonstrate the child's sophisticated knowledge of different insects, amphibians, and reptiles that the child could fluently and eloquently describe to the adult listener. This interaction is also supported by Machado (2007) and Oken-Wright (1998) because open-ended questions result in more than one fixed and short response. As this particular question starting with a word "what" was posed to the child, the child's mind was quickly working and his active thinking then enabled the child to use language to inform the adult of much that he knew about nature.

Reading

The young participants acquired a science concept initially through a book reading. While interacting with the young participants, the adults read either an entire book or selective pages closely related to the science concept to assist the science concept inquiry. All the children's books used in this study were informational picture books. In light to Machado (2007), non-fiction books can be of great assistance in offering science concepts or precise vocabulary. According to Machado, McViker (2007), Otto (2006), and Strasser and Seplocha (2008), reading enhances language and literacy competencies as children are exposed to the progression of texts from left to right and book reading enables them to understand that a book is read from the front to the back. Children may also become aware that it is the print, rather than pictures in the book, that carries real information about the story. Reading aloud supports children's observation of how written language works and how one goes about reading (Otto, 2006). As children become involved in reading or begin reading aloud wholeheartedly, they are well on their way to become committed readers (Johnson, 2009).

Thinking while reading

While listening to an adult reading aloud, children commented on things that related to their life experiences or background knowledge to aid their comprehension. When talking about the physical features of an ant, 4-year-old MyKaila shared with Heather what she knew about the care of her eyes: "Eyes. Don't touch the eyes." The book was appropriate to this young child's level of understanding. She was able to decipher the adult's oral language that assisted her in understanding the book content. The appropriateness also was reflected through the child's ability to attempt to understand the reading content by linking her life-experience. This is encouraging to the child, who may want to learn more from books in her future endeavors: "When children can make a connection between what they hear when adults read aloud and their personal lives, they are more likely to be involved, interested, and constantly learning from their books" (Johnson, 2009, p. 48).

In Silina's reading only two pages of the book, "Baby Whales Drink Milk" by Barbara Juster Esbensen, a six-year-old Geron, could say five or six sentences by commenting on things that were familiar to him. S denotes the teacher and G represents Geron.

S: [S reads] Humans are mammals. Cats, dogs, and horses, and pigs are mammals too.

G: I got two dogs. [P child]
G: Every time we take the little one for a walk, she gets hyper. [P child]
G: Then we put her back into the house. [P child]
G: She tries to bite my ankle off! [P child]
S: Oh no! That is not good! [P adult]
. . .
S: [S continues to read] They all feed their babies milk that comes from their bodies. Whales are mammals. Whale babies drink milk too.
G: My little sister used to drink milk, but she doesn't now. [P child]

Geron tried to make sense of what he was hearing by relating it to his own experiences and observations. The child's inner-world was clearly manifested through his self-talk. A carefully selected book, suited to the child's individuality and cognitive capacity, elicited so many comments from the child (P child) concerning his background knowledge. Experiences of this type are supported by Johnson (2009), Machado (2007), and Ruddell (2004). The interaction between adult and child provides a scaffold for the child to construct meaning, which helps enhance their comprehension if the book offers content relates to the child's daily experience (Machado, 2007).

In studying what snakes need to survive, Katie, a seven-year-old child, read a book, "All About Snakes," by Martha E. H. Rustad." Her interest and a high degree of concentration made her stop the reading several times. The book engaged her in active thinking: "Do snakes really do this?" Or "do snakes really need that?" Even though her second drawing fully reflected her mastery of the science concept, Katie was also able to self-correct herself on the shape of a snake's tongue: "I made sure to get the tongue right this time (see Figure 4).

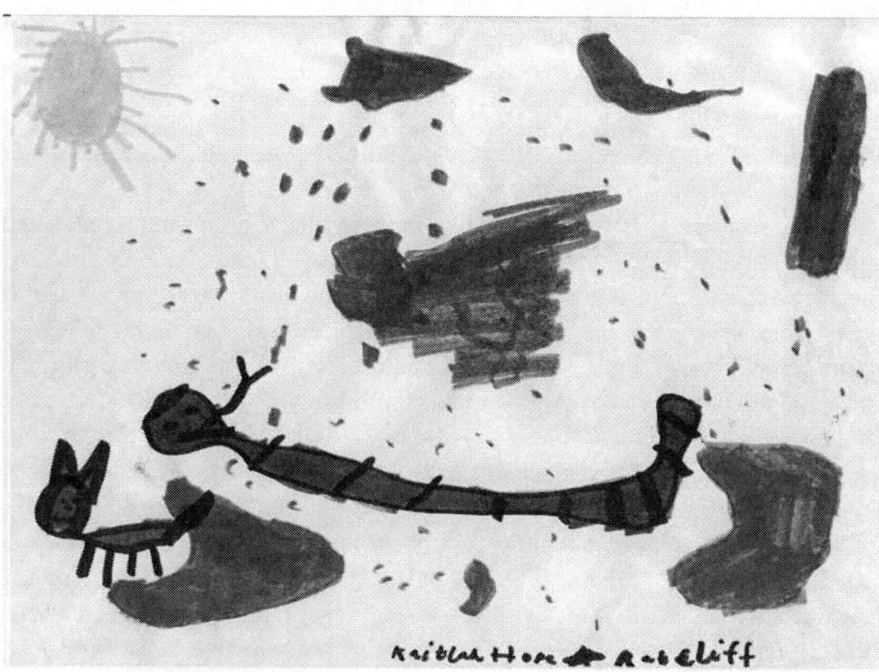

Figure 4. Katie's awareness of the appearance of a snake's tongue

I saw in the book that I didn't draw it right the first time" (see Figure 5). This book meticulously selected by the adult based on the child's interest and her prior knowledge enabled the child to build new knowledge on what she already knew. It is consistent with the strategies supported by Johnson (2009) to improve comprehension through making connections by combing new with old after the child synthesizes recently encountered information. Communicating the science concept, verbally describing it, graphically writing it down, and talking about the drawing were a sufficient base for the child to grasp the newly acquired concept (Paquett et al., 2007).

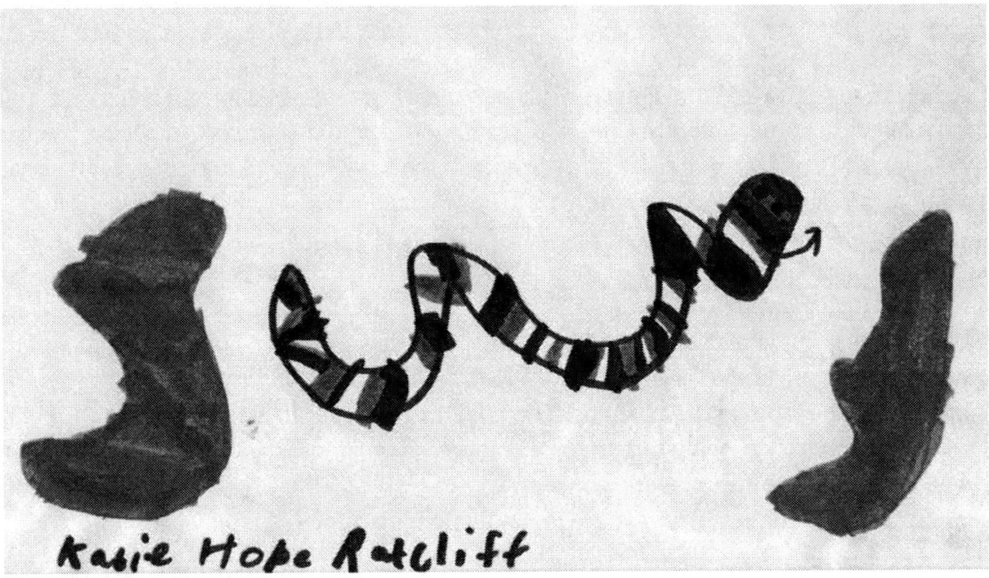

Figure 5. Katie's understanding of the snake's tongue prior to learning

Voluntary Repeating

Silina, an adult, read the title: "Baby Whales Drink Milk" Geron, a six-year-old child, voluntarily repeated, "Baby whales drink milk." In this way, Geron was able to begin to establish a science concept about one characteristic of a mammal. In a different case, Hilina reported that MyKaila, four years old, was very much interested in what was being read to her. Listening to a book, "Ants" by Coughlan, Mykaila kept repeating the key words off of each page. For example, page 7 says, "Ants are black and brown." MyKaila repeated, "Black and brown."

These two young children were engrossed in the books. The title or the content of the book captivated their attention. Their willingness to repeat after the adults provided them with practice involving semantic, syntax, phonetic, and phonological knowledge (Machado, 2007; Otto, 2006). In Geron's case, the book title of "Baby whales drink milk" includes a plural noun and a complete sentence structure with a subject, verb, and an object." In MyKaila's case, the child was exposed to four aspects of language as the sentence, "Ants are black and brown," contains a complete sentence with a subject and predicate adjectives. In addition, with the aid of picture, the child might have enhanced her concept of colors, black and brown.

The verbal imitation helps enhance the child's phonologic knowledge and provided a way for a child to increase language acquisition. Repeating new words is an attempt for the child to become familiar with them (Machado, 2007). In this sense, book reading opens the door to literacy and is an opportunity for the child to gain new vocabulary and information. Clay (1991a) and Machado (2007) believed that, most likely, children would use the language heard or acquired from book reading in their futures book talks.

Requested Repeating

Sometimes, an adult asked a child to repeat words during reading aloud. The following is an example showing how Ashley asked the child, Tyler, a five-year-old child, to read after her.

A: That's right, there are three body parts. They are called the head, thorax, and abdomen. Can you repeat those words after me?
A: Head (pointing to the head)
T: Head
A: Thorax (pointing to the thorax)
T: Thorax
A: Abdomen (pointing to the abdomen).
T: Abdomen.
. . .

Repeating after an adult enabled the child to practice pronouncing new words and to sustain the child's listening. The child had to pay attention to the reading aloud in order to follow the direction. The words, such as "thorax" and abdomen," are relatively hard to say and are rarely used in a child's daily life. Reading after the adult served as a signal to the child that these words were important. While saying these words, the child would intentionally look at the corresponding pictures to try to comprehend the meaning of these words. While the child was able to enhance her phonological skills, she also had a chance to increase vocabulary and pragmatic knowledge (Otto, 2006). In addition, this is a technique for an adult to encourage the child to learn new words. This strategy was also supported by Machado (2007) in that repetition is necessary in teaching a new word to a child.

Book Impact on Learning

Anna intentionally drew the attention of Olivia, a six-year-old child, to the book reading with the following words after listening to the child's explanation of her first drawing (see Figure 6):

A: Do you think dolphins eat other things besides seaweed and fish?
O: [Thinking] I don't know
A: Well why don't we find out. I brought a book to read to you today that talks about dolphins and what they eat.

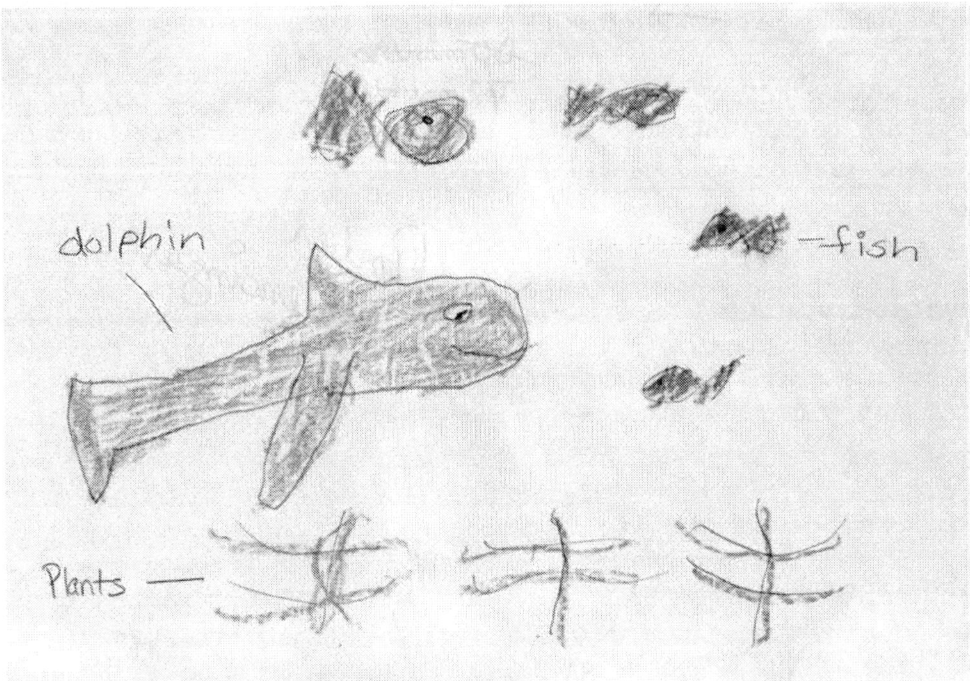

Figure 6. Book impact

With intrigued interest in what a dolphin eats, the child paid undivided attention to the book reading. Concept or informational picture books tell a story about a specific concept through pictures or illustrations, helping children think about ideas (Johnson, 2009). The effect of the book reading was reflected evidently in a hands-on activity. Olivia was asked to choose among several cut-outs, such as apples, carrots, doughnuts, cakes, fish, shrimp, squid, seaweed, turkey, and chicken, to glue on a piece of blue construction paper that represented the sea to demonstrate and construct the science concept of the diet of a dolphin. When asked to rationalize why apples, carrots, doughnuts, cakes, seaweed, turkey, and chicken were not the candidates for the construction paper, Olivia responded very loudly, "Because that's not what the book said!"

The empowerment of the book on a child's learning can also be demonstrated through the following instance. After Mindi (a six-year-old child) answered all the questions about the growth cycle of a plant, Nina asked her how she was so knowledgeable of the topic. Mindi attributed her knowledge to the book:

N: . .[C]ould you tell the stages of a seed growing, starting with the seed? [IQ adult LLQ adult]

M: Yep! First, there is the seed that is in the ground under the dirts and soils, then it gets fat and the roots and hair roots grow, it comes out of ground and grows leaves. [I child]

N: That's right, and how did you know all of that? [IQ adult LLQ adult]

M: Cuz I learned it in that book. [I child]

These two examples demonstrate the children's mastery of the concepts. Additionally, reading aloud not only was a remarkable source of listening activity to a child, but also an important first step for a child to move to literacy (Machado, 2007). These two children benefited from the book reading by having an opportune time for building vocabulary and extending phonological awareness. Book reading also enabled them to be exposed to morpheme, syntax, semantics, and a literate form (Machado, 2007; Snow & Tabors, 1993).

The child's comprehension was consistent with the belief held by Cullinan (1992) and Machado (2006) that picture books could have a long lasting effect, helping children remember events by the meaningful framework the books offer.

Learning to Value Books and the Library

When Brenda was ready to read a book to Jasmine, the six-year-old girl requested, "Can I read it?"

B: Sure. As you read it, pull on your string to see the different stages the seed goes through to become a pumpkin. [P adult]
J: How about you read it and I'll pull the string. [P child]

Brenda knew that Jasmine could read and comprehend the poem. With that knowledge kept in mind, Brenda suggested they would both read it.

B: How about we take turns reading? [P adult]
B: You start with the first line, and then I'll read the next. [P adult]
J: OK. [Y child]

Jasmine read first. After reading the first line, she decided to keep going. As she arrived at the parts where the seed changed into a plant, she tugged on the string to make the leaves appear. She read some more until the orange pumpkin appeared.

J: This is cool! I am going to show this to my teacher. [P child]
B: That's a good idea and you can tell her what you have learned about the lifecycle of pumpkins. [P adult]
J: Can I take the book too? [LLQ child]
B: How about I write down the title and who wrote it, then she can get it at your school library? [P adult]
J: Yeah and I am going to check the book out when we go to the library. [P child]

In this interactive communication, negotiation led the child to have an opportunity to read the book while an adult was listening. The dialogue modeled for the child the social skills in making a request and a suggestion, if viewed necessary: "Can I read it?" "How about you read it and I'll pull the string." In this interactive dialogue, the child did not only express her own thoughts, but also asked a question. In addition, she demonstrated her capability to use somewhat complex sentence structure in unveiling her thinking: "How about you read it and I'll pull the string." This idea was confirmed by the adult with a similar sentence structure: "How about we take turns reading?" It further taught the child about turn-taking. Toward the end, the child's utterance is more advanced, showing a complex sentence structure: "I am going to check the book out when we go to the library." The enjoyable discovery by the child heightened her interest in books and fed her with the knowledge of how interesting information can be found and how books can be used in searching for answers. The joy of book reading frivolously paves the way for establishing a formal literal form as books contain complete sentences with correct semantics and syntax (Machado, 2007). In addition, the interaction reinforced the idea of the usefulness of a library: "Yeah and I am going to check the book out when we go to the library." This learning opportunity not only enabled the child to develop the science concept, but also exposed her to the value of the book and the usefulness of a library.

Writing

Literacy involves a series of strategies young children use in their attempts to comprehend and produce oral and written language (Machado, 2007; Teale, 1995). It is imperative that adults help young children increase their awareness that both written or pictorial marks and print words carry meaning (Machado, 2007; Wells, 1981).

Phonological Learning

Ruby emphasized phonological awareness while helping Austin (a five-year-old child) acquire a science concept by soliciting information and by legibly writing down what the child told her.

R: Oh. I see. [P adult]
R: Alright, I'll write and you tell me what to say. [P adult]
A: (points to the largest elephant)
R: You want to tell me about this elephant first? [LLQ adult]
A: Happy. Happy Elephant. Happy Elephant [I child]
R: You want it to say Happy… [CQ adult]
A: This, is, a, ha-ppy, el-e-phant. [I child]
R: (writes) Okay. Anything else? [LLQ adult IQ adult]
A: (points to the smallest elephant) on this one…um, mad. This, is, a, mad, el-e-phant. [I child]
R: (writes)
A: (points to the middle sized elephant) Okay, on this one it's a sad el-e- phant. Sad. [I child]
R: (writes) This, is, a…. [P adult]
A: (joins in) sad, el-e-phant. I child
R: Elephant. Okay. Any other words you want on your paper? [LLQ adult IQ adult]
R: No. [I child]

Ruby was dictating the child's utterances, facilitating the child's phonological awareness by working as a scribe (Machado, 2007; Oken-Wright; 1998; Otto, 2006). While writing down the child's utterances, Ruby deliberately sounded out each of the syllables to facilitate the child's phonemic awareness (Machado, 2007).

Requested Matching of Printed Labels to Pictures

Engaging Abbi (an eight-year-old child) in the learning of the ladybug's life cycle, Melissa invited the child to not only draw, but also label her drawing.

M: Abbi will you please draw me another picture of what the life cycle of a ladybug is? [LLQ adult]
A: You mean will I draw you a picture of what I KNOW the life cycle of a ladybug is? [CQ child LLQ child]
M: Yes, that's what I mean. [P adult]
M: If you could please label what you are drawing, that would be of great help. [P adult]
[five minutes later]
A: Okay, here is the picture, and it is labeled too. [P child]

Melissa creatively incorporated literacy skill building into this content learning opportunity. The learning of the science concept apparently was a suitable opportunity for the child to use both types of written languages (drawing and conventional writing) to express what she knew. This palatable technique is consistent with Machado's (2007) suggestion to intentionally incorporate skill building into daily conversations and daily activities.

When engaging the child in learning, Jaime invited McKenzie (a six-year-old child) not only to place cards with visual images, but also to place, in order, those cards with printed words only:

J: Now let's try an activity I brought along for you to try. [R adult]
J: On these cards are [pictures of] the different stages of the life cycle of a pumpkin. [P adult]
J: Can you put them in the correct order of how a pumpkin grows? [LLQ adult]
M: O.K. (put cards in order after 18 seconds). [Y child]
J: Good job! [P adult]
J: On these cards is the name for every stage. [I adult]
J: Do you think you can put them above the right picture? [LLQ adult]
M: [In 21 seconds, she puts the cards above the correct stage as Jaime reads her the different words]

This was a meaning-centered activity (Puckett & Diffily, 2004), in which the child not only was exposed to listening and was encouraged to think, but also had an opportunity to increase the awareness of print and phonetic awareness. Jaime's explanation of this activity was fairly long. The three whole sentences were comprised of two statements and one question. Without paying attention and having the ability to comprehend the requests, this young child would not have been able to respond when it was her turn to speak: "O.K," nor would she have manipulated the cards according to the instructions. Visual representations are a semi-abstract means (Charlesworth & Lind, 2006) for a child to acquire knowledge conceptually, a step closer to abstract thinking and learning. The child's capability of ordering these cards in a sequential order represented her complete grasp of concepts as a result of corresponding mental pictures that she had established in the process of learning. It also shows that she was at the threshold of being able to think semi-abstractly. Her way of thinking further was promoted by the cards printed with words only. At this point, the child must listen carefully to each of the words and must then quickly relate to a just acquired concept, in order, to make a decision of where this particular card should be placed. This activity matched Machado's (2007) recommendation concerning the integration of language arts into daily activity and conversation. Again, this is consistent with the notion made by Machado and Otto (2007) that literacy development is enhanced when children are provided with opportunities to connect images and words.

Requested Labeling of Pictures

When Shannon was asking Erik, age 7, if she could take his drawing with her to show her teacher, Erik's desire to write became evident (see the ensuing dialogue shown below):

S: You have made a beautiful picture Erik and you have gotten all the stages of the lifecycle correct. [P adult]
S: Would you mind if I took this to school and showed my teacher? [LLQ adult IQ adult]
E: Nope. You can. [P child]
E: But let me write something down here (opens the book that Shannon just has read to him to a page with the names of different butterflies and starts to write down a specific type). [P child]
E: What does this say? (He points to a dragonfly). [IQ child LLQ child]
S: That is an island paradise dragonfly and [it lives] in Madagascar. [I adult]
E: Okay, well! That's the kind that I drew so I want to put its name on the paper. [I child]
E: Can I do that? (Erik adds colors to his adult dragonfly that resembles a dragonfly shown in the book). [IQ child LLQ child] (see Figure 7)

His immense interest in the dragonfly urged him to examine closely dragonflies shown on every page while listening to the book being read aloud. The visual image of the Island Paradise dragonfly captivated the child's attention. The uniqueness of this dragonfly, from the child's perspective, inspired him to want to write. Even though the dragon's name is fairly complex, it did not seem to deter this seven-year-old child. This is consistent with the position of Caswell and Duke (1998) and Johnson (2009) that a child's desire to read and write enlarges, if a non-fiction book caters to a child's interest.

In a similar case, Tracy's child partner, Kolton, at the age of 5, labeled each figure he just drew, such as "egg, tadpole, frog leg, and adult frog" (see Figure 8). When interviewed by the adult about why he went a few "extra miles" to do the writing, Kotlon responded confidently, "Because the cards had some labeling." The cards that Tracy designed were used to enable Kolton to construct the science concept of the dragonfly's life cycle. Impacted by the words in addition to pictures printed on these cards, the child was motivated to write. This demonstrates that if a strategy employed by an adult is well suited to a child's background knowledge and daily life experience, the eagerness of learning becomes a catalyst in inspiring the child to move beyond what had been expected by the adult. The "extra miles" strode as it were by the child benefited his literacy inquiry. It was due to the appropriateness and meaningfulness of this activity that this child became an active learner who delighted in the activity, which further intensified an early literacy foundation (Gundling, 2002, Machado, 2007).

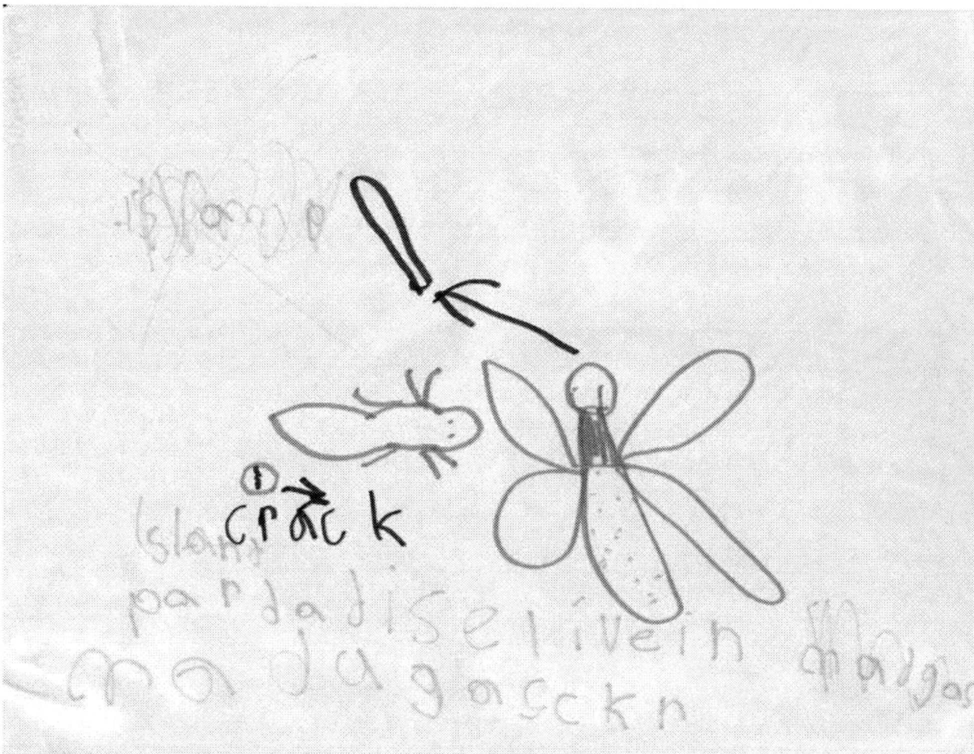

Figure 7. Voluntary writing

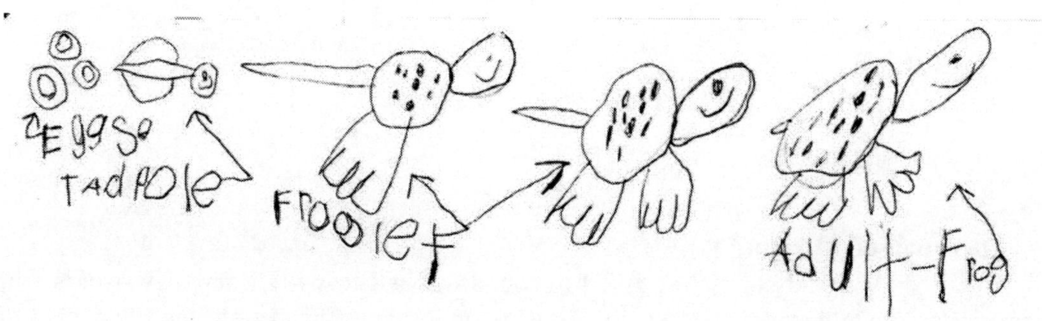

Figure 8. Voluntary labeling

Megan's child partner, Rylee (a four-year-old child), voluntarily wrote, "To Megan From Rylee" on her second bug picture. The act of a drawing promoted this young child to practice her writing skills (see Figure 9). The child's liking for her teacher encouraged her to write, an attempt to engage in early literacy (Machado, 2007; Oken-Wright, 1998).

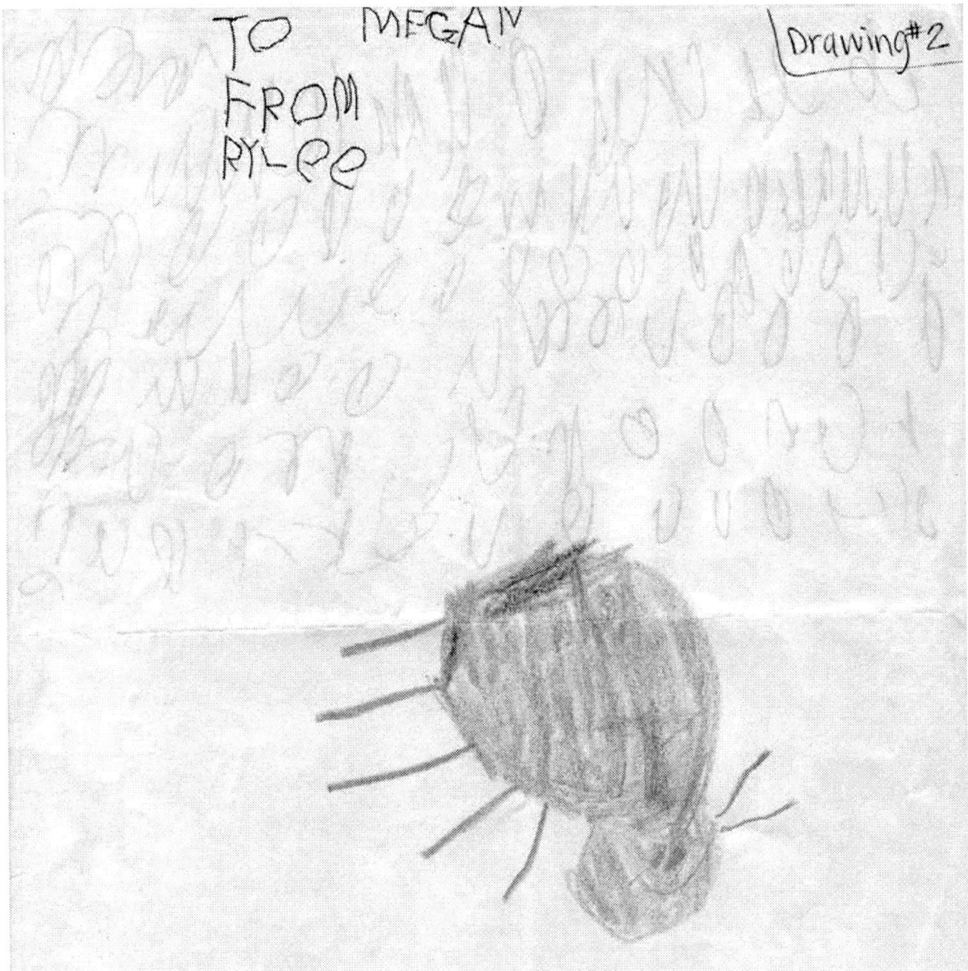

Figure 9. Voluntary Writing

Encouraged Writing

Alie, a six-year-old child, was asked to sound out and to write a few new words with Jennifer's help while explaining her first drawing on a science concept of the life cycle of a frog:

J: Can you tell me about your picture? [LLQ adult]
A: This is a baby frog. *(She pointed to the smallest frog)* [I child]
J: Do you think that you could write "baby frog?" [IQ adult LLQ adult]
A: Yep *(She writes 'baby.')* [Y child]
J: Great! [P adult]
A: This is a frog growing up. *(She points to the medium frog.* [I child]
J: I bet you could write 'growing up' with my help. [P adult]
A: Yep *(She writes 'gr' and Jennifer helps her with the rest.)* [Y child]
A: This is the mommy frog. *(She points to the largest frog.)* [I child]
J: Let's write it. *(She writes 'mom.')* [R adult] (see Figure 10)

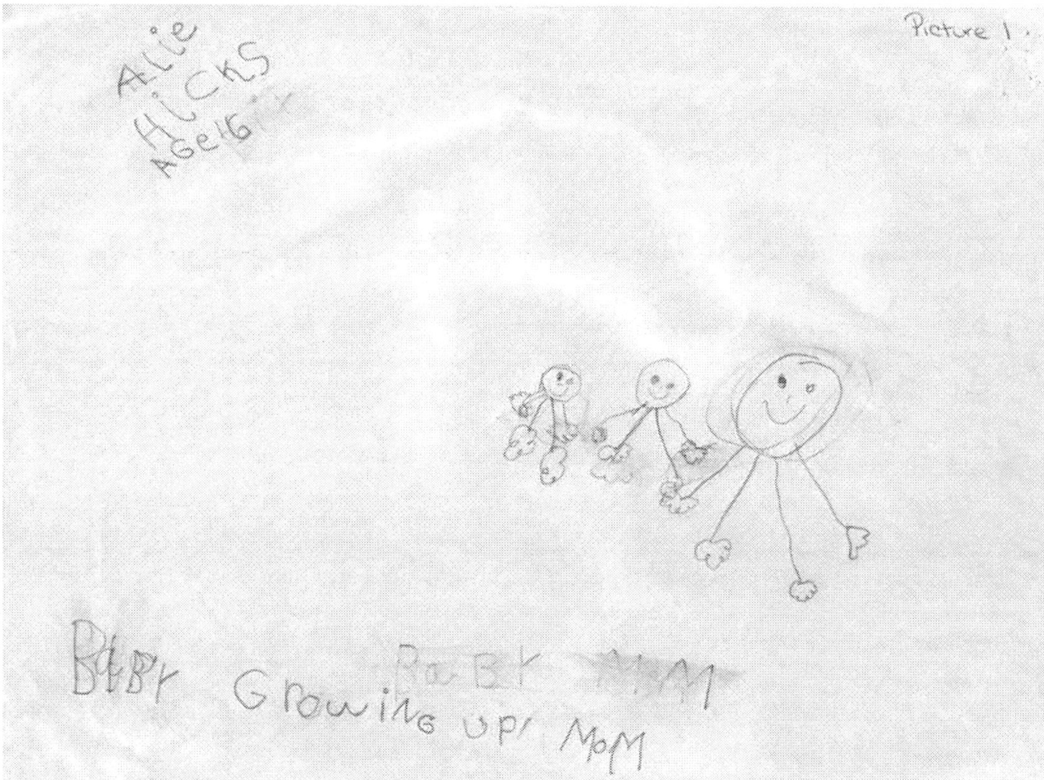

Figure 10. Encouraged Writing

The visual images played an important role in the child's inquiry of a science concept that kept the child's attention and promoted her conceptual learning in science. Simultaneously, Jennifer capitalized on the child's deep interest in the topic to advance her literacy competency by encouraging her to label her pictorial language. This first drawing, used as an assessment tool to gauge the child's prior knowledge (Chang, 2007), not only showed how much the child knew of this science concept, but also enabled the child to be aware of quite a number of new written words. This opportunity helped increase Alie's semantic and phonemic knowledge (Otto, 2006).

Requested Name Writing

When her child partner completed a drawing, Jessica encouraged Anthony, a 5-year-old child, to write his name and a number:

> J: Can you put your name on it? [LLQ adult]
> A: Is that a good N? [I child LLQ child]
> J: That's great. [P child]
> J: Can you put a one on the picture so we know that it's your first drawing? [LLQ adult] (see Figure 11).

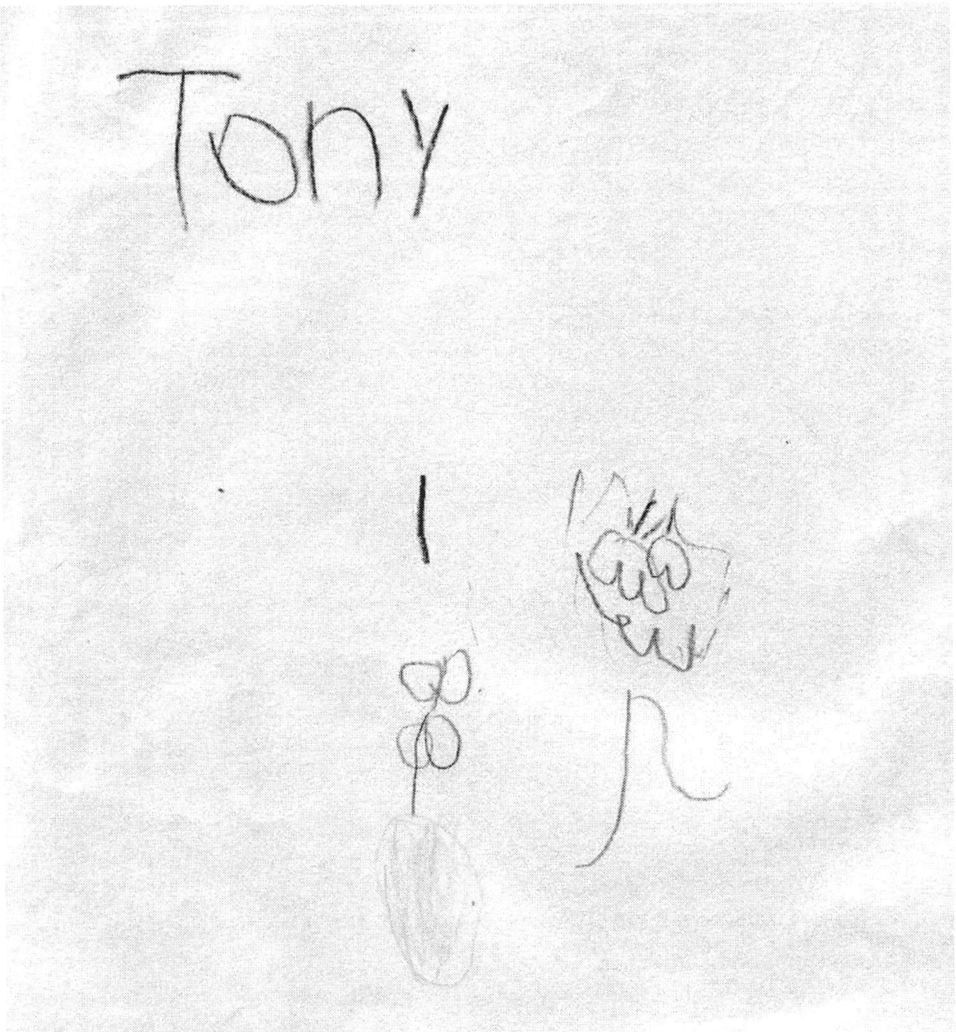

Figure 11. Requested name writing

Printing a child's own name on artwork is one of the beneficial activities that are fully endorsed by researchers and factually practiced by many early childhood teachers as this activity helps lead young children to the path of early literacy (Machado, 2007; Otto, 2006)

Recognizing and Enlarging Vocabulary

The learning process not only afforded an opportunity for a child to talk about the concept just learned, but to listen to the instructions in order to know how to engage in the activity provided. In the meantime, this was also an opportunity for a young child to check his level of understanding about what he knew with an adult's presence while acquiring new words and increasing the awareness of phonology. Sabrina put out a series of cards for Josiah (a six-year-old child) to place in a sequential order to represent the grow cycle of a tree. Soon after the cards were shown, Josiah immediately pronounced what he knew:

S: Now, you are going to put the labels where they go. [R adult]
J: Okay. I think I know what this spells: seeds. [P child]
S: You are right. [P adult]
S: Can you put it with its picture? [LLQ adult]
[Josiah glues the word SEEDS under the picture of the seeds. Sabrina helps Josiah read the rest of the labels. Josiah glues them with the corresponding pictures without assistance.] [see Figure 12]

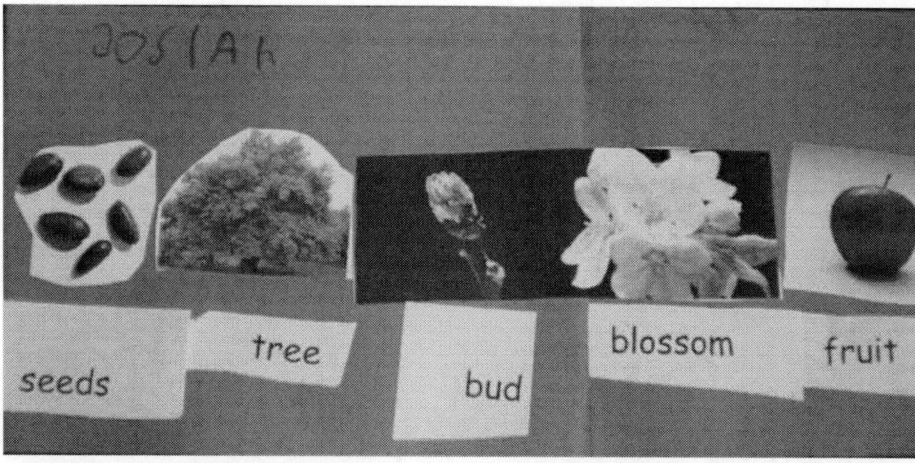

Figure 12. Recognizing vocabulary

In the process of learning the science concept of the water cycle, Dominic, a six-year-old child, learned how to say three big words: evaporation, condensation, and precipitation with Bridges, a caring adult:

B: . . . Will you explain what's happening in your picture? [IQ adult LLQ adult]
D: Yup! Water, cloud, rain. (Points to each part) It goes like this see (Traces the order with his finger) [I child] (see Figure 13)
B: What are those stages called again? [RQ adult LLQ adult]
D: Vaprtization, condentration, and precipitation. [I child]

Although Bridges was satisfied with the child's mastery level of the concept, as Dominic was able to describe it with the words that he felt comfortable using, the adult utilized the moment to talk about the child's drawing to reinforce the three newly acquired words she did this despite the fact that the adult knew it was very challenging for the child to master these words within this lesson. Assisting a child in learning new words is one of commonly identified critical behaviors that a teacher has in facilitating the child's language acquisition (Machado, 2007).

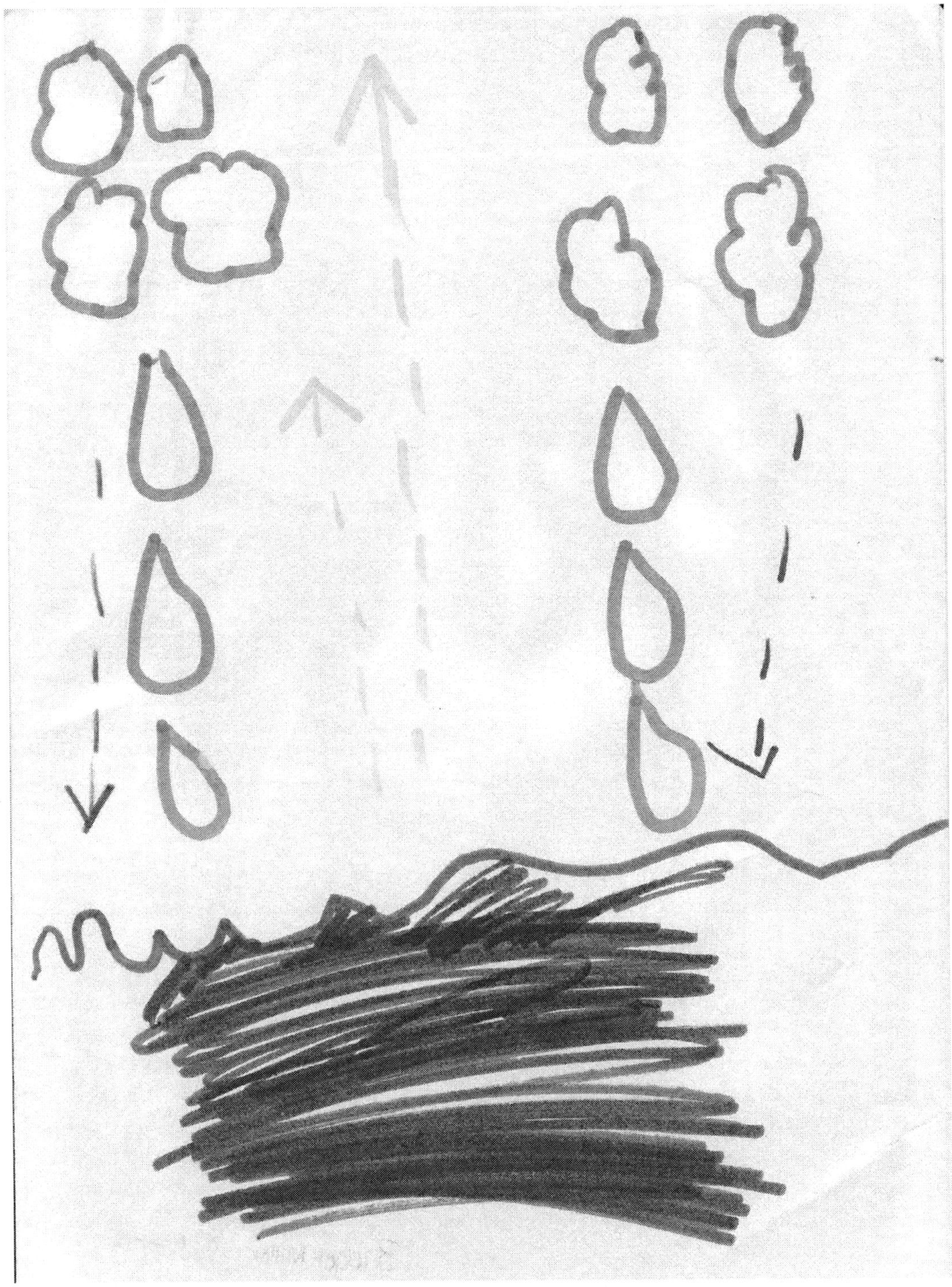

Figure 13. Enlarging vocabulary

Visual Literacy/Viewing

The young participants were requested to produce two drawings throughout a lesson with one at the very beginning as a pre-assessment tool and with the other at very end as a post-assessment tool (Chang, 2007). Drawing is viewed as part of the visual arts, which is also termed, visual literacy. Visual literacy or viewing is the fifth language arts area. It concerns a child's perception of the world and how he or she sees and interprets viewed images. ". . .art offers a rich and easily accessible way to express meaning" (Soundy, Guha, & Qin, 2007, p. 82). The ability to understand and produce visual messages involves visual literacy (Machado, 2007).

Drawings

The first drawing made by Kevin (a five years old child) increased the child's desire to know more about physical characteristics of a spider. Following his explanation of the drawing, Hannah, the adult, was ready to read aloud a relevant book to him. While she was reading the book title and its author and illustrator, the spider on the cover of the book immediately caught Kevin's attention and spurred him into action. He immediately grabbed his picture and drew another circle for the body (see Figure 14) Kevin's reaction toward the visual image presented on the book cover demonstrates the child's ability to think visually. Visual thinking is useful in "improving children's cognitive, reading, writing, and creative skills" (Machado, 2007, p. 164).

Jennie worked with Samantha, a four year old child, on the life cycle of a pumpkin. Samantha volunteered to turn every page while the book was being read. Jennie observed that the child was able to visually think of the picture on each page and to interpret its content (see the conversation below):

J: Do you know what you will find when you cut the top part off of the pumpkin?
S: Duh! Seeds! [Laughing]
J: How did you know that?
S: From the picture in the book.

The act of page turning assists a child in his or her literacy development (Machado, 2007). In this interaction, turning pages focused the child on listening to the book reading, which, in turn, was advantageous to her knowledge building about the relationship between pictures and print. Visual images in the book are a language (Machado, 2006), helping to formulate mental pictures in a child's mind. Incorporating visual literacy into other language arts areas, such as listening, speaking, reading, and writing, has been advocated by Machado (2007) and Morrow and Asbury (2003).

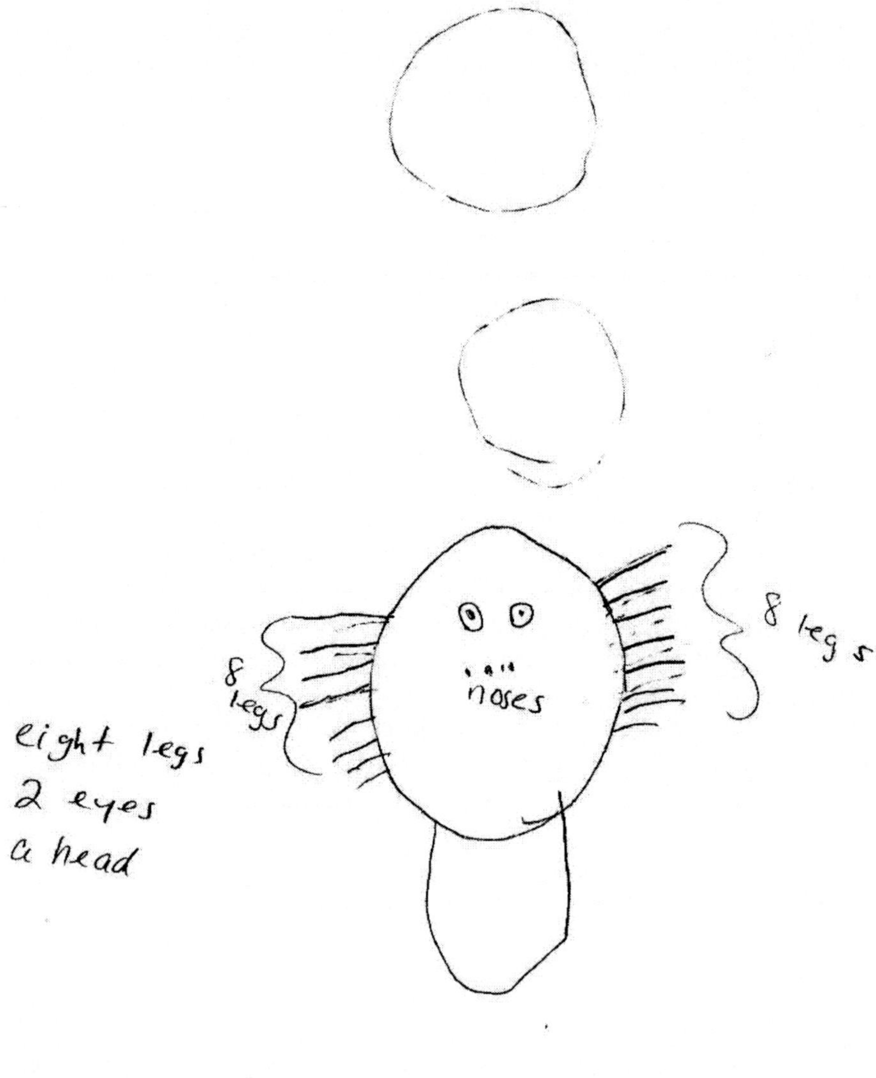

Figure 14. *Drawing*

Talking About Drawing

Kate (an eight years old child) was very articulate about what a snake needs to survive. Her explanation of the drawing also explicitly displayed that the child had a clear idea of what color a snake was portrayed by the book. Even though the color purple dominated this drawing, the adult understood that the noticeable dominance of purple did not represent the child's misunderstanding of the color of a snake, because purple was one of the child's favorite colors. H denotes the adult and K denotes Kate, the child.

H: Can you tell me . . . about what you have drawn this time? [LLQ adult]

K: Sure! I drew the sun in the corner, because snakes need heat. [I child]

K: Then, I drew some rain, lots and lots of rain, because snakes need a lot of water. [I child]

K: This time I made my snake purple, because in the book it showed an orange snake, and well, I like the color purple. [I child]

In comparison with her first drawing (see Figure 5), Kate's second drawing (see Figure 4) shows the child's increased listening and reading comprehension. An analysis of the child's verbal representation showed that Kate had mastered the science concept. The finding was consistent with Paquett et al.'s (2007) research conclusion: "Listening and reading comprehension can be assessed by analyzing children's visual, verbal, and written representations of their understandings" (p. 65). Talking about drawings is a strategy for assisting learners in combining their prior knowledge with the new information, stemming from the use of a non-fiction book and being presented by symbol systems, such as verbal discussion and drawing. Responding through art develops young children's language skills (Short, Kauffman, & Kahn, 2000; Soundy, Guha, & Qin, 2007). The finding is consistent with Snow, Burns, and Griffin's (1998) notion that activity, such as drawing, could provoke and direct children's attention to the relationship between print and speech. A kind of exploratory play, drawings and scribbling are used by young children to communicate with others, as they convey their underlying understandings and represent their awareness about print (Machado, 2007, Sulzby, 1996). It paves the way to early printing and reading attempts, as children are helped to be aware that print symbolizes oral language and written marks hold meaning (Machado, 2007). Once "it is written, it can be read" (Kalmar, 2008, p. 89). Through their ability to decipher the created symbols verbally, their acquisition of speaking and visual literacy competencies are facilitated (Machado, 2007).

Drawing to Know

Abbi (an eight-year-old child) was asked to draw the life cycle of a ladybug at the beginning of a lesson. It took the child about five minutes to complete the drawing. Melissa then invited the child to share the drawing verbally with her: "Okay, so that is what you think the life cycle of a ladybug is?" The child replied with great confidence: "Yes, I know what the life cycle of a ladybug is." As the adult encouraged the child to say more about her drawing, the child interrupted, "Okay, wait a minute. Let me label them for you." She wrote, "egg," "with out spots," "with spots," and "steeped on" either above or beneath a symbol she created (see Figure 15). Yet, the full confidence about this particular science concept soon was questioned by the adult's statement, urging the child to pay close attention to the book that was about to be read.

M: Okay, so you think that ladybugs start as an egg, then it turns into a ladybug without spots, then it is a ladybug with spots, and then it gets killed by being stepped on? [I child]

A: Yes, that is what the ladybug's life cycle is. [P adult]

M: Okay. How about I read you a book on the life cycle of a ladybug? [LLQ adult]

A: Alright. Wait does that mean? [IQ child LLQ child]

A: You are telling me I'm wrong? [IQ child LLQ child]

M: I'm not saying you are wrong, but I don't think you are completely correct. [P adult]

A: Okay, let's read the book, so I can learn about the life cycle and get it right. [P child]

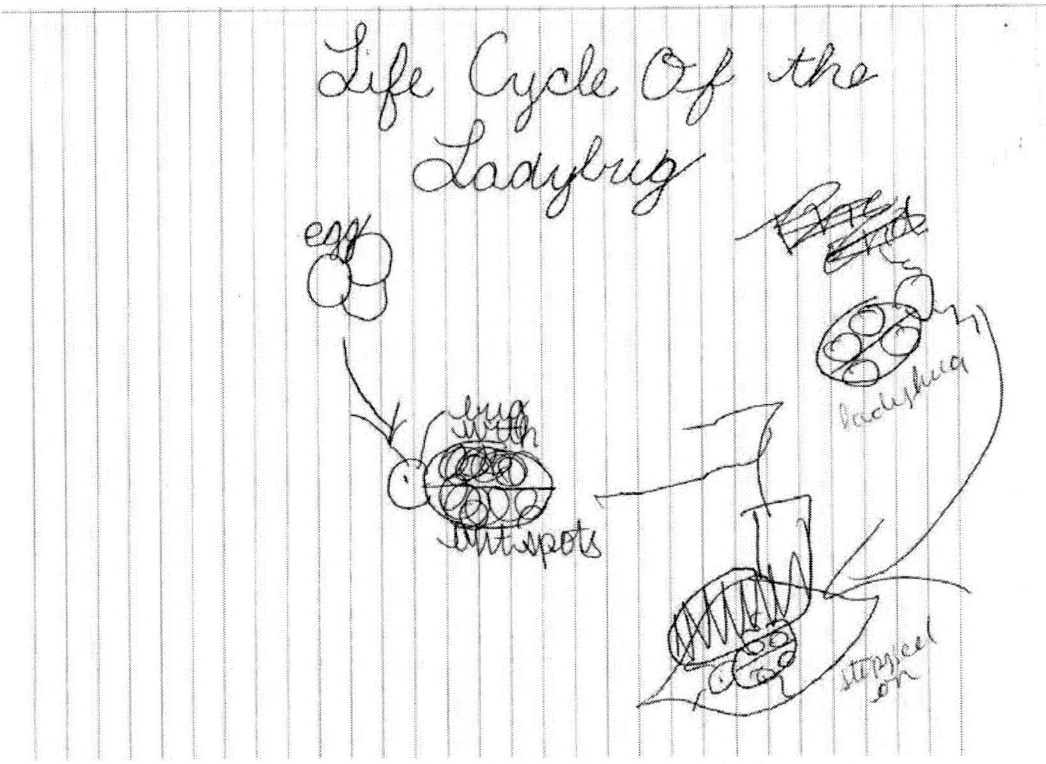

Figure 15. Learning to write

The book reading was followed by discussion, questions and answers, and a hands-on activity focused on this science concept. The child was then invited to produce another drawing:

M: Abbi will you please draw me another picture of what the life cycle of a ladybug is? [LLQ adult]
A: You mean will I draw you a picture of what I KNOW the life cycle of a ladybug is? [CQ child LLQ child]
M: Yes, that's what I mean. [P adult]
A: Okay, here is the picture, P child and it is labeled too. [P child]
. . .
M: Thanks, Abbi. [P adult]
A: Alright. Thanks for asking me. P child
A: I really enjoyed doing that, and learning about the life cycle of a ladybug. [P child]

The analysis of the pre- and the post-drawings reveals the mastery of the science concept, which was also evident in the findings of Paquett et al. (2007). The researchers upheld the strategy of Talking Drawing (McConnell, 1993) as it increased reading and listening comprehension. The strategy is comprised of several steps from having children unveil their prior knowledge of a topic that has been selected for instruction. The created graphic representations are verbally shared by the child artists. Instruction on the specific topic ensues that is followed by the production of a second drawing and by the comparison of two drawings made by the children during the process. It is believed that this is an effective framework for organizing, remembering, and constructing meaning from text, as one makes visual images within the mind while reading or being read to (Paquett et al., 2007; Reutzel, 2003). The functionality of the first drawing works as an avenue to exhibit children's created mental pictures. The visual representations then are orally explained by the children, so the listener will know the real meaning of the graphic language. It is an essential step for a viewer to undertake, which is fully supported by Church (2005) and Paquett et al. (2007). The conceptual development demonstrated through the post-drawing primarily is attributable to book reading and discussion, which enhance student comprehension skills and broaden knowledge bases. Verbal exchanges about the content scaffolds children's topical understanding (Paquett et al., 2007), thinking, language uses, and writing (Machado, 2007; Otto, 2006). In Abbi's case, the child's disequilibrium, derived from her pre-drawing, oral elaboration of the drawing, and the way Melissa invited the child to the book reading, stimulated the child's thinking and encouraged the child to pay closer attention to the book. Resulting discussion about the book content furthered the topic understanding, extending her confidence to express what she knew about the science concept pictorially. She also had a chance to develop her writing and vocabulary; she was able to add "s" to "egg" and to correctly spell "larva" and "pupa" in her second drawing. The strategy of Talking Drawings is beneficial to enhancing emergent literacy as it involves talking and drawing. They both also may provide an opportunity to those who have difficulty reading to taste the fruit of success (Paquett et al., 2007).

CONCLUSION

This study was intended to explore the opportunities that an integrated curriculum offered to facilitate language learning and how an integrated curricular approach mediated children's language and literacy competencies while children were engaged in learning a science concept. The findings show that the children's listening and speaking primarily was facilitated by answering questions posed by the adult participants. Questions were largely recitation questions (RQ) and information questions (IQ), which provided a basis for maintaining an ongoing conversation (Pine, 1994; Otto, 2006) and encouraged language development (Otto, 2006). Adults' personal speech (P adult) also worked as another source of language to enhance children's listening and speaking acquisition.

In their acquisition of a science concept via a lesson that incorporated language arts and the visual arts, the young participants were offered many opportunities that could increase their language and literacy skills. The lesson included introduction, a request for a first drawing as an assessment means to determine prior knowledge, follow-up discussion after reading aloud a book, hands-on activity, and a request for a second drawing as an assessment means to formally gauge the learning outcome. The entire process of interaction is in line with Otto's (2006) notion that language development activities need to be integrated into the curriculum. The integration was also in correspondence with the principles of developmentally appropriate practices in that teachers need to provide many opportunities for children to hear and to use language for different purposes (Bredekamp & Copple, 1997).

This study also examined the facilitation of language and literacy competencies through discretely exploring each of the five language arts areas, namely, listening, speaking, reading, writing, and visual literacy. It was found that there were various opportunities available to the young children, assisting their acquisition of language and literacy skills. The young children's listening acquisition was facilitated through following directions and learning mathematics, such as counting and ordinal numbering, recognizing words, and reading aloud in addition to listening to questions posed by adults.

Even though speaking was a result of responses to the adults' recitation questions (RQ), information questions (IQ), and the adults' personal speech (P adult), it was also facilitated through discussing book content (a book walk), turn-taking and vocabulary learning, and through the investigation of a topic of interest to the particular child.

During the time of book reading, the young participants displayed various behaviors which were conducive to literacy development, including thinking while reading, voluntary repeating, requested repeating, book impact on learning, and learning to value books and the library. The act of reading aloud nonfiction texts increases conceptual development and vocabulary (Elster, 1994; Otto, 2006) as picture and/or story books expose children to more precise and varied vocabulary than other sources do.

Children's written language was facilitated over the course of the integrated lesson through the following aspects: phonological learning, requested matching of printed labels to pictures, requested labeling of pictures, encouraged writing, requested name writing, and recognizing and enlarging vocabulary. The children's visual literacy acquisition was facilitated through drawings, talking about drawing, and drawing to know.

The findings suggest that teachers should read pictures to children in a children's book, provide opportunities for children to arrange pictures in a sequence that tells a story (Machado, 2007), pique children's interest in libraries, use new words with children, extend children's comments through questioning, focus children's attention on an analysis of books read to them, engage children in intellectual challenging conversations (Dickinson & Tabors, 2001), obtain and maintain children's attention (Dickinson & Tabors, 2001), support children's writing attempts (Dickinson, 2001), give individual children adequate time to speak (Schickendanz, 2003), engage children in extensive conversations (Schickendanz, 2003).

A body of literature recognizes the importance of infusing the visual arts into the curriculum, because it assists young children to visually express themselves and to communicate with others. Yet, when communicating with young children, the focus often seems to be placed on concepts, such as shapes, colors, and texture.

> Language goals for art activities focus on encouraging children to develop conceptual knowledge related to art and to be able to verbally describe the colors, textures, or shapes with which they are working. . . . Children should also learn the concept name of the particular technique they are using. Rather than labeling the technique as simply "painting," a teacher should explain the type of painting involved, such as sponge painting, string painting, finger painting, block painting, or brush painting. Otto, 2006, p. 203

This study points to a different direction when it comes to the use of art center or visual arts. In enhancement of language and literacy skills, "talking about drawing" is a form of visual arts conversation taking place at the art center, which enables the child to express her thoughts and mental images verbally. Considering young children share their inner world in a symbolic manner, children's paintings can represent meaning, which, in turn, can be talked about. This behavior is more appropriate than simply placing its focus on experimenting with different colors or novice art tools when children are engaged in painting. This study shows it is possible to create an art center and visual art experiences to serve more than one purpose. Through this study, the young participants were able to put words to their experiences via visual art/drawings, the symbolic language, because young children express and learn through symbols (Edwards, Gandini, & Forman, 1998; Otto, 2006). If texture, shapes, and colors are part of the curriculum goal, creative adults or teachers can flexibly integrate the concepts into the children's learning process. At times, the exploration of various mediums of artistic expression can be artfully linked with subject areas-related inquiry. If children are encouraged to use writing throughout the curriculum for various purposes in different learning centers in an early childhood classroom setting, integration of visual arts then makes a lot of sense. Drawing should take place not only in a writing center, where the exploration of communication through symbols takes place (see Otto, 2006), but also in other locations and occasions as well. Dialogic interactions then widen learning scope and spectrum, making learning meaningful, purposeful, interesting, and educational.

Implications for Education

This study offers several educational implications for teachers and adults working with young children. Children's learning experiences should be meticulously and thoughtfully planned in light of their prior knowledge (Kalmar, 2008), interest (William, Hedrick, & Tuschinski, 2008), and present conceptual understandings in order to motivate them to learn (William et al., 2008). Inquiry of science concepts can be integrated into curriculum with the premises that children's interests are clearly underscored and understood and that the topic of study is interesting to the majority of the children involved in the learning process. The lesson should be orchestrated and organized such that it is coherent and logical, and considers all possible subject areas that will support and buttress the curriculum. "To promote literacy, teachers think about how each theme activity involves listening, speech, reading, and writing and how to logically connect these areas during ongoing activities" (Machado, 2007, p. 191). The national Reading Panel Report (2000) and Morrow and Asbury (2003) urged teachers in early literacy to organize instruction in a systematic way.

Planning also involves the consideration of a meticulously and thoughtfully selected book that is accurate in science content. The decision of book selection should be in line with the child's prior experience (Otto, 2006), age, interests, and background knowledge (Chang, 2007). Professional literature stresses the importance of the impact that an integrated approach to language arts has on outcomes for learning and recommends a literature-based curriculum for both elementary and preschool settings (see Machado, 2007). Informational or non-fiction books, employed in the literacy/literature-based approach, are supportive of thematic teaching in the early childhood field, and are of great value to literacy development (Machado, 2007). Early childhood teachers can use this teaching strategy to start discussion, drama, art, and other language arts activities to strengthen various concepts inquiries, which can, in turn, spark children's desire to explore what interests them, to seek out answers, to ponder questions, or to provide a response (Machado, 2007).

Engaging children in reading is equally important in the child's acquisition of a science concept and language and literacy competencies. Motivation is the heart and soul of engagement: "[a]s motivation increases, students want to spend more time reading" (Johnson, 2009, p. 48). It is an adult's responsibility to create and seek out strategies suitable for reaching this end. An excellent book selection is the key to motivating young children to participate in learning actively.

Considering that a child is a novice communicator, an adult needs to play a crucial role in supporting language acquisition in a dialogic dyad (Brunner, 1990; Vygotsky, 1978; Otto, 2006) to make a scafffolded conversation successful. After a read-aloud, a discussion is useful to enhance the child's listening, speaking, thinking, comprehension, phonetic, and phonemic acquisition. It would be helpful for the adult to ask question about the child's learning, including what the child is thinking, how further learning experience be built on as a result of this interaction.

Listening to children throughout a lesson, emphasizing what is said rather than how it is said, is essential and valuable to the continuation of discourse between adult and child. With intimate listening, adults are able to be on the same wavelength with children. The absence of the adult who monopolizes verbal interactions not only encourages children to talk about what they know, but also assists them in putting ideas into words. Conversations are likely to be sustained when adults try to talk and pose questions pertaining to children's lines of thought.

To maintain children's attention to an ongoing conversation and an inquiry regarding a science concept, shared reference between an adult and a child should be one of the key elements (Otto, 2006; Tronick, Als, & Adamson, 1979). A jointly interesting object or event, such as drawing and a science concept, can gain the attention of both the adult and the child (Otto, 2006), making conversation meaningful and purposeful.

Having children use drawings to express what they know and what they have learned plays an important role in an integrated learning process. Arts "are visually expressive and communicative by nature, they also provide opportunities to enhance language development" (Otto, 2006, p. 203). Children are able to experiment with and explore how written language is used in specific contexts (Otto, 2006). Displaying drawings or art products in the classroom or storing them in the students' journals for later reference would allow teachers to gain very little information about children's insights and their learning. Asking students to demonstrate their inner thoughts through a unique drawing is much more meaningful and beneficial than having them produce a paragraph in writing about a particular topic determined by the teacher (Paquett, Fellow, & Jalongo, 2006/2007). Talking about drawing is useful and necessary as the pictures may represent very different meaning to children, compared to an adult's interpretation of the same drawing. While talking with the child about his or her drawing, the adult provides a scaffold for the child's language and literacy acquisition and helps those who struggle with reading to experience success (Paquett et al., 2006/2007) while, at the same time, obtaining some knowledge of the child's mental picture.

Recommendation for Future Research Effort

Research on visual literacy as a means of support to children's learning in language arts and other subject areas should continue in its scope and depth as more and more children are attracted by TV, videos, and computer games and many early childhood teachers pay more attention to oral language and written text than to visual thinking and learning (Karchmer,

Mallette, & Leu, 2003). Research is also needed to examine the effect of visual literacy on later elementary reading achievement (Roskos, Christie, & Richgels, 2003) and on the relationship between non-fiction books and children's learning (Casergue & Plauche, 2003). The effect resulting from the well-selected book on children's science concept inquiry and the development of language and literacy acquisition should also be an area of further investigation.

The replication of this study is useful and necessary. Future effort may also be exerted to examine the effect of the same approach employed by this study on a small group of children.

Significance of the Study

While the public eye is focusing on children's reading and writing achievement and classroom instruction in reading and writing, the focus on instructional time to enhance children's reading and writing skills is inappropriate, as it is not the remedial solution for children's reading deficiency in US schools (Hirch, 2004). Researchers (Machado, 2007; Morrow & Asbury, 2003; Otto, 2006) and the National Reading Panel Report (2000) mutually emphasized the essence of systematic and well-orchestrated instruction concerning early literacy. Equally recognized by the professional literature is the important role that an integrated approach to language arts plays in children's learning achievement, because children benefit from the exposure to background information in history, science, literature, and arts. Literacy instruction should be seamlessly blended into subject matter learning with reading and writing working as a tool for students' content learning (Fisher & Ivey, 2005; Lacina & Watson, 2008). It is, therefore, recommended that a literature-based curriculum be employed in both elementary and preschool settings, as students make sense of content knowledge with the use of listening, speaking, reading, writing, and viewing (Fisher & Ivey, 2005) and as the acquisition of language and literacy skills derives from content-rich-reading-selection curricula (Hirch, 2004; Machado, 2007) as well as from situating children in a meaningful learning context (Machado, 2007). Moreover, Kalmar (2008) and Pappano (2008) called on early childhood educators to give children something to talk in order to develop their literacy. On the basis of aforementioned reasons, the results of this study answer all these calls. In this learning experience, the young participants acquired a science concept with the support of a combination of five areas of language arts, including listening, speaking, reading, writing, and visual literacy. The children had ample opportunities to express thoughts verbally. In addition, this study makes a contribution to learning a science concept in an enjoyable and somewhat lighthearted manner. This study can be helpful to elicit a more promising discussion about ways to facilitate young children's acquisition language and literacy competencies while assisting them in learning a science concept through an integrated curriculum.

Limitation

A limitation about this means of data collection might be that the researcher was unable to engage in follow-up interviews with the adults who were teaching the children. An additional limitation relates to the fact that the transcription might contain errors due to typos or careless mistakes. This limitation was minimized, to a degree, by the prolonged data collection and by additional means used in the data collection, such as drawings and communication notes between the researcher and the participants. This study also is limited in its generalizability to all children due to its small size and because the sample lacks diversity. The study, however, did make a contribution to the children's learning in that they were exposed to five language arts and had opportunities to use language and to gain literacy competencies through an integrated curriculum that was systematically planned and organized and that was designed to help young children develop a science concept.

REFERENCES

Allington, R., Guice, S., Li, S., Michelson, N., & Baker, K. (1995). *Patterns of implementation of literature-based curriculum* (Report Series 1.14). National Research Center on Literature Teaching and Learning, Albany, NY. (ERIC Document Reproduction Service No. ED ED386731)

Beals, D. E. (1993). Explanatory talk in low-income families' mealtime conversations. *Applied Psycholinguistics, 14*, 485-513.

Bredekamp, S. & Copple, C. (Eds.). (1997). *Developmentally appropriate practice in early childhood programs serving children from birth through age 8.* Washington D.C.: National Association for the Education of Young Children.

Bruner, J. (1978). The role of dialogue in language acquisition. In A. Sinclair, R. Jarvella, & W. Levelt (Eds.), *The child's conception of language* (pp. 241-256). New York: Springer-Verlag.

Burmark, L. (2002). *Visual literacy: Learn to see, see to learn.* Alexandria, VA: Association for Supervision and Curriculum Development.

Camarata, S. (1995). A rationale for naturalistic speech intelligibility intervention. In M. Fey, J. Windsor, & S. Warren (Eds.), *Language intervention: Preschool through the elementary years* (pp. 63-84). Baltimore, MA: Paul H. Brookes.

Cabergue, R. M., & Pauche, M. B. (2003). Immersing children in nonfiction: Fostering emergent research and writing. In D. M. Barone & L. M. Morrow (Eds.), *Literacy and young children: Research-based practices.* (pp. 243-260). New York: The Guilford Press.

Caswell, L., & Duke, N. K. (1998). Non-narrative as a catalyst for literacy development. *Language Arts, 75*(2), 108-117.

Chang, N. (2007, October). A Medium for nurturing the development of language and literacy skills of young children at home. Paper presented at the meeting of the National Association of the Education of Young Children, Chicago, IL.

Chang, N. (1996). *The role of the teacher in children's acquisition of concepts based on Reggio principles and related theories.* Unpublished doctoral dissertation, Vanderbilt University of Nashville, TN.

Charlesworth, R., & Lind, D. (2006). Science and math for young children. Cincinnati, OH: Delmar.

Cho, B. K., & Kim, J. J. (1998, April). *Literature based science activities in kindergarten through children's picture book.* Paper presented at the Annual Conference of Association for Childhood Education International, Tampa, FL.

Church, E. B. (2005). Learning from children's art and writing. *Early Childhood Today, 19*(5), 35-42.

Clay, M. (1991a). *Becoming literate: The construction of inner control.* Portsmouth, NH: Heinemann.

Creswell, J. W. (2002). *Educational research: Planning, conducting, and evaluating quantitative and qualitative research.* Columbus, OH: Upper Saddle River.

Cullinan, B. E. (1992). Whole language and children's literature. *Language Arts, 69*(6), 426-430.

Duke, N., & Pearson, P. D. (2002). Effective practices for developing teaching comprehension. In A Farstrup & S. J. Samuels (Eds.), *What research has to say about reading instruction* (3rd ed.). Newark, NJ: International Reading Association.

Edwards, C., Gandini, L., & Forman, G. (1998). *The hundred languages of children: The Reggio Emilia Approach-advanced reproach* (Eds.). Greenwich, CT: Ablex.

Fisher, D., & Ivey, G. (2005). Literacy and language as learning in content-area classes: A departure from "every teacher a teacher of reading." *Action n Teacher Education, 27*(2), 3-11.

Fries, P. (n.d.). *Systemic approaches to child language.* Retrieved August 1, 2007, from Developmenthttp://www.isfla.org/Systemics/Definition/ChildDev.html

Fu, V. R., Stremmel, A. J., & Hill, L. T. (2002). *Teaching and learning: Collaborative explorations of the Reggio Emilia Approach.* Columbus, OH: Merrill/Prentice-Hall.

Gambrell, L. B., & Mazzoni, S. A. (1999). Principles of best practice: Finding the common ground. In L. B. Gambrell, L. M. Morrow, S. B. Neuman, & M. Pressley (Eds.), *Best practice in literacy instruction.* New York: The Guilford Press.

Gandini, L. (2002). The story and foundations of the Reggio Emilia approach. In V. Fu, Stremmel, & L. Hill (Eds.), *Teaching and learning: Collaborative exploration of the Reggio Emilia approach* (pp. 13–21). Columbus, OH: Merrill/Prentice-Hall.

Genishi, C., & Dyson, A. (1984). *Language assessment in the early years.* Norwood, NJ: Ablex.

Gundling, R. (2002). Promoting early literacy in early childhood program. *Child Care Bulletin, 27*, 7-8.

Halliday, M. A. K. (1973). *Explorations in the functions of language.* London: Edward Arnold.Homeschool-curriculum-for-life.com (n.d.) *Why read aloud to your child.* Retrieved January 28, 2008, from http://www.homeschool-curriculum-for-life.com/why-read-aloud.html

Huck, C.S. (1992). Literacy and literature. *Language Arts, 69*(7), 520-526. International Reading Association and National Council of Teachers of English (2006-2007). *Literacy engagements.* Retrieved November 14, 2007, from http://www.readwritethink.org/literacy/index.html International Reading Association and National Council of Teachers of English (2006-2007). *IRA/NCTE standards for the English Language Art* Retrieved November 14, 2007, from http://www.readwritethink.org/standards/index.html

Johnson, D. (2009). *The joy of children's literature.* New York: Houghton Mifflin Harcourt Publishing Company.

Kalmar, K. (2008). Let's give children something to talk: Oral language and preschool literacy. *Young Children, 63*(1), 88-92.

Karchmer, R. A., Mallette, M. H., & Leu, D. J. Jr. (2003). Early literacy in a digital age: Moving from a singular book literacy to the multiple literacties of networked information and communication technologies. In D. M. Barone & L. M. Morrow (Eds.), *Literacy and young children: Research-based practices*. (pp. 175-194). New York: Guilford.

Katz, L. G., & Chard, S. C. (1996). The contribution of documentation to the quality of early childhood education. (ERIC Documentation Reproduction Services No. EDO-PS-96–2).

Lacina, J., & Watson, P. A., (2008). Focus on literacy: Effective content teachers for the middle grades. *Childhood Education, 84*(3), 159-162.

Lincoln, Y. S., & Guba, E. G. (1985). *Naturalistic inquiry*. Newbury Part, CA: Sage.

Machado, J. M. (2007). *Early childhood experiences in language arts: Early Literacy*. (8th Ed.). Clifton Part, NY: Thomson Delmar Learning.

Malaguzzi, L. (1993). History, ideas, and basic philosophy. In C. Edwards, L. Gandini, & G. Forman (Eds.), *The hundred languages of children: The Reggio Emilia Approach to early childhood education*, (pp. 41–89). Norwood, NJ: Ablex.

McCormick, T. W. (1988). *Theories of reading in dialogue: An interdisciplinary study*. New York: University Press of America.

McConnell, S. (1993). Talking drawings: A strategy for assisting learners. *Journal of Reading, 36*(4), 260-269).

McVicker, C. (2007). Young readers respond: The importance of child participation in emerging literacy. *Young Children, 62*(3), 18-22.

Morrow, L. M., & Asbury, E. (2003). Current practices in early childhood literacy development. In L. M. Morrow, L. B. Gambrell, & M. Pressley (Eds.), *Best practices in literacy instruction* (pp. 43-63). New York: The Guilford Press.

National Reading Panel (2000). *Teaching children to read: An evidence-based assessment of the scientific research literature on reading and its implications for reading instruction* (NIH Publication No. 00-4769). Washington, DC: National Institute of Child Health and Human Development.

National Research Council (1996). National Science Education Standards. Washington, D.C.: The National Academy Press.

Oken-Wright, P. (1998). Transition to Writing: Drawing as a Scaffold for Emergent Writers. *Young Children, 53*(4), 76-81.

Otto, B. V. (2006) *Language development in early childhood*. 2nd Edition. New Jersey: Upper Saddle River.

Pappano, L. (2008). The power of family conversation: School and community programs help parents build children's literacy from birth. *Harvard Education Letter*. Retrieved May 22, 2008, from http://www.edletter.org/insights/familyconversation.shtml

Paquette, K. R., Fello, S. E., & Jalongo, M. R. (2006/2007). Talking drawings: Improving intermediate sutdents' comprehension of expository science text. *Childhood Education*, 83(2), 80-86.

Pine, J. (1994). The language of primary caregivers. In C. Gallaway & B. Richards (Eds.), *Input and interaction in language acquisition* (pp. 15-37). Cambridge, London: Cambridge University Press.

Puckett, M., & Diffily, D. (2004). *Teaching young children: An introduction to the early childhood profession* (2nd Ed.). New York: Harcourt Brace.

Reich, P. (1986). *Language development*. Upper Saddle River, NJ: Prentice Hall.

Reutzesl, R. D. (2003). *Teaching children to read: Putting the pieces together*. New York: Prentice Hall.

Rinaldi, C. (1998). Projected curriculum constructed through documentation Progettazione: An interview with Lella Gandini. In C. Edwards, L. Gandini, & G. Forman (Eds.), *The hundred languages of children: The Reggio Emilia Approach-advanced reproach*, (pp. 113–126). Greenwich, CT: Ablex.

Roskos, K. A., Christie, J. F., & Richgels, D. J. (2003). The essentials of early literacy instruction. *Young Children, 58*(2), 52-60.

Royce, A., & Wiley, D. (2005). The common ground. *Science and Children, 42*(5), 40-42.

Ruddell, R. (2004). Researching the influential literacy teacher: Characteristics, beliefs, strategies, and new research directions. In R. Ruddell & N. Unrau (Eds.), *Theoretical models and processes of reading* (5th ed.) (pp. 979-997). Newark, DE: International Reading Association.

Short, K. G., Kauffman, G., & Kahn, L. H. (2000). "I just need to draw:" Responding to literature across multiple sign system. *The Reading Teacher, (54)*, 160-171.

Snow, C. E., & Tabors, P. O. (1993). Language skills that relate to literacy development. In B. Spodek & O. Sracho (Eds.), *Yearbook in early childhood education* (pp. 222-246). New York: Teachers College Press.

Snow, C., Bruns, S., & Griffin, P. (Eds). (1998). *Preventing reading difficulties in young children.* Washington, DC: National Academy Press.

Soundy, C. S., Guha, S., & Qin, Y. (2007). Picture power: Placing artistry and literacy on the same page. *Young Children, 62*(3), 82-88.

Stauffer, R. C. (1970). *The language experience approach to the teaching of reading.* New York: Harper and Row.

Stegelin, D. A. (2003). Application of the Reggio Emilia approach to early childhood science curriculum. *Early Childhood Education Journal, 30*(3), 163-169.

Stieglitz, M. G. (1972). *The visual differential: An experimental study of the relation of varied experiences with visuals to shape discrimination.* Unpublished doctoral dissertation. University of Wisconsin.

Strasser, J., & Seplocha, H. (2008). Using picture books to support young children's literacy. *Childhood Education, 83*(4), 219-224.

Strickland, D. S. (1990). Family literacy: Sharing good books. *Young Children, 43*(7), 518-519.

Sulzby, E. (1996). Roles of oral and written language as children approach conventional literacy. In C. Pontevecorvo, M. Orsolini, B. Burge, & L. B. Resnick (Eds.), *Children's early text construction* (pp. 25-46). Mahwah, NJ: Lawrence Erlbaum. Teale, W. H. (1995). Introduction. In T. Harris & R. Hodges (Eds.), *The literacy dictionary.* Newark, DE: International Reading Association.

Tizard, B. (1981). Language at home and at school. In C. Cazden (Ed.). *Language in early childhood education* (pp. 17-27). Washington, DC: National Association for the Education of Young Children.

Trousdale, A. (1990). Interactive storytelling: Scaffolding children's early narratives. *Language Arts, 67*(2), 164-173.

Weismann, D. (1970). *The visual arts as human experience*. Englewood Cliffs, NJ: Prentice Hall.

Wells, G. (1981). *Learning through interaction: The study of language development.* Cambridge, MA: Cambridge University Press.

Wells, G. (1986). *The meaning makers: Children learning language and using language to learn*. Portsmouth, NH: Heinemann.

William, L. M., Hedrick, W. B., & Tuschinski, L. (2008). Motivation: Going beyond testing to a lifetime of reading. *Childhood Education, 84*(3), 135-141.

In: Children and Language: Development, Impairment … ISBN 978-1-60692-395-5
Editor: Michael A. Reed

Chapter 4

READING IMPAIRMENT IN CHILDHOOD: OVERVIEW OF THE ELECTROPHYSIOLOGICAL CORRELATES OF DEVELOPMENTAL DYSLEXIA

***Barbara Penolazzi*[1], *Chiara Spironelli*[1] *and Alessandro Angrilli*[1, 2]**
[1]Department of General Psychology, University of Padova,
Via Venezia 8, 35131 Padova, Italy
[2]CNR Institute of Neuroscience, Padova section, Italy

ABSTRACT

Electrophysiological measurements enabled us to greatly increase our knowledge on the most spread learning disability in childhood represented by the Developmental Dyslexia (DD). The present chapter reviews the most relevant studies, which used either Event Related Potentials (ERPs) or Electroencephalographic (EEG) bands to investigate reading disabilities in developmental age. Several studies are here described, which succeeded in showing processing abnormalities not only in dyslexics, but also in children genetically at risk of dyslexia, through the analysis of both the "classical" electrophysiological components (i.e., MMN, P300, N400) and earlier evoked potentials. The electrophysiological markers of neuronal dysfunctions found in these children, helped scientists to uncover the psychophysiological mechanisms chiefly involved in this language disorder. These are: deficits in speech sound processing and impairment in manipulating the phonological features of grapheme strings. A considerable advance in the field has been recently reached by using EEG bands, traditionally used for detecting group differences in resting state, but currently extended to the measure of cognitive activation obtained through different experimental tasks. Such studies revealed functional differences in both fast and slow EEG rhythms between dyslexics and controls. The use of two functionally distinct EEG rhythms, theta and beta bands, in line with several ERP results, supports the view that dyslexics' reading difficulties are related to a linguistic impairment which is represented essentially at phonological level. Similar conclusions were further supported by the analysis of delta rhythm - a functional marker of cortical inhibition - during the performance of different linguistic tasks. Group differences in delta activation points to a delay in dyslexics' brain maturation. The review of recent literature on electrophysiological correlates of DD, on one hand supports the view that ERPs, with their excellent time resolution, can represent an optimal tool for investigating language disorders mainly along time domain. On the other hand, EEG bands are able to show both functional and maturational aspects of dyslexics' brains, thus representing a distinct measurement with respect to ERPs. These two electrophysiological methods provide complementary information for a better understanding of the neural and cognitive mechanisms involved in DD. In conclusion, electrophysiological measures could represent an effective tool for making early diagnoses of dyslexia or for predictions of future reading problems in infants at risk, but they could also be valuable for testing the efficacy of rehabilitative trainings.

1. Developmental Dyslexia

1.1 Main Features of Developmental Dyslexia

Developmental Dyslexia, or Specific Reading Disability (hereafter often referred to as *DD*, or simply *dyslexia*) is a clinic syndrome classified among developmental learning disorders. It consists of a pronounced and persistent difficulty in learning to read, despite normal intelligence and motivation, spared sensory acuity, and adequate educational and socioeconomic opportunities [World Health Organization, 1993].

Both incorrect and non-fluent decoding of written language mark dyslexics' reading performance, which, in order to diagnose the disability, must be significantly inferior (two standard deviations or more, in standardized reading tests) compared with the performance of normal readers matched for age or reading age. In dyslexia (as well as in the other developmental learning disorders) the main dysfunction is characterised by a relative "specificity", that is, despite the presence of the reading disability, the general intelligence is rather preserved (IQ, assessed with standardized intelligence tests, is in these children typically less than two standard deviations from the average IQ). In regard to this issue, it is noteworthy that, although dyslexics can sometimes show comprehension and reasoning problems during reading, these must be considered as secondary deficits, due to their low-level decoding disability [Shaywitz, 1998]. Further, individuals suffering from DD must be free from other severe sensory or neurological impairments, which can englobe reading disability as secondary symptom (e.g., even if individuals suffering from deafness or from mental retardation can show reading deficits, these have to be interpreted as a mere consequence of their primary sensory or neurological disturb, and therefore, in these cases, a diagnosis of DD would result inadequate). Finally, as last diagnostic criterion, reading disability must interfere not only with scholastic career, but also with every daily activity involving reading skills, and the interference must be persistent. Indeed, dyslexia does not represent a transient developmental lag, rather it is a chronic condition [Shaywitz, 1998]: accuracy, speed, and automation of dyslexics' reading will always show a gap with respect to those of matched normal readers, although early and continuative rehabilitative trainings can allow them to achieve high levels of education.

A large amount of evidence, especially coming from twin studies [DeFries, Fulker, & LaBuda, 1987; Stevenson, Graham, Fredman, & McLoughlin, 1987] and surveys showing familial clustering of dyslexia [Smith, Gilger, & Pennington, 1996] has confirmed that DD is a phenotypically heterogeneous neurological syndrome with a genetic aetiology [Schulte-Körne, Deimel, Müller, Gutenbrunner, & Remschmidt, 1996; Pennington, 1997; Smith, Kelley, & Brower, 1998; Castles, Datta, Gayan, & Olson, 1999; Flint, 1999; Francks, MacPhie, & Monaco, 2002]. Although dyslexia does not commonly segregate in families in a simple mendelian way, it shows a strong genetic involvement, and familiarity for reading impairment is considered one of the most reliable predictor for the following development of the disorder. Further, the high comorbidity of dyslexia with oral or written language developmental disabilities, which is another main risk factor of future reading deficits, supports a particular vulnerability of many linguistic brain areas to hereditary factors [Geschwind & Galaburda, 1985]. Genetic linkage analyses have identified loci on several chromosomes (e.g. 1, 2, 3, 13, 15 and, above all, chromosomes 6 and 18), which have shown strong and replicable effects on reading skills. The neural anomalies, determined by these genetic alterations (and producing, in turn, decoding dysfunctions at cognitive and behavioural level), are still under investigation. However, although opinions are not unanimous on this issue, many data (especially from animal studies, see paragraph 1.3) suggest that genetic factors would cause reading impairment by producing focal anomalies in the cerebral regions specifically involved in language processing, that are left perisylvian areas [Ramus, 2004].

It is necessary to underline that, even assuming genetic bases of dyslexia, people suffering from this disorder differ in their individual profiles for many features (at neurobiological, cognitive and behavioural levels), also produced by a complex set of environmental factors. For instance, the presence of certain hormonal environments during the prenatal period (i.e., high levels of foetal testosterone) can be crucial in producing a wide range of sensorimotor deficits often associated to the reading impairment [Rosen, Herman, & Galaburda, 1999], and contributes in this way to enormously vary the phenotypic manifestations of dyslexia (see, paragraph 1.3). At the same time, environmental factors external to the specific individual histories of dyslexics have been shown to add variations in the occurrence and severity of the reading disability. Among these factors, the intrinsic structure of the language to which the individual is exposed is decisive for the prevalence of the disability. Indeed, it has been demonstrated that DD occurrence is much higher in language with an irregular (or deep) orthography (i.e., English, French, etc.), than in language with a regular (or shallow) orthography (i.e., Italian, German, etc.), the latter showing more transparent correspondence between graphemes and phonemes, and thus being easier to learn [Lindgren, De Renzi, & Richman, 1985]. Therefore, considering the complex relationships between inherited and environmental factors at the origin of the different phenotypic subtypes of DD, we should consider this disorder as an extremely heterogeneous and multifarious syndrome.

Epidemiological data [for a review see Shaywitz & Shaywitz, 2005], indicate that the specific reading disability, which can be seen as the extreme inferior limit of a normal distribution of reading skills, is probably the most frequent neurobehavioral disorder in developmental age and its prevalence rates range from ~ 5 to ~17.5%, depending on several factors (i.e., diagnostic criteria, assessment tests, regularity of the language orthography, etc.). Although someone reported that DD affects males and females equally [Wadsworth, DeFries,

Stevenson, Gilger, & Pennington, 1992; Flynn & Rahbar, 1994; Shaywitz, 1998], by ascribing the classical sexual differences in its occurrence to a sampling bias (following this hypothesis, dyslexic males should be easily identified with respect to females, and therefore included in the sample, because of their more disruptive behaviour), DD is most typically reported in males, with a variable sex ratio depending on different factors (i.e., IQ, phenotypic sub-type of dyslexia, impairment severity, etc. [Olson, 2002; Ramus, 2004]).

Children affected by this disorder show often other deficits in many linguistic and non-linguistic domains: oral and/or written language (at the basis of specific language impairment, dysphasia and/or dysgraphia), mathematical skills (dyscalculia), motor coordination (dyspraxia), temporal orientation (dyschronia), visuospatial skills (developmental right hemisphere syndrome), attentional capabilities (attentional deficit disorder with hyperactivity) [Dewey, 1995; Gross-Tsur, Shalev, Manor, & Amir, 1995; Fawcett, Nicolson, & Dean, 1996; Rapin & Allen, 1998]. This comorbidity of dyslexia with many other developmental disorders proves their partially common origins, involving both genetic factors and environmental influences, and contributes to produce a complex syndrome in which a combination of several other deficits can complicate or worsen the main disadvantageous condition. Just because of this phenotypical variability of the syndrome, many efforts have been made in the attempt to classify its different subtypes. The distinction which mirrors the classification of acquired dyslexia (i.e., reading impairment with a lesional origin), based on dyslexics' error patterns, distinguishes a *phonological* type of dyslexia (alteration of the reading mechanisms which use the grapheme-phoneme conversion rules typical of each language), a *surface* type (impairment of the reading mechanisms which retrieve the phonology starting from a visual identification of the global lexical unity), and a *mixed* type (impairment of both the previous reading mechanisms) [Castles & Coltheart, 1993]. A different classification of dyslexia subtypes, made on the basis of aetiological assumptions, differentiates, instead, between a *dysphonetic* type and a *dyseidetic* type of reading disability, involving phonological/speech discrimination deficits or visual perceptual impairments, respectively [Boder, 1973]. Despite these not much fruitful classificatory attempts, at present, it is more prudent and useful a characterization, rather than a categorization, of dyslexic syndrome. In this view, only an early and complete assessment of cognitive, sensory and motor functions, going over taxonomic purposes, may allow to identify the severity of decoding problems and the presence of other kinds of dysfunctions. This characterization of the deficit, targeted on individual's symptoms and features will permit to create the basis for its treatment, expected to be as much effective as much early and specific.

1.2 Causal Hypotheses of Developmental Dyslexia

In spite of the general consensus on the genetic component of DD, after many years of research, theorists are still in disagreement about the neurological and cognitive mechanisms which, defective and dysfunctional not only on genetic basis, can have a causal role in explaining the reading disability. Thus, researchers' efforts are directed to find the common factors which account for most symptoms, and to characterize this disorder by uncovering causal relationships between different levels of explanation (i.e., genetic, neurobiological and cognitive).

The *phonological deficit theory* of DD supports its purely linguistic origin, referring to a specific deficit in representation (or in the access of representation) and processing of the smallest speech sounds: the phonemes [Bradley & Bryant, 1983; Shaywitz, 1998; Snowling, 2001; Shaywitz, Shaywitz, Pugh, Mencl, Fulbright, Skudlarski et al., 2002; Ramus, Rosen, Dakin, Day, Castellote, White et al., 2003; Shaywitz, Shaywitz, Fulbright, Skudlarski, Mencl, Constable et al., 2003; Ramus, 2004; Shaywitz et al., 2005]. This deficit is usually characterized by at least three main components [Wagner & Torgesen, 1987]: the first is low phonological awareness or metaphonology (difficulty in understanding the relationships between the phonemes of spoken language and the corresponding graphemes of written language, which causes further difficulties to consciously manipulate these sublexical units); the second component is limited verbal short-term memory (both considering the span of the memory store, and the functioning of the working memory); the third component is slow lexical retrieval (particularly clear-cut for rapid naming tasks). As direct consequence of the above deficits, dyslexics show a general impairment in decoding processes (especially when based on grapheme-phoneme conversion rules), which produces very inadequate reading performance and other common linguistic deficits as well. In this perspective, the sensorimotor symptoms, often associated to decoding impairments, are thought as simple comorbid factors, without causal relationships with the reading disability.

Starting from evidence showing the presence of several auditory deficits in the dyslexic population, an alternative theoretical approach, the *temporal (or rapid) processing deficit theory* of DD [Tallal & Piercy, 1973; Tallal, 1980; Merzenich, Schreiner, Jenkins, & Wang, 1993; Stein & Walsh, 1997], assumes a basic impairment in the perceptual processing of stimulus temporal features as the main cause of reading disability. According to this theory, dyslexics are unable to process stimuli, especially in acoustic modality, when these are presented briefly or in rapid temporal succession (as in the case of normal speech). In this view, dyslexics' phonological deficits are considered secondary to the main deficit in the temporal processing of auditory stimuli.

Based on a reversed causal scenario, the *visual processing deficit theory* of DD, even admitting a common defective phonology in dyslexics, assumes that this component is accessory in decoding impairment and that a dysfunction in brain visual mechanisms of reading is the core deficit [Stein, 1993; Stein & Talcott, 1999]. The hypothesis that reading disorder is pre-linguistic in nature arose from a number of studies showing additional visual abnormalities in many dyslexics: slow processing of visual information, longer visual persistence for stimuli with low spatial frequencies, impaired contrast sensitivity, binocular fixation instability, reduced sensitivity to visual motion [Lovegrove, Bowling, Badcock, & Blackwood, 1980a; Lovegrove, Heddle, & Slaghuis, 1980b; Martin & Lovegrove, 1987; Eden, VanMeter, Rumsey, & Zeffiro, 1996; Cornelissen, Hansen, Hutton, Evangelinou, & Stein, 1998; Stein, 2001]. Since all these symptoms specifically pertain to the magnocellular (or transient) visual system, this hypothesis, presuming a dysfunction of visual information processing by this sensory pathway (supported by neurobiological evidence, see paragraph 1.3), is often called *magnocellular (or magnosystem) visual theory* of DD [Anderson, Essick, & Siegel, 1985; Livingstone & Hubel, 1988].

One attractive and parsimonious interpretation of available evidence, in which all quoted theories could converge, points to dyslexia as a general sensorimotor syndrome. The unification of the different approaches has been made by extending the hypothesis of a magnocellular visual deficit to a general multisensory deficit in the whole magnocellular sensory system. In this view, the phonological deficit, considered as a part of a more general sensorimotor syndrome, has been ascribed to a more general auditory impairment and is considered to have the same neurobiological origin as the visual impairment: a sensory dysfunction of the magnocellular system, which is also evident in the tactile domain [Galaburda, 1999; Grant, Zangaladze, Thiagarajah, & Sathian 1999]. Since the magnosystem reaches the cerebellum, via the posterior parietal cortex, this *extended magnocellular theory* of DD provides a possible explanation also for the motor deficits frequently associated with the reading disability, thus including the *cerebellar/motor dysfunction hypothesis* of DD as well [Nicolson & Fawcett, 1990; Nicolson, Fawcett, & Dean, 2001]. Further, as the magnocellular system is also important for directing visual attention and for visual search processes, in virtue of its wide connections with the posterior parietal cortex, some authors have argued, as a variant, that a *visuo-spatial attentional deficit*, indirectly mediated by the magnocellular deficit, may cause reading disorders [e.g., Valdois, Gèrard, Vanault, & Dugas, 1995].

Currently, most theories on the causes of DD coexist, and have not been falsified as each one is supported by a whole body of empirical evidence. Nevertheless, the amount and strength of experimental data in favour of either the one or the other approach varies, leading to theories with different degree of scientific value. However, at present, the strongest evidence converges in identifying the phonological deficit as the core dysfunction of the reading disability [Bradley et al., 1983; Paulesu Frith, Snowling, Gallagher, Morton, Frackoviak et al., 1996; Shaywitz, 1998; Snowling, 2001; Ramus, 2003, 2004; Shaywitz et al., 2005; Ramus & Szenkovits, 2008]. Indeed, after the initial great interest and enthusiasm generated by the extended magnocellular deficit hypothesis of dyslexia, we are currently observing a reversed trend in favour of the phonological hypothesis, due to the inherent problems that the magnosystem theory presents. The first big limit of this theory is that dyslexia has been defined as a complex sensorimotor syndrome, but many recent empirical data have shown that, even thought the prevalence and the significance of the sensorimotor deficits remain uncertain, these non-linguistic deficits involve only one third of dyslexic population [Ramus, 2003]. Indeed, whereas phonological impairment characterized all dyslexics, the other frequently reported deficits (in visual, auditory, attentional and motor domains), considered relevant for theories of the magnosystem, are actually present only in a small subsample of impaired readers, and therefore they can not be considered the primary cause of reading difficulties. The second important trouble of magnocellular hypothesis is that, even in the case in which one or more sensorimotor deficits are co-occurring with the reading disability, they do not always meet the requirements made on the basis of the theory. Indeed, dyslexics can present sensory deficits also for stimuli in frequency domains which not exclusively pertain to the magnosystem pathway; similarly, their auditory impairment, when present, can also be extended, in addition to rapid frequency changes, to slow frequency changes, or can even regard only these latter [Amitay, Ben-Yehudah, Banai, & Ahissar, 2002; Chiappe, Stringer, Siegel, & Stanovich, 2002; Ramus et al., 2003]. Finally, another critical issue for the magnocellular theory of DD is that, whenever present, simple sensory deficits can hardly be connected by causal links to reading disability, and this is confirmed by the fact that visual or auditory deficits are not reliable predictors of reading disturbance as much as phonological impairments [Kronbichler, Hutzler, & Wimmer, 2002; Share, Jorm, MacLean, & Matthews, 2002]. Taken together, these lines of evidence suggest a clear weakness of the magnocellular dysfunction theory of DD in favour of the phonological deficit theory.

Someone could argue that ascribing a linguistic disability, like reading impairment, to a purely linguistic cause, like phonological deficit, can sound tautological, rather than explanatory. This because phonological awareness has been demonstrated to be positively correlated with reading skills, but the causal direction between the two factors is not so clear. However, Ramus [2003] suggested some arguments in favour of this issue: first, since phonological awareness has been proved to be a good pre-school predictor of later reading skills [Pennington & Lefly, 2001; Lyytinen, Guttorm, Huttunen, Hämäläinen, Leppänen, & Vesterinen, 2005], the causal direction is far from being ambiguous (i.e., phonological awareness enhances reading skills, even though these can produce a positive feedback on the phonological awareness itself); second, as already mentioned, the phonological impairment can not be ascribed to the phonological awareness deficit only, as other components (i.e., poor verbal short-term memory and lexical retrieval) have been demonstrated to be, although related, quite independent from phonological awareness [Compton, DeFries, & Olson, 2001; Wolf, Goldberg O'Rourke, Gidney, Lovett, Cirino, & Morris, 2002]. Therefore, although impaired phonological components in dyslexics deserve further investigations, the phonological alteration remains the most consistent factor capable of explaining the core of this reading disability.

The sensorimotor syndrome, instead, is considered optional with respect to reading dysfunction, and it has been hypothesized [Ramus, 2004, 2006] that sensory and motor deficits may be present only in the less pure cases of dyslexia, when the written language decoding impairment is associated with other developmental disorders (i.e. specific language impairment, attentional deficit, autism, etc.). In this view, these deficits should be interpreted as consequent and secondary to other comorbid disorders, with limited causal links with reading skills, but able to enormously worsen the primary disability, by adding new dysfunctions. For these reasons, DD should be considered a multiform syndrome, characterized by different sub-types, in which, side by side with the phonological deficit (the main and sole symptom in the "pure dyslexia"), sensorimotor and attentional dysfunctions can additionally contribute, in different ways, depending on individual differences, to make the basic disability more severe and complex.

1.3 Neurobiological Abnormalities in Developmental Dyslexia

A considerable amount of data confirmed the presence of structural and functional abnormalities in dyslexics' brains [for reviews see Habib, 2000; Démonet, Taylor, & Chaix, 2004; Eckert, 2004]. The first neuropathological examinations and the following neuroimaging studies run on dyslexics showed several microscopic cerebral structural anomalies (i.e., ectopias, microgyri, neurons with small cell bodies or scarce dendritic ramification), which for the first time led to hypothesize a possible abnormality in specific stages of their prenatal brain maturation [Galaburda & Kemper, 1979; Galaburda, Sherman, Rosen, Aboitiz, & Geschwind, 1985; Kaufmann & Galaburda, 1989; Humphreys, Kaufmann, & Galaburda, 1990; Livingstone, Rosen, Drislane, & Galaburda, 1991; Galaburda, Menard, & Rosen, 1994; Robichon & Habib, 1998]. These neural anomalies were identified in the left perisylvian cortex, in the white matter, in the magnocellular layers of thalamus (both in the lateral, and in the medial geniculate nuclei, in the corpus callosum and in the cerebellum. Structural hemispheric anomalies due to incomplete cerebral lateralization were found in dyslexics at a more macroscopic cerebral level as well, and these consisted in absent or reversed asymmetry of the planum temporale [Geschwind & Levitsky, 1968], decreased asymmetry of the parietal operculum [Habib & Robichon, 1996], and bilateral or reversed asymmetry of inferior frontal gyrus [Jernigan, Hesselink, Sowell, & Tallal, 1991; Robichon, Lévrier, Farnarier, & Habib, 2000].

Functional brain imaging studies supported many of the above structural findings, showing dysfunctions in a broad cortical network of dyslexics' brains, mainly distributed in the left hemisphere, which includes perisylvian and temporo-parieto-occipital brain areas (i.e., planum temporale, inferior frontal gyrus, superior, middle and inferior temporal gyri, fusiform gyrus, angular gyrus and supramarginal gyrus). In particular, evidence suggested an impairment of the left posterior brain system for reading, that is, the disruption of the connections between dorsal (parietal) and ventral (occipito-temporal) circuits, related to grapheme-phoneme mapping and to global lexical entry recognition [Helenius, Tarkiainen, Cornelissen, Hansen, & Salmelin, 1999; Simos, Breier, Fletcher, Bergman, & Papanicolaou, 2000; Paulesu, Démonet, Fazio, McCrory, Chanoine, Brunswick et al., 2001; Temple, Poldrack, Salidis, Deutsch, Tallal, Merzenich et al., 2001; Démonet et al., 2004]. As a consequence, to overcome this failure of left posterior reading system, in dyslexics the neural activity has been found shifted towards more anterior left regions (which are sometimes overactivated compared with normal readers), or right perisylvian areas (typically not involved in low-level decoding processes) [Shaywitz et al., 1998; Brunswick, McCrory, Price, Frith, & Frith, 1999; Simos et al., 2000; Georgiewa, Rzanny, Gaser, Gerhard, Vieweg, Freesmeyer et al., 2002; Shaywitz et al., 2002; Démonet et al., 2004].

All these neurobiological abnormalities are open to many interpretations, especially because, depending on the study (with its peculiar variables: i.e., dyslexic samples, experimental tasks, neurobiological methods for measuring neural structure or activity, etc.), the set of detected anomalies is always partial with respect to the whole set of anomalies above reported. Therefore, on the basis of the theoretical approach, different subsets of abnormalities have been used to support each explicative hypothesis of DD. More precisely, structural and functional anomalies in left perisylvian areas have been typically used in favour of linguistic/phonological deficit theory of DD, as these regions have a main role in linguistic and phonological processing [Price, 1998]. On the contrary, the structural alteration of thalamus have been used to claim the magnosystem theory of DD, in such a direction that thalamic anomalies in the magnocellular layers of lateral geniculate nucleus are considered to cause dyslexics' visual deficits, and anomalies in the medial geniculate nucleus are expected to cause auditory deficits. The crucial question is related to the discovery of the causal direction between these two kinds of anomalies (i.e. cortical versus thalamic). A top-down explanation, consistent with phonological deficit theory of DD, supposes that genetically driven cortical abnormalities in the left perisylvian cortex (responsible for phonological impairment) are able to start a retrograde degeneration till the sensorial thalamic nuclei (which are responsible for sensory deficits), which in turn can extend to the posterior parietal cortex and to the cerebellum (responsible for motor and attentional deficits, respectively). Conversely, a bottom-up explanation, consistent with magnosystem dysfunction theory of DD, supposes an opposite scenario: genetically driven thalamic anomalies are able to propagate in all the areas connected to the thalamus (i.e. perisilvian cortex, and possibly also posterior parietal cortex and cerebellum). Data on this issue are provided by animal studies and suggest, in agreement with behavioural data attesting the phonological origin of DD, a top-down explanation. This top-down theory is based on experimental evidence that mice and rats with spontaneous or experimental induced cortical abnormalities subsequently develop thalamic anomalies [Herman, Galaburda, Fitch, Carter, & Rosen, 1997; Peiffer, Rosen, & Fitch, 2002]; in addition, these animal exhibit a variety of learning deficits, whereas sensory dysfunctions are present only depending on whether specific hormonal condition are met [Rosen et al., 1999]. Based on these finding, it has been proposed a neurobiological model which, although originally thought to explain causal factors of DD, can be applied to other developmental disorders as well (starting from the assumption that the kind of disorder is strictly related to the cortical abnormality location) [Ramus, 2004, 2006]. According to this model (see Figure 1), which currently offers the most plausible framework with a considerable amount of explanatory arguments, genetically driven focal anomalies in the left perisilvian cortex cause the phonological impairment which characterized all individuals with DD. Depending on environmental influences, especially the prenatal exposure to certain hormonal factors (e.g., sex hormones like androgens), cortical anomalies can drive thalamic anomalies, which in turn are responsible for the sensorimotor syndrome sometimes associated to reading disability.

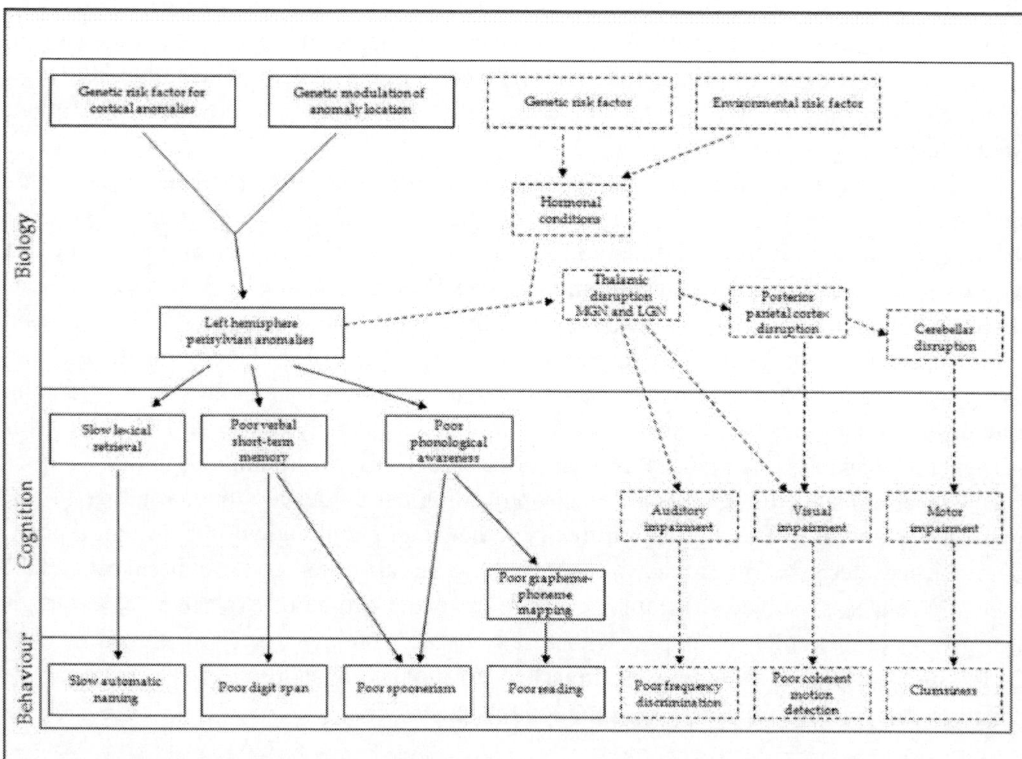

Figure 1. Neurobiological model proposed by Ramus to explain the aetiology of Developmental Dyslexia. Solid lines represent core traits of developmental dyslexia, dashed lines represent associated traits, not necessarily present in each affected individual. LGN: lateral geniculate nucleus, MGN: medial geniculate nucleus (redrawn from Ramus, 2004).

2. Electrophysiological Correlates of Developmental Dyslexia

2.1 Event Related Potentials in the Study of Developmental Dyslexia

Event-related potentials (ERPs) are voltage fluctuations evoked from specific synchronously active neuron assemblies, which are temporally associated to some kind of external (i.e., physical stimulation) or internal (i.e., cognitive processing, motor preparation) events. They are usually recorded from the human scalp and extracted from the electroencephalographic spontaneous rhythmic oscillations (typically much larger in amplitude) through an averaging procedure time-locked to the specific eliciting event [Fabiani, Gratton, & Federmeier, 2007]. ERP components span a continuum between the exogenous, or early, potentials (i.e., obligatory responses evoked by the physical features of the eliciting event) and the endogenous, or late, potentials (i.e., responses evoked by cognitive processes associated to external events, but without a necessary direct link between the former and the physical features of the latter). Despite a limited spatial resolution, ERPs, with their ability to determine the sequence of events closely occurring in time (on the order of milliseconds), can be used in paradigms specifically designed either to understand how the brain process the various cognitive functions (referring in particular to their time-course and constitutive subcomponents) or to make specific diagnoses of physical and mental dysfunctions.

For its excellent time resolution, ERP technique turns out to be particularly suitable to investigate both reading (a complex cognitive function consisting of many subprocesses, hard to be investigated with behavioural methods) and reading disability, especially when the latter manifests itself with a time-based symptom, like decoding dysfluency. In recent years, the use of evoked potentials for studying reading disability, allowed the collection of many results (briefly reported in the next sub-paragraphs, following the order of component latencies), which suggested a wide range of ERP anomalies in dyslexics. Although the most frequent anomalies are related to the auditory evoked components (namely to the MMN), which point to a general weakness of auditory processing at the basis of reading disability, it is still difficult to establish, on the bases of electrophysiological evidence alone, whether this can support the temporal processing deficit theory rather than phonological impairment theory of DD. A correct interpretation of the available findings should take into account many variables (especially related to subjects' sample selection or to the choice of experimental paradigm). Thus, given the difficulty to support with a reasonable certainty a specific causal theory of DD, it is more useful to use these ERP markers for achieving more effective diagnoses and detailed phenotypical profiles of the examined readers.

Early Evoked Components

Event related positive or negative deflections peaking around the first 100 ms following an acoustic or visual stimulus are usually called "early" evoked components. They are fast and obligatory (i.e., not dependent on attentional resources) responses of the physiological system to stimulus physical features. Considering the use of these early components to investigate DD in the auditory domain (which was more investigated than the visual one), several studies reported results mainly related to the hemispherical asymmetries. A group of dyslexic children characterized as dyseidetics showed left lateralization in early evoked components to musical and speech stimuli, whereas a group of dysphonetics failed to show any asymmetry [Fried, Tanguay, Boder, Doubleday, & Greensite, 1981]. Similar results were found in a sample of adult dyslexics, classified into similar sub-groups (i.e., dyseidetics and dysphonetics) [Rosenthal, Boder, & Callaway, 1982]. In line with this evidence, Brunswick and Rippon [1994] observed larger N1 amplitudes over the left hemisphere in normal readers during dichotic presentation of syllables, and the reversed asymmetry in children with reading disability. To our knowledge, only one study [Yingling, Galin, Fein, Peltzman, & Davenport, 1986] was not able to find differences between dyslexics and controls in response to simple acoustic stimuli. Many other studies reported smaller amplitudes, longer latencies, reduced or inverse hemispherical lateralization of early obligatory components in children with developmental disorders, but these findings will be not reported in the present review as participant selection did not meet the specific criteria for a clear diagnosis of DD (and very often the samples investigated were constituted by children with reading impairments mixed to children with more general learning or language disabilities).

MMN

The mismatch negativity (MMN) is a middle-latency negative component, with a fronto-central distribution, peaking between 100 and 250 ms after an acoustic stimulus, which is evoked by infrequent and physically deviant stimuli (in one of several features: i.e., pitch, duration, intensity, rise time, etc.) with respect to the sequence of homogeneous stimuli in which it randomly occurs. Since it is generally evoked by unattended stimuli, the MMN is considered to reflect automatic change detection [Kraus, McGee, Carrell, & Sharma, 1995], and therefore can be used to test the pre-attentive discriminatory skills within the auditory system. There are many studies which employed MMN to investigate reading impairments, however, with a few exceptions, findings are quite consistent on the whole and attest alterations in amplitude, latency and hemispherical lateralization of this evoked potential in dyslexic readers. In particular, depending on the study, reduced, delayed or inversely lateralized MMNs have been shown to mark acoustic discrimination impairments in dyslexics. On one hand, several studies reported this discriminatory deficit in response to all kinds of deviant auditory stimuli, comprising simple pure tones [Baldeweg, Richardson, Watkins, Foale, & Gruzelier, 1999; Maurer, Brem, Bucher, & Brandeis, 2003a; Maurer, Bucher, Brem, & Brandeis, 2003b]. On the other hand, other studies found discrimination impairments for deviant speech-related sounds, thus supporting a pre-attentive, linguistic explanation of reading disabilities [Schulte-Körne, Deimel, Bartling, & Remschmidt, 2001]. As Lyytinen at al. [2005] have suggested, MMN differences between normal and impaired readers appear more related to complexity and processing demands, rather than just mere speech vs. non-speech distinction of the used stimuli. This viewpoint was supported by the findings of Kujala and colleagues [Kujala, Alho, & Näätänen, 2000], who found MMN differences between adult dyslexics and controls only for deviant stimuli occurring within complex (not speech-related) sound patterns, whereas deviant sounds failed to differentiate groups when occurring within simple sound patterns.

Overall, results have suggested that impairments in implicit (or pre-attentive) auditory processing (often so small that escape behavioural measurements) could give rise to dyslexics' deficits. In details, altered MMN can be explained by deficits both at the lowest level of auditory discrimination processing and at the highest level of auditory (and in particular phonological) short term memory processing. Therefore MMN anomalies have been considered to support, depending on the theoretical orientation, either the auditory (temporal processing or magnocellular) deficit hypothesis of DD, or the phonological deficit hypothesis. Taking out the theoretical implications, it should be reminded that a very important applicative aspect of MMN is represented by its predictive value for the future occurrence of reading disabilities in infants with familial risk for DD [for a review see Lyytinen et al., 2005]. Indeed, it was largely proved that, with respect to other ERP markers, a reversed hemispherical asymmetry of this component (which in normal controls is wider in the left hemisphere) to acoustic and speech sounds, represents a reliable predictor for later development of dyslexia in children at-risk, even before the first year of age (see the last paragraph for a more detailed report). In addition, Kujala e colleagues [Kujala, Karma, Ceponiené, Belitz, Turkkila, Tervaniemi et al., 2001] demonstrated that audio–visual training (not specifically based on speech sounds) improves the reading skills of the treated dyslexics and that this behavioural advance was correlated with greater MMN amplitude. Therefore, despite the relatively few conclusive findings concerning the significance of auditory processing in dyslexia, important advances can be expected in future from the use of ERP markers, like MMNs, as basis for the diagnosis, prognosis and evaluation of training efficacy in reading disorders.

N200

The N200 is a middle-latency negative deflection whose scalp distribution and functional significance vary according to modality and experimental manipulations. It can be detected both in auditory (with maximum amplitude at fronto-central sites), and in visual modality (with maximum at occipital locations). In many experimental paradigms, the N200 amplitude appears to reflect the detection of some kind of mismatch between the entering stimulus and the representations of the prior stimuli, actively generated and stored in short term memory. This component diverges from the MMN since, differently from the latter, it is usually elicited when subjects orient attention and must respond in active tasks of mismatch detection [Fabiani et al., 2007]. Differently from the above reported findings on MMN, an interesting research of Kujala et al. [Kujala, Halmetoja, Näätänen, Alku, Lyytinen, & Sussman, 2006] did not find MMN differences between impaired and normal readers, during a passive condition in which deviant speech sounds (of different duration compared with standard ones) must be ignored. On the contrary, in the active target condition (requiring a response to deviant stimuli) the N200 amplitude was considerably lower in the group of poor readers. For authors, this would demonstrate an association between reading difficulty and deficits in a conscious (i.e., attentive, rather than pre-attentive) stage of stimulus processing. By using a completely different paradigm, in which written words and letter strings have to be processed by normal and impaired readers, a result in the opposite direction has been found [Bergmann, Hutzler, Klimesch, & Wimmer, 1995]. In detail, increased N200 (which authors named N220) were found in impaired readers specifically for word processing. This was interpreted as reflecting dyslexics' compensatory mechanisms aimed to face a reduced anticipatory activation of cortical regions involved in word processing. This was indexed by a decreased Contingent Negative Components (CNV), measured in an interval preceding the N200. It is evident, from the few examples of N200 here reported, that the modulation of this component is strictly related to the experimental variables and can be functionally interpreted only by a careful examination of each specific paradigm.

P300

The P300 is a middle-latency positive component, peaking around 300 ms after an infrequent and deviant task-relevant stimulus, interspersed within a series of more frequent and standard stimuli (the classical "odd-ball" paradigm). This component is considered related to conscious processing and evaluation of stimuli in the working memory, as subjects must attend and actively respond to the odd-ball stimuli [Fitzgerald & Picton, 1983]. In impaired readers, it has been generally found P300 with reduced amplitude [Lovrich & Stamm, 1983; Holcomb, Ackerman, & Dykman, 1986; Erez & Pratt, 1992], delayed latency [Mazzotta & Gallai, 1992] or with an altered lateralization (i.e. earlier latencies to speech stimuli in the right hemisphere with respect to controls' left dominance [Brezniz & Misra, 2003]) in many studies, all results suggesting an inefficient processing of task-relevant information [Taylor & Keenan, 1990]. This observation has generally been used by the theorists who support an attentional deficit at the basis of reading disability, as a proof in favour of their explicative theory. However, more controlled studies revealed altered P300s only in specific sub-samples of dyslexics, who in addiction suffered for attentional disorders [Duncan, Rumsey, Wilkniss, Denckla, Hamburger, & Odou-Potkin, 1994]. This finding undermines attentional deficit theory of DD and raises a crucial point in the employment of this component to study reading disorder. Since attentional deficits are often associated to reading disability (as reported in the first section of this chapter), anomalies in P300 can be considered to index attentional impairment as one of the possible causes of reading deficits (and not as a comorbidity factor) only when the samples of dyslexics under investigation are clearly diagnosed as free from specific attentional disorders, like in the case of the well controlled research of Holcomb and coworkers [Holcomb, Ackerman, & Dykman,1985]. However, even in the mentioned study, the relationships between attentional and reading deficits, based on dyslexics' reduced P300, can be open to an alternative explanation: dyslexics' repeated experiences of scholastic failures could produce more general and diffuse difficulties in attention engaging tasks, therefore attentional problem would be a consequence more than a cause of reading disorders.

N400

The N400 is a negative endogenous component, peaking around 400 ms after the eliciting stimulus, with a posterior distribution, and a tendency to right lateralization. Since N400 amplitude has proved to be inversely correlated with many variables of a stimulus, in relation to its context (i.e., stimulus probability of occurrence, stimulus repetition, stimulus congruency with the context, subjective expectation of stimulus occurrence based on individual's semantic memory, etc.), this component has been interpreted to reflect high level processing, such as meaning extraction and semantic integration of a stimulus within the context [Kutas & Federmeier, 2000].

Anomalous N400s during sentence comprehension have been reported in many studies on developmental reading disabilities, unfortunately findings are not univocal, and this makes their interpretation quite difficult. Some authors reported decreased N400 amplitude in dyslexics children [Stelmack, Saxe, Noldy-Cullum, Campbell, & Armitage, 1988; Helenius, Salmelin, Service, & Connolly, 1999], which was interpreted as a failure to engage semantic memory during linguistic comprehension. On the contrary, other studies reported increased N400 amplitude in impaired readers [Neville, Coffey, Holcomb, & Tallal, 1993; Robichon, Besson, & Habib, 2002], which was considered to reflect their compensatory effort to extract word meaning and integrate it within the sentence. As reported in the first part of the present chapter (paragraph 1.1), many behavioural data demonstrated that impaired readers can sometimes show comprehension and reasoning deficits during text reading [Shaywitz, 1998]. However, it is noteworthy that such high–level cognitive problems must be regarded as secondary deficits, due to dyslexics' main impairment in low-level decoding. Therefore, text comprehension dysfunctions, as indexed by altered N400s, should be considered as a common natural consequence of more basic decoding impairments, and, as such, not very informative with regard to the causal mechanisms possibly involved. In other words, since high-order impairment in reading can be expected with elevated probability in dyslexics, as a consequence of their basic low-order deficits, the investigation of earlier ERP components appears more effective in our opinion, being these indexes more strictly related to the primary impaired mechanisms of DD.

Conversely, the so-called N420 detected by Penolazzi and colleagues [Penolazzi, Spironelli, Vio, & Angrilli, 2006] has to be considered in a completely different way. In fact, although this component has been found within a time interval roughly corresponding to that of the traditional N400, its different spatial distribution suggested to authors a completely different functional meaning. Within a linguistic paradigm in which the same set of words were processed on the basis of various linguistic criteria, the N420 was considered as related to a low-level processing phase, common to all the different experimental tasks: i.e., the grapheme-phoneme conversion during reading. In addition to spatial distribution and the paradigm used, this interpretation was supported by the mean reading times of the sample investigated, which showed that, during the N420 interval, both normal and impaired readers were still engaged in the basic processes of word decoding, a condition which makes the execution of a more high–level linguistic processing (like semantic elaboration) very unlikely. Indeed, whereas in controls this component was left lateralized, in disabled readers it was more distributed across hemispheres. Dyslexics' lack of lateralization, found also in a later slow negative wave (700-1500 ms time interval), points to an altered cerebral asymmetry of the basic mechanisms necessary for reading the most important of which is the orthography-phonology mapping. In this view, these findings would therefore support the hypothesis of a phonological deficit underlying developmental reading disabilities.

2.2 Electroencephalographic Bands in the Study of Developmental Dyslexia

Electroencephalography (EEG) is the measurement of electrical activity (post-synaptic currents) generated by neuronal assemblies, as recorded from electrodes placed on the scalp. Brain electrical oscillations cover a large range of values in amplitude (~ 5-200 μV) and frequency (~ 0.5- 100 Hz), and the constituent waves of EEG are usually characterized by specific ranges of such frequencies, giving rise to the well-known electroencephalographic (EEG) bands. These rhythms are classically linked to particular states of cortical arousal. As a general rule, waves with low frequency and large amplitude, typical of slow bands (i.e., delta and theta), have been traditionally associated to absent or decreased cognitive processing, whereas high frequency and small amplitude waves, characteristic of fast bands (e.g., beta and gamma) have been related to active cognitive processing [Pizzagalli, 2007]. However the more recent employment of EEG in experimental paradigms appropriately created to test task- and stimulus-related linguistic processing, has contributed to enrich (and sometime partially change) the functional significance of many bands, which therefore can be used nowadays as markers of more specific processes. Like ERPs and despite a low spatial resolution, EEG band analysis offers the possibility to study brain functions with a time resolution in the middle between fMRI and ERPs.

In the study of dyslexia, EEG bands have been traditionally investigated, under resting condition, in order to detect basic brain activity differences between impaired and normal readers. Although data are not univocal, most of such studies found an overall increase in slower rhythms (i.e., delta and theta bands) and a decrease in mid range frequencies (especially alpha) in children with reading disabilities associated or not to other learning disorders [Sklar, Hanley, & Simmons, 1972; Colon, Notermans, DeWeerd, & Kap, 1979; Ahn, Prichep, John, Baird, Trepetin, & Kaye, 1980; John, Prichep, Ahn, Easton, Friedman, & Kaye, 1983; Harmony, Hinojosa, Marosi, Becker, Rodríguez, Reyes et al., 1990a; Fonseca, Tedrus, Chiodi, Cerqueira, & Tonelotto, 2006]. Only a few studies were not able to find any electrophysiological differences between impaired and normal readers in resting periods [Fein, Galin, Yingling, Johnstone, Davenport, & Herron, 1986; Yingling et al., 1986]. However these findings are the minority and many reasons probably account for these inconsistent results, above all confounded variables related to sample selection (e.g., few participants, phenotypic variability, comorbidity) and experimental setting (e.g., different parameters of EEG recording and analysis). Focusing on to the majority of the studies which found differences between groups, it is critical to note that they showed in dyslexics abnormal EEG patterns (i.e., relative preponderance of slower rhythms over faster ones), analogous to those which typically mark infancy and early childhood with respect to adulthood [Matoušek, M., & Petersén, 1973; John, Ahn, Prichep, Trepetin, Brown, & Kaye, 1980; Gasser, Verleger, Bacher, & Sroka, 1988; Harmony, Marosi, Díaz de León, Becker, & Fernández, 1990b]. For this reason, the main interpretation of the EEG abnormalities observed in impaired readers, especially in the case of less severe disabilities, has been often limited to a general, more or less persistent, maturational lag in brain development.

Although EEG studies under resting state provided important information about basic differences between normal and impaired readers, a significant advance in the research on electrophysiological correlates of DD has been reached only recently, by using experimental paradigms aimed at stressing (through specific stimuli or tasks) the functional cognitive processes assumed to be potentially impaired in dyslexics (i.e., linguistic, perceptual, attentional). Within this new perspective of event related EEG studies, which will be briefly reviewed in the present paragraph, a further progress has been reached by shifting the focus from a more coarse band or spectral analysis, performed on the entire task period [Ackerman, McPherson, Oglesby, & Dykman, 1998; Rippon & Brunswick, 1998, 2000], to a more fine-grained analyses based on time intervals corresponding to different processing phases required by the task [Klimesch, Doppelmayr, Wimmer, Gruber, Röhm, Schwaiger et al., 2001a; Klimesch, Doppelmayr, Wimmer, Schwaiger, Röhm, Gruber et al., 2001b; Spironelli, Penolazzi, Vio, & Angrilli, 2006; Spironelli, Penolazzi, & Angrilli, 2008; Penolazzi, Spironelli, & Angrilli, in press]. With such strategy, differences between dyslexics and controls, actively engaged in different experimental tasks, have been found particularly in beta, alpha and theta bands [Klimesch et al., 2001a, 2001b; Milne, Hamm, Kirk, & Corballis, 2003; Spironelli et al., 2006, 2008], and, more recently, in delta rhythm as well [Penolazzi et al., in press]. This new approach to the issue allowed to greatly enlarge the restrictive maturational lag hypothesis of reading disabilities, by detecting precise impaired mechanisms in specific brain regions at the basis of dyslexics' behavioural deficits.

In agreement with the fact that the functional significance of ***alpha*** rhythm (8-12 Hz) is heavily debated (particularly in studies investigating evoked EEG activity), and it is still difficult to clearly define its physiological role [Pizzagalli, 2007] the many studies which used it to investigate DD have led to different and inconsistent results [Duffy et al.1980; Harmony et al., 1990a; Ortiz, Exposito, Miguel, Martin-Loeches, & Rubia, 1992; Rippon & Brunswick, 2000] Depending on the study, dyslexics showed increased or diminished alpha levels compared with controls, possibly because different alpha sub-bands may be functionally dissociated [Klimesch, 1999]. Therefore, given that studies which used alpha band did not allow to deepen the dynamics involved in reading disorders, they will be not treated in the present review on event related EEG correlates of dyslexia.

On the contrary, the research on reading disability has recently received a great impulse by the employment of ***theta*** band in several experimental paradigms. This EEG rhythm, characterized by wide and slow waves (4–8 Hz), prevails (together with the delta rhythm) in infancy also during waking, and gradually decreases over developmental age. Whereas traditional EEG studies reported theta activity in adults prominently during sleep, or drowsiness state, more recent findings have associate the increase of this rhythm with enhanced effective cognitive processing, improved ability to focus and sustain attention, and increased mental effort or task difficulty [Gevins & Smith, 2000]. In addition, increased theta activity has been interpreted as reflecting the extensive use of specific mechanisms, like information retention or scanning in working memory [Gevins, Smith, McEvoy, & Yu, 1997; Klimesh, 1999; Gevins et al., 2000; Jensen & Tesche, 2002; Sauseng, Klimesch, Dopplemayr, Hanslmayr, Schabus, & Gruber, 2004; Sauseng, Klimesch, Schabus, & Dopplemayr, 2005]. Since the most robust explicative hypothesis of DD narrows the reading disorder mainly to deficits in phonological working memory (see paragraph 1.2), the use of theta band as proved functional marker of verbal working memory and linguistic executive functions involvement turned out to be natural. Ackerman et al. [Ackerman, Dykman, Oglesby, & Newton, 1995] found increased theta (and decreased beta) power in poor readers with respect to controls during letter and word reading. In line with this result, Rippon and Brunswick [1998, 2000] reported an increase of frontal theta activity in impaired compared with normal readers, selectively during a phonological processing, contrasted with a visual task. This finding, which confirmed the discriminative power of theta band in relation to different cognitive tasks (whereas, in the same investigation, alpha and beta band analyses failed to reveal task-dependent differences in dyslexics), was interpreted as reflecting dyslexics' decreased task automaticity and increased effort to compensate the basic phonological deficit. Klimesh et al. [2001a] investigated tonic and basic levels of theta band in a sample of dyslexic children, engaged in number, word and pseudo-word reading tasks. The authors found, in the patient sample, a bilateral increase in theta activity specifically during word reading, conversely controls showed a highly selective left lateralized activation for words. Interestingly, results on dyslexics' anomalous language-related theta lateralization have been confirmed by a series of studies, which, extending the investigation to other bands, succeeded in correlating specific altered EEG patterns to particular phases of dyslexics' word reading [Spironelli et al., 2006, 2008; Penolazzi et al., in press]. These studies, using a well-tested linguistic CNV paradigm, based on word-pair visual presentation [Angrilli, Dobel, Rockstroh, Stegagno, & Elbert, 2000; Angrilli, Elbert, Cusumano, Stegagno, & Rockstroh, B., 2003; Penolazzi et al., 2006;

Spironelli & Angrilli, 2006; Spironelli et al., 2006, 2008], engaged dyslexics and age-matched controls in different kinds of linguistic tasks. In detail, children were asked to judge word pairs on the basis of different criteria (each corresponding to an experimental task), appositely employed to test different mechanisms of written word processing: from the low level visuo-perceptual processing (in the control Orthographic task), to the higher level rhyming and semantic association processes (in the Phonological and Semantic tasks, respectively). Besides the possibility to test several subprocesses potentially impaired in dyslexics, an innovative feature of this paradigm consisted in the use, in all tasks, of the same set of words as first stimulus of each pair, to exclude interfering effects related to the features of the specific selected words (e.g., length, frequency, lexical category, etc. [Penolazzi, Hauk, & Pulvermuller, 2007]). Thus, the adopted paradigm allows to attribute all significant effects only to the specific processes engaged by the task and not to possible confounding factors. This allowed authors to find in dyslexics an altered pattern of theta activation (4-8 Hz), both in the temporal dimension and in the cortical space [Spironelli et al., 2006]. Analyses performed on three different phases of word processing (i.e., "W1": word encoding interval; "iISI" and "tISI": respectively initial and terminal parts of the inter-stimulus-interval between words of each pair), compared with a baseline interval, showed in controls a time-dependent and task-related cortical activation: a peak of theta activity during word encoding interval, and, always during this processing phase, a greater theta amplitude on the left hemisphere for the Phonological task, compared with the more bilateral activity of the Semantic task. On the contrary, dyslexics showed a peak of theta activity which was delayed to the first inter stimulus interval, and shifted to the right hemisphere during all phases of the Phonological task, and in some intervals of the Semantic task. Therefore dyslexics' dysfunctional, unspecific and anomalous (in both time course and hemispherical asymmetry) theta activation to language has been interpreted as due to a defective recruitment of left hemisphere structures during the verbal working memory phase, especially in the Phonological task.

Similar results were found, using the same linguistic paradigm on a different sample of impaired readers, in a following study [Spironelli et al., 2008] which added to previous findings with the novel contribution of ***beta*** band (13-30 Hz), a more classical index of cortical activation. Evidence of dysfunctional beta band alteration in dyslexic children has recently been provided by several studies. Klimesch et al. (2001b), by comparing alpha (8-12.5 Hz) and beta (12.5-16 Hz) band activations in the same experimental paradigm above described, found a selective deficit in dyslexics' word processing. Controls showed a task-dependent beta activation: i.e., higher beta percentages during word reading in left hemisphere locations roughly corresponding, for authors, to Broca's area and angular gyrus, and increased right/midline beta amplitude during number processing. Instead, dyslexics showed a complete lack of task selectivity. Therefore, beta band was interpreted, by Klimesh and colleagues, as a cortical index able to measure the capability to process specific stimuli (i.e., words, numbers, etc.), and, in particular in linguistic paradigms, to reflect grapheme-phoneme processing only in normal readers. Further evidence of dysfunctional beta band alteration in dyslexic children was also provided by Milne et al. (2003). These authors compared two subsamples of compensated dyslexics, i.e., dysphonetics and dyseidetics children, with a control group, during a lexical decision task on visually presented words and pseudo-words, and found no overall differences in mean beta power between normal and impaired readers. However, a significant interaction group by anterior-posterior axis was found: whereas dysphonetic children showed increased beta activity over anterior sites, and dyseidetics over posterior ones, controls revealed a different pattern without antero-posterior differences. In agreement with most neuroimaging studies (see paragraph 1.3), Milne et al. interpreted these findings as a demonstration of the segregation of different word subprocesses in anterior and posterior regions of linguistic areas, thus confirming the capability of beta as a marker able to locate specific cognitive functions. In their study, Spironelli and colleagues (2008) introduced EEG beta band with the aim to collect more detailed topographical information on reading impairment. Indeed, whereas theta band is controlled by the deep subcortical structures of the temporal lobe, involved in working memory [Leung, 1998; Tesche & Karhu, 2000; Vertes, 2005], beta band is essentially produced by highly confined superficial cortical activity, depending by many independent generators typically recruited by high-level cognitive processing [Pantev, Makeig, Hoke, Galambos, Hampson, & Gallen, 1991; Tallon-Baudry & Bertrand, 1999]. Results revealed that the two EEG bands had very similar patterns of activation (see Figure 2), and were therefore, to some extent, functionally correlated, as previously demonstrated for working memory processes [Leung, 1992; Sarnthein, Petsche, Rappelsberger Shaw, & von Stein, 1998; Slotnick, Moo, Kraut, Lesser, & Hart, 2002; Sarnthein, Morel, von Stein, & Jeanmonod, 2003]. Thus, beta band helped to interpret theta band as an effective index of complex cognitive processes implemented on the cortical surface. Indeed, whereas controls showed greater theta and beta activation at left frontal sites during the Phonological task, dyslexics showed at anterior locations a dysfunctional right lateralization in all tasks. On the contrary, at posterior sites, impaired readers showed greater left lateralization during both Phonological and Orthographic tasks, possibly indicating an altered and difficult phonological transcoding process during verbal working memory phases of word processing. Therefore, also results of the last study, by linking dyslexics' defective verbal working memory to the altered patterns of EEG activity, supports phonological deficit hypothesis of DD. Further, it promotes the use of theta and beta bands as useful instruments for assessing task-related language lateralization and its impairment in developmental age, being enough sensitive to task manipulation and to different phases of word processing.

In the last study, the use of the same CNV linguistic paradigm [Angrilli et al., 2000] for measuring ***delta*** band (0-4 Hz) has not only strengthened previous results, but also represented a positive evolution for the investigation of the developmental disorder by means of EEG rhythms [Penolazzi et al., in press]. Since delta waves predominantly characterise EEG in developmental age, it marks cerebral immaturity, but, at the same time, delta waves are present in adulthood during the deepest stages of sleep, or in severe pathological conditions [De Jongh, de Munck, Baayen , Jonkman, Heethaar, & van Dijk, 2001; Wienbruch, Moratti, Elbert, Vogel, Fehr, Kissler et al., 2003; Babiloni, Frisoni, Steriade, Bresciani, Binetti, Del Percio et al., 2006]. Thus, this rhythm is generally considered a clear-cut index of cortical inhibition. The study of Penolazzi et al. [in press] aimed at investigating DD by using delta band both for detecting group differences in brain maturation and for measuring, with an innovative approach, functional differences in task-related linguistic brain asymmetry.. Results of this study are in line with past findings of the same research group [Spironelli et al., 2006, 2008]: indeed delta activity, a clear marker of cortical inhibition, showed a specular pattern with respect to the previously investigated theta and beta bands, used as markers of functional activation (see Figure 3).

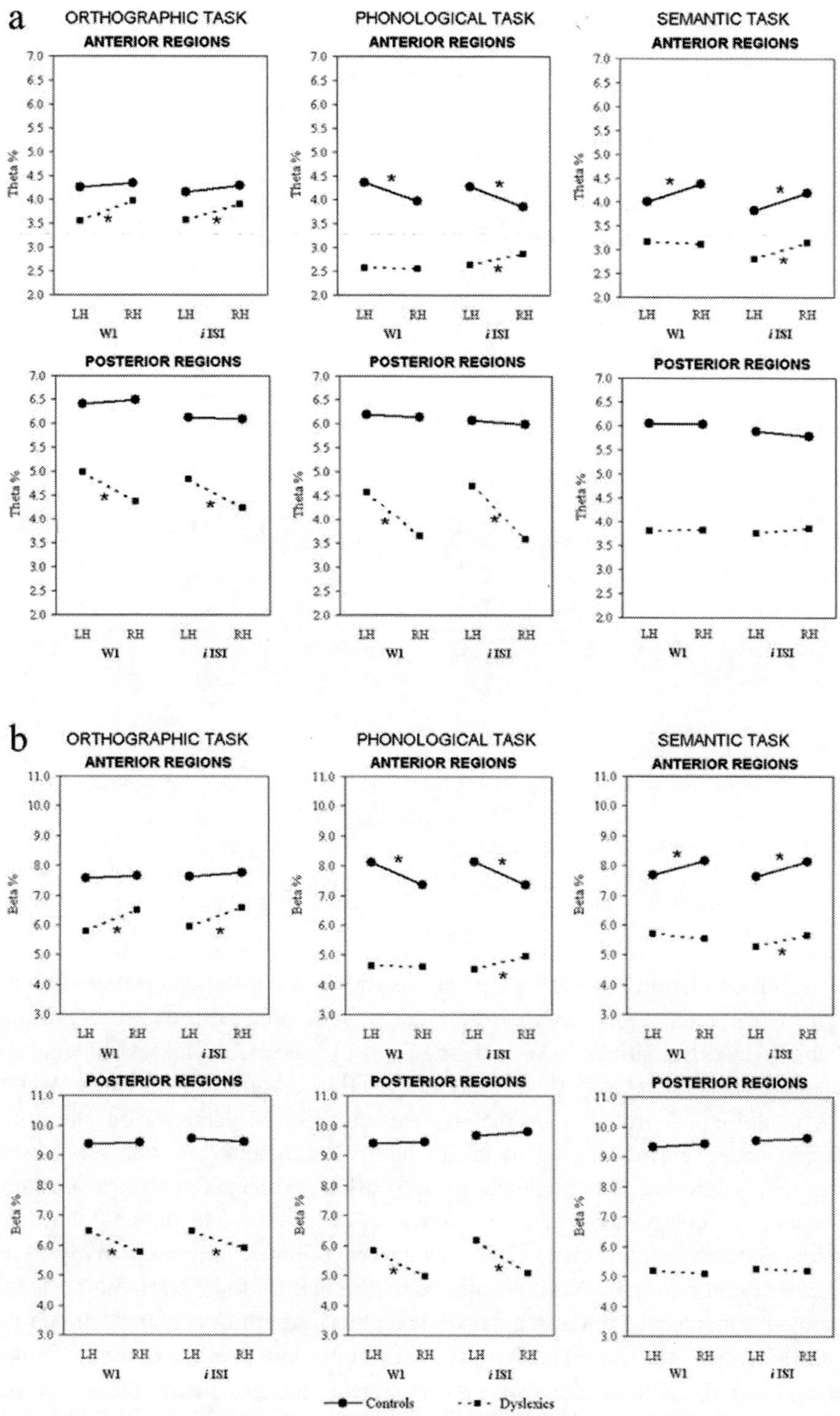

Figure 2. Percentages of normalized Theta (a) and Beta (b) bands in dyslexics and controls (dashed and full lines, respectively) during W1 and *i*ISI intervals throughout three linguistic tasks in the four cortical quadrants. Asterisks indicate significant post-hoc test results (redrawn from Spironelli, et al., 2008).

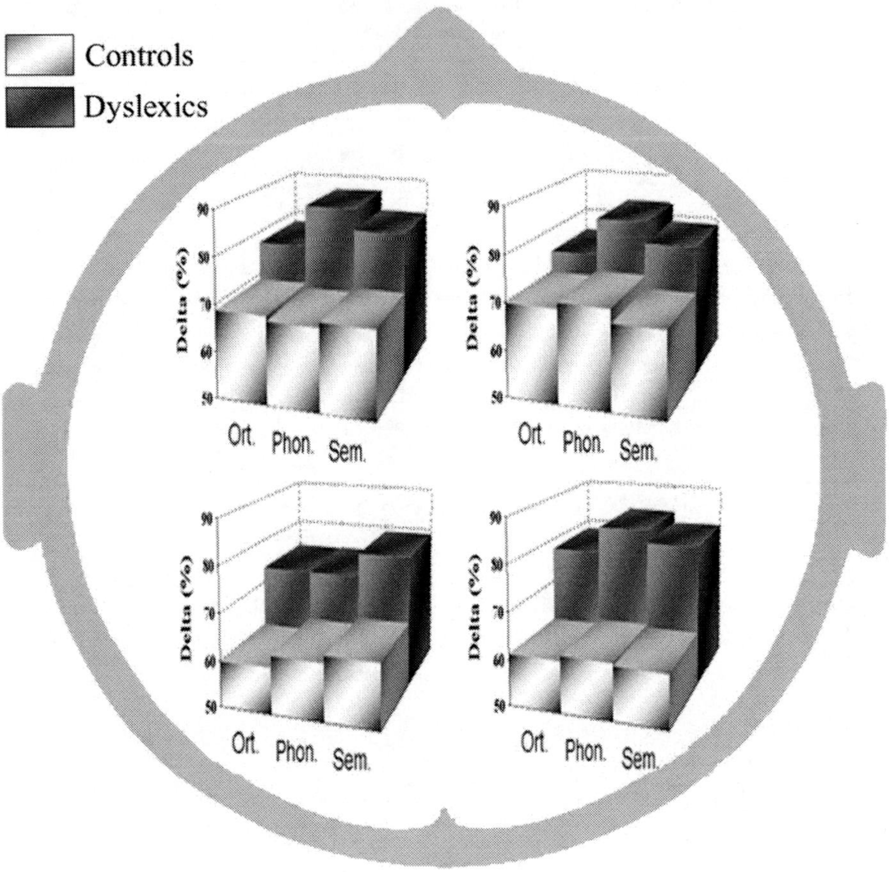

Figure 3. Percentages of Delta band in dyslexics and controls (dark and light bars, respectively) throughout three linguistic tasks in the four cortical quadrants (from Penolazzi et al., in press).

A first result concerning dyslexics' greater overall delta amplitude represented a clearcut evidence of their greater brain electrical immaturity compared with controls. Further, unlike controls' ability to differentiate tasks and linguistic processes, dyslexics showed essentially the same pattern of delta activity in all tasks (although the highest delta values were reached during the phonological processing): that is, greater delta percentages on anterior left and posterior right areas (corresponding to the disinhibition of anterior right and posterior left cortical regions). Therefore, these data confirmed both a greater brain electrical immaturity of impaired readers compared with controls, and a specific deficit in phonological processing mediated by anterior left linguistic networks (more severely impaired in dyslexics' with respect to other brain regions). With this approach, the maturational lag hypothesis of DD has been integrated with that of phonological deficit, thus providing a more detailed picture of impaired readers' main features. Turning the attention to delta band, its classical employment in measuring basic differences between groups appears at least restrictive, given its proven ability to discriminate different kinds and phases of linguistic processes in normal readers. Thus, side by side to more popular and traditional EEG rhythms sensitive to cognitive processing, a more extensive use of delta band is encouraged, being this last one of the few tools suited to investigate cognitive functioning and brain maturational lags, at the same time.

3. Why to Use Electrophysiological Measures in The Study of Developmental Disabilities

Electrophysiological methods are relatively non-invasive and less expensive compared with other brain functional imaging techniques, and, although they do not stand out for spatial resolution, provide multidimensional measures (i.e., which can be characterized for amplitude, latency/ frequency, scalp distribution) of neural activity, with an excellent temporal resolution of the processes induced by specific stimuli or tasks. This makes electrophysiological measures particularly suitable to investigate cognitive processes, which generally consist of several substages, hardly detectable with behavioural measures. The possibility of disentangle the subcomponents of a process, offered by ERPs and EEG measures, becomes even more important for studying cognitive disorders, especially when different explicative theories on the underlying impaired mechanisms still coexist (like in the case of DD). Further, electrophysiological methods can become unrivalled instruments to identify, through specific markers or patterns of electrical activity, all cases in which deficits are present, although not completely (or not yet) manifest at the behavioural/clinical level, and could worsen without an immediate treatment (i.e., light disorders; infants or child genetically at risk for some disability, but still not able to be identified by behavioural assessments). Thanks to all the above described features, electrophysiological methods represent the elective tool for a more comprehensive understanding of the cognitive and neural mechanisms underlying DD.

Focusing on a more clinical/practical perspective, the first prominent benefit, which electrophysiological methods can provide to the study of DD, is the facilitation and acceleration of the diagnostic process. The improved detection of impaired readers can be favoured by electrophysiological measures at least in three ways. First, although behavioural testing will probably remain the simplest and less expensive way of screening preschool and school children, electrophysiological measures can contribute to anticipate and strengthened the diagnosis of reading disability delineated with the behavioural assessment. In particular, the power of neurobiological data, when supported by behavioural ones, could be very important for reaching a correct diagnosis, especially in transparent orthographies, where reading impairment is more difficult to detect in comparison with deep orthographies [Landerl, Wimmer, & Frith, 1997; Zoccolotti, De Luca, Di Pace, Judica, Orlandi, & Spinelli, 1999]. Indeed, whereas in the latter the reading impairment is identified without difficulty for deficits in both accuracy and speed (because of the high percentage of irregular words), in the former a slower reading speed is often the only symptom easily detectable (since more regular grapheme-phoneme correspondences hide a part of the disorder). For this reason, reading disabilities in regular orthographies are frequently underestimated or exchanged for normal developmental delays in reading skill acquisition, and therefore their diagnosis would greatly gain from additional electrophysiological evidence. Second, whereas in many cases behavioural testing fails to identify marks or precursors of reading impairments, electrophysiological measures can be particularly suited to isolate predictive cues of future reading problems in infants or children, genetically at risk for dyslexia [for a review see Lyytinen et al., 2005]. Many prospective studies indeed have found that, at a very early age (6 months or even earlier) several ERP patterns (overall, pointing to an anomalous right hemisphere dominance of children at-risk, during low level processing of auditory and speech-related stimuli, instead of the left typical dominance of controls) can differentiate children with and without familial risk of dyslexia [Molfese & Molfese, 1997; Molfese, 2000; Molfese, Molfese, & Modglin, 2001]. Further, it has been shown that these brain responses have a reliable predictable value, since they correlate with the delayed interval of acquisition and development of language and reading skills [Leppänen, Pihko, Eklund, & Lyytinen, 1999; Pihko, Leppänen, Eklund, Cheour, Guttorm, & Lyytinen, 1999; Guttorm, Leppänen, Richardson, & Lyytinen, 2001; Guttorm, Leppänen, Tolvanen, & Lyytinen, 2003]. Third, electrophysiological methods, being able to distinguish the subcomponents of a process which can be selectively impaired, can contribute, more than behavioural measurements, to make differential diagnoses among the various sub-types of dyslexia. As stressed in the first paragraph, DD must be considered an extremely heterogeneous and multifactorial syndrome, in which side by side to the decoding impairment, a combination of several other deficits can complicate or worsen the disadvantageous condition. In this view, an electrophysiological paradigm, specifically created to assess the various cognitive components which could be impaired (i.e., linguistic, perceptual, attentional), can provide a detailed picture of the individual's symptoms and features, favouring, in turn, more personalized (and, thus, more effective) treatment procedures.

The improvement in the diagnostic process, which can be boosted by electrophysiological data, is aimed, first of all, at allowing the immediate implementation of a supportive training, since treatment efficacy is successful as much it occurs early and is individually targeted. In this view, besides the diagnosis, the second main applicative contribution of electrophysiological methods to the study of DD concerns its ability to test and compare the efficacy of different rehabilitative therapies. Indeed, by repeatedly measuring electrophysiological activity (for instance to coincide with the beginning and the end of the treatment, or with regular follow-up examinations), it can be possible to test the efficacy of specific remediation trainings (or eventually of coping strategies naturally developed with experience, when specific trainings are missing). Starting from the assumption that a wider neural reorganization after the training is associated, with high probability, to a more extensive and long-lasting behavioural improvement in reading performance, the comparison of electrophysiological recordings in succession may allow to evaluate behavioural progresses by the extent and the localization of cortical reorganization. From a theoretical perspective this will increase our current knowledge on cerebral plasticity phenomena related to linguistic processes, and from a clinical viewpoint it will drive the selection of the most effective treatments suited for a variety if individuals affected by dyslexia.

In conclusion, ERPs, with their excellent time resolution, represent an ideal tool to study and detect language disorders, especially when the reading disability manifests itself mainly along time domain. EEG bands, being able to show not only functional, but also maturational features of dyslexics' brains, represent a distinct complementary method with respect to ERPs. Therefore, from a theoretical point of view, these two electrophysiological methods, less invasive and expensive compared with other brain imaging techniques, provide complementary information for a better understanding of the neural and cognitive mechanisms involved in DD. In addition, from a clinical/practical point of view, electrophysiological measures promise to be an effective instrument for making early diagnoses of dyslexia. Used together with behavioural testing, they can help to achieve an early detection of reading disorder, and, more crucial, they promise to offers, in future, reliable markers able to identify the risk of developing future reading disabilities in infants genetically at-risk (sample on whom, for obvious reasons, behavioural tests are still inapplicable). Finally, electrophysiological measures, indirectly favouring early and personalized linguistic trainings (naturally resulting from early diagnoses), can provide a valuable support to test their efficacy, by means of periodically repeated examinations of neural reorganizations underlying behavioural progresses. Therefore, addressing the initial question of this paragraph, there are good reasons to encourage, in the next future, a more extensive use of electrophysiological methods in the study of dyslexia (and the other developmental disorders as well): besides the possibilities they give to increase our theoretical knowledge on reading disabilities, they promise to become an effective tool to make early and differentiated diagnoses/prognoses, to predict future problems in infants with familial risk of DD, to test the efficacy of the therapy, by correlating neural reorganization phenomena to behavioural advances promoted by the therapy itself.

REFERENCES

Ackerman, P.T., Dykman, R.A., Oglesby, D.M., & Newton, J.E.O. (1995). EEG power spectra of dysphonetic and nondysphonetic poor readers. Brain and Language 49, 140-152.

Ackerman, P.T., McPherson, W.B., Oglesby, D.M., & Dykman R.A. (1998). EEG Power spectra of adolescent poor readers. Journal of Learning Disabilities, 31, 83-90.

Ahn, H., Prichep, L., John, E.R., Baird, H., Trepetin, M., & Kaye, H. (1980). Developmental equations reflect brain dysfunctions. Science, 210, 1259-1262.

Amitay, S., Ben-Yehudah, G., Banai, K., & Ahissar, M. (2002). Disabled readers suffer from visual and auditory impairments but not from a specific magnocellular deficit. Brain, 125, 2272-2285.

Anderson, R.A., Essick, G.K., & Siegel, R.M. (1985). Encoding of spatial location by posterior parietal neurons. Nature, 301, 419-421.

Angrilli, A., Dobel, C., Rockstroh, B., Stegagno, L., & Elbert, T. (2000). EEG brain mapping of phonological and semantic tasks in Italian and German languages. Clinical Neurophysiology, 111, 706-716.

Angrilli, A., Elbert, T., Cusumano, S., Stegagno, S., & Rockstroh, B. (2003). Temporal dynamics of linguistic processes are reorganized in aphasics' cortex: An EEG mapping study. Neuroimage, 20, 657-666.

Babiloni, C., Frisoni, G., Steriade, M., Bresciani, L., Binetti, G., Del Percio, C., Geroldi, C., Miniussi, C., Nobili, F., Rodriguez, G., Zappasodi, F., Carfagna, T., & Rossini, P.M. (2006). Frontal white matter volume and delta EEG sources negatively correlate in awake subjects with mild cognitive impairment and Alzheimer's disease. Clinical Neurophysiology, 117, 1113–29.

Baldeweg, T., Richardson, A., Watkins, S., Foale, C., & Gruzelier, J. (1999). Impaired auditory frequency discrimination in dyslexia detected with mismatch evoked potentials. Annals of Neurology, 45, 495–503.

Bergmann, J., Hutzler, F., Klimesch, W., & Wimmer, H. (2005). How is dysfluent reading reflected in the ERP? Journal of Neurolinguistics, 18, 153-165.

Boder, E. (1973). Developmental dyslexia: a diagnostic approach based on three atypical reading-spelling pattern. Developmental Medicine and Child Neurology, 15, 663-687.

Bradley, L., & Bryant, P.E. (1983). Categorizing sounds and learning to read: a causal connection. Nature, 301, 419-421.

Brezniz, Z., & Misra, M. (2003). Speed of processing of the visual-orthographic and auditory-phonological systems in adult dyslexics: The contribution of asynchrony to word recognition deficits. Brain and Language, 85, 486–502.

Brunswick, N., McCrory, E., Price, C.J., Frith, C.D., & Frith, U. (1999). Explicit and implicit processing of words and pseudowords by adult developmental dyslexics: A search for Wernicke's Wortschatz? Brain, 122, 1901-1917.

Brunswick, N., & Rippon, G. (1994). Auditory event-related potentials, dichotic listening performance and handedness as indices of lateralisation in dyslexic and normal readers. The International Journal of Psychophysiology, 18, 265–275.

Castles, A., & Coltheart, M. (1993). Varieties of developmental dyslexia. Cognition, 47, 149-180.

Castles, A., Datta, H., Gayan, J., & Olson, R.K. (1999). Varieties of developmental reading disorders: genetic and environmental influences. Journal of Experimental Child Psychology, 72, 73-94.

Chiappe, P., Stringer, R., Siegel, L.S., & Stanovich, K.E. (2002).Why the timing deficit hypothesis does not explain reading disability in adults. Reading and Writing, 15, 73-107.

Colon, E.J., Notermans, S.L., DeWeerd, J.P.C., & Kap, J. (1979). The discriminatory role of EEG power in dyslexic children. Journal of Neurology, 221, 257-262.

Compton, D.L., DeFries, J.C., & Olson, R.K. (2001). Are RAN- and phonological awareness-deficits additive in children with reading disabilities? Dyslexia, 7, 125-149.

Cornelissen, P.L., Hansen, P.C., Hutton, J.L., Evangelinou, V., & Stein, J.F. (1998). Magnocellular visual function and children's single word reading. Vision Research, 38, 471-482.

De Jongh, A., de Munck, J., Baayen, J., Jonkman, E., Heethaar, R., & van Dijk, B. (2001). The localization of spontaneous brain activity: First results in patients with cerebral tumors. Clinical Neurophysiology, 112, 378–385.

DeFries, J.C., Fulker, D.W., & LaBuda, M.C. (1987). Evidence for a genetic aetiology in reading disability of twins. Nature, 329, 537–39.

Démonet, J.F., Taylor, M.J., & Chaix, Y. (2004). Developmental dyslexia. The Lancet, 363, 1451-1460.

Dewey, D. (1995). What is developmental dyspraxia? Brain and Cognition, 29, 254-274.

Duffy, F.H., Denckla, M.B., Bartels, P.H. & Sandini, G. (1980). Dyslexia: regional differences in brain electrical activity by topographic mapping. Annals of Neurology, 7, 412-420.

Duncan, C.C, Rumsey, J.M., Wilkniss, S.M., Denckla, M.B., Hamburger, S.D., & Odou-Potkin, M. (1994). Developmental dyslexia and attentional dysfunction in adults: brain potential indices of information processing. Psychophysiology, 31, 386-401.

Eckert, M. (2004). Neuroanatomical markers for dyslexia: a review of dyslexia structural imaging studies. The Neuroscientist 10, 362–371.

Eden, G.F., VanMeter, J.W., Rumsey, J.M., & Zeffiro, T.A. (1996). The visual deficit theory of developmental dyslexia. Neuroimage, 4, 108–117.

Erez, A., & Pratt, H. (1992). Auditory event-related potentials among dyslexic and normal-reading children: 3CLT and midline comparisons. International Journal of Neuroscience, 63, 247–264.

Fabiani, M., Gratton, G., & Federmeier, K.D. (2007). Event-Related Brain Potentials: Methods, Theory, and Applications. In J. Cacioppo, L.G. Tassinary, G.G. Bernstom (Eds.), The handbook of psychophysiology (pp.85-119). Cambridge: Cambridge University Press.

Fawcett, A.J., Nicolson, R.I., & Dean, P. (1996). Impaired performance of children with dyslexia on a range of cerebellar tasks. Annual Dyslexia, 46, 259-283.

Fein, G., Galin, D., Yingling, C.D., Johnstone, J., Davenport, L., & Herron, H. (1986). EEG spectra in dyslexic and control boys during resting conditions. Electroencephalography and Clinical Neurophysiology, 63, 87-97.

Fitzgerald, P.G., & Picton, T.W. (1983). Event-related potentials recorded during the discrimination of improbable stimuli. Biological Psychology, 17, 241–276.

Flint, J. (1999). The genetic basis of cognition. Brain, 122, 2015-2032.

Flynn, J.M., & Rahbar, M.H. (1994). Prevalence of reading failure in boys compared with girls. Psychology in the Schools, 31, 66-71.

Fonseca, L.C., Tedrus, G.M.A.S., Chiodi, M.G., Cerqueira, J.N., & Tonelotto, J.M.F. (2006). Quantitative EEG in children with learning disability. Arquivos de Neuropsiquiatria, 64, 376-381.

Francks, C., MacPhie, I.L., & Monaco, A.P. (2002). The genetic basis of dyslexia. The Lancet neurology, 1, 483-490.

Fried, I., Tanguay, P. E., Boder, E., Doubleday, C., & Greensite, M. (1981). Developmental dyslexia: Electrophysiological evidence of clinical subgroups. Brain and Language, 12, 14–22.

Francks, C., MacPhie, I.L., & Monaco, A.P. (2002). The genetic basis of dyslexia. The Lancet neurology, 1, 483-490.

Galaburda, A.M. (1999). Developmental dyslexia: A multilevel syndrome. Dyslexia 5, 183–191

Galaburda, A.M., & Kemper, T.L. (1979). Cytoarchitectonic abnormalities in developmental dyslexia: a case study. Annals of Neurology, 6, 94-100.

Galaburda, A. M., Menard, M.T., & Rosen, G.D. (1994). Evidence for aberrant auditory anatomy in developmental dyslexia. The Proceedings of the National Academy of Sciences of the U.S.A., 91, 8010-8013.

Galaburda, A. M., Sherman, G.F., Rosen, G.D., Aboitiz, F., & Geschwind, N. (1985). Developmental dyslexia: four consecutive patients with cortical anomalies. Annals of Neurology, 18, 222- 233.

Gasser, T., Verleger, R., Bacher, P., & Sroka, L. (1988). Development of the EEG of school-age children and adolescents. I. Analysis of band power. Electroencephalography and Clinical Neurophysiology, 69, 91-99.

Georgiewa, P., Rzanny, R., Gaser, C., Gerhard, U.J., Vieweg, U., Freesmeyer, D., Mentzel, H.J., Kaiser, W.A., & Blanz, B. (2002). Phonological processing in dyslexic children: a study combining functional imaging and event related potentials. Neuroscience Letters, 318, 5–8.

Gevins, A., & Smith, M.E. (2000). Neurophysiological measures of working memory and individual differences in cognitive ability and cognitive style. Cerebral Cortex 10, 829–839.

Gevins, A., Smith, M.E., McEvoy, L., & Yu, D. (1997). High-resolution EEG mapping of cortical activation related to working memory: effects of task difficulty, type of processing and practice. Cerebral Cortex, 7, 374– 385.

Geschwind, N., & Galaburda, A.M., (1985). Cerebral lateralization. Biological mechanisms, associations, and pathology: II. A hypothesis and a program for research. Archives of Neurology, 42, 521-552.

Geschwind, N., & Levitsky, W. (1968). Human brain: left-right asymmetries in temporal speech region. Science, 161, 186-187.

Grant, A.C., Zangaladze, A., Thiagarajah, M.C., & Sathian, K. (1999). Tactile perception in developmental dyslexia: a psychophysical study using gratings. Neuropsychologia 37, 1201–11.

Gross-Tsur, V., Shalev, R.S., Manor, O., & Amir, N. (1995). Developmental right-hemiphere syndrome: clinical spectrum of the nonverbal learning disability. Journal of Learning Disabilities, 28, 80-86.

Guttorm, T. K., Leppänen, P.H.T., Richardson, U., & Lyytinen, H. (2001). Event-related potentials and consonant differentation in newborns with familial risk for dyslexia. Journal of Learning Disabilities, 34, 534–544.

Guttorm, T. K., Leppänen, P.H.T., Tolvanen, A., & Lyytinen, H. (2003). Event-related potentials in newborns with and without familial risk for dyslexia: Principal component analysis reveals differences between the groups. Journal of Neural Transmission, 110, 1059–1074.

Habib, M. (2000). The neurological basis of developmental dyslexia: an overview and working hypothesis. Brain, 123, 2373-2399.

Habib, M., & Robichon, F.(1996). Parietal lobe morphology predicts phonological skills in developmental dyslexia. Brain and Cognition, 32, 139-142.

Harmony, T., Hinojosa, G., Marosi, E., Becker, J., Rodríguez, M., Reyes, A., & Rocha, C. (1990a). Correlation between EEG spectral parameters and an educational evaluation. International Journal of Neuroscience, 54, 147-155.

Harmony, T., Marosi, E., Díaz de León, A.E., Becker, J. & Fernández, T. (1990b). Effect of sex, psychosoeial disadvantages and biological risk factors on EEG maturation. Electroencephalography and Clinical Neurophysiology, 75, 482-491.

Helenius, P., Salmelin, R., Service, E., & Connolly, J.F. (1999). Semantic cortical activation in dyslexic readers. The Journal of Cognitive Neuroscience, 11, 535-550.

Helenius, P., Tarkiainen, A., Cornelissen, P., Hansen, P.C., & Salmelin, R. (1999). Dissociation of normal feature analysis and deficient processing of letter-strings in dyslexic adults. Cerebral Cortex 9, 476–83.

Herman, A.E., Galaburda, A.M., Fitch R.H., Carter, A.R., & Rosen, G.D. (1997). Cerebral microgyria, thalamic cell size and auditory temporal processing in male and female rats. Cerebral Cortex, 7, 53–464

Holcomb, P. J., Ackerman, P. T., & Dykman, R. A. (1985). Cognitive event-related brain potentials in children with attention and reading deficits. Psychophysiology, 22, 656–667.

Holcomb, P. J., Ackerman, P. T., & Dykman, R. A. (1986). Auditory event-related potentials in attention and reading disabled boys. International Journal of Psychophysiology, 3, 263–273.

Humphreys, P., Kaufmann, W.E., & Galaburda, A.M. (1990). Developmental dyslexia in women: neuropathological findings in three patients. Annals of Neurology, 28, 727-738.

Jensen, O., & Tesche, C.D. (2002). Frontal theta activity in humans increases with memory load in a working memory task. European Journal of Neuroscience 15, 1395– 1399.

Jernigan, T.L., Hesselink, J.R., Sowell, E., & Tallal, P.A. (1991). Cerebral structure on magnetic resonance imaging in language- and learning-impaired children. Archives of Neurology, 48, 539-545.

John, E.R., Ahn, H., Prichep, L., Trepetin, M., Brown, D., & Kaye, H. (1980). Developmental equations for the EEG. Science, 210, 1255- 1258.

John, E.R., Prichep, L., Ahn, H., Easton, P., Friedman, J., & Kaye, H. (1983). Neurometric evaluation of cognitive dysfunctions and neurological disorders in children. Progress in Neurobiology, 21, 239-290

Kaufmann, W.E., & Galaburda, A.M. (1989). Cerebrocortical microdysgenesis in neurologically normal subjects: a histopathologic study. Neurology, 39, 238-244.

Klimesch, W. (1999). EEG alpha and theta oscillations reflect cognitive and memory performance: A review and analysis. Brain Research Reviews, 29, 169-195.

Klimesch, W., Doppelmayr, M., Wimmer, H., Gruber, W., Röhm, D., Schwaiger, J., & Hutzler, F. (2001a). Alpha and beta band power changes in normal and dyslexic children. Clinical Neurophysiology, 112, 1186-1195.

Klimesch, W., Doppelmayr, M., Wimmer, H., Schwaiger, J., Röhm, D., Gruber, W., & Hutzler, F. (2001b). Theta band power change in normal and dyslexic children. Clinical Neurophysiology, 112, 1174-1185.

Kraus, N., McGee, T., Carrell, T.D., & Sharma, A. (1995). Neurophysiologic basis of speech discrimination. Ear and Hearing, 16, 19-37.

Kronbichler, M., Hutzler, F., & Wimmer, H. (2002). Dyslexia: verbal impairments in the absence of magnocellular impairments. Neuroreport, 13, 617-620.

Kujala, T., Alho, K., & Näätänen, R. (2000). Cross-modal reorganization of human cortical functions. Trends in Neurosciences, 23, 115–120.

Kujala, T., Halmetoja, M. A., Näätänen, R., Alku, P., Lyytinen, H., & Sussman, E. (2006). Speech- and sound-segmentation in dyslexia: evidence for a multiple-level cortical impairment. European Journal of Neuroscience, 24 , 2420–2427

Kujala, T., Karma, J., Ceponiené, R., Belitz, S., Turkkila, P., Tervaniemi, M., & Näätänen, R., (2001). Plastic neural changes and reading improvement caused by audiovisual training in reading-impaired children. Proceedings of the National Academy of Sciences, 98, 10509–10514.

Kutas, M., & Federmeier, K.D. (2000). Electrophysiology reveals semantic memory use in language comprehension. Trends in Cognitive Sciences, 4, 463-470.

Landerl, K., Wimmer, H., & Frith, U. (1997). The impact of orthographic consistency on dyslexia: A German-English comparison. Cognition, 63, 315–334.

Leppänen, P. H. T., Pihko, E., Eklund, K. M., & Lyytinen, H. (1999). Cortical responses of infants with and without a genetic risk for dyslexia: II. Group effects. Neuroreport, 10, 901–905.

Leung, L.S. (1992). Fast (beta) rhythms in the hippocampus: A review. Hippocampus 2, 93-98.

Leung, L.S. (1998). Generation of theta and gamma rhythms in the hippocampus. Neuroscience and Behavioral Reviews 22, 275-290.

Lindgren S. D., De Renzi E., & Richman L. C., (1985). Cross national comparisons of developmental dyslexia in Italy and the United States. Child Development, 56, 1404-1417.

Livingstone, M.S., & Hubel, D.H. (1988). Segregation of form, color, movement and depth: anatomy, physiology and perception. Science, 240, 740-749.

Livingstone, M.S., Rosen, G.D., Drislane, F.W., &, Galaburda, A.M. (1991). Physiological and anatomical evidence for a magnocellular defect in developmental dyslexia. The Proceedings of the National Academy of Sciences of the U.S.A., 88, 7943–7947.

Lovegrove, W.J., Bowling, A., Badcock, D., & Blackwood, M. (1980a) Specific reading disability: differences in contrast sensitivity as a function of spatial frequency. Science, 210, 439–440.

Lovegrove, W.J., Heddle, M., & Slaghuis, W. (1980b). Reading disability: spatial frequency specific deficits in visual information store. Neuropsychologia, 18, 111-115.

Lovrich, D., & Stamm, J. S. (1983). Event-related potential and behavioral correlates of attention in reading retardation. Journal of Clinical Neuropsychology, 5, 13–37.

Lyytinen, H., Guttorm, T.K., Huttunen, T., Hämäläinen, J., Leppänen, P.H.T., & Vesterinen, M., (2005). Psychophysiology of developmental dyslexia: a review of findings including studies of children at risk of dyslexia. Journal of Neurolinguistic, 18, 167-195.

Martin F., & Lovegrove, W. (1987). Flicker contrast sensitivity in normal and specifically disabled readers. Perception, 16, 215-221.

Matoušek, M., & Petersén, I. (1973). Frequency analysis of the EEG in normal children and in normal adolescents. In P. Kellaway & I. Petersén (Eds.), Automation of Clinical Electroencephalography (pp. 75-102). New York: Raven Press.

Maurer, U., Brem, S., Bucher, K., & Brandeis, D. (2003a). Altered tone and phoneme mismatch negativity in children at risk for dyslexia. Neuroreport, 14, 2245–2250.

Maurer, U., Bucher, K., Brem, S., & Brandeis, D. (2003b). Development of the automatic mismatch response: From frontal positivity in kindergarten children to the mismatch negativity. Clinical Neurophysiology, 114, 808–817.

Mazzotta, G., & Gallai, V. (1992). Study of the P300 event-related potential through brain mapping in phonological dyslexics. Acta Neurologica, 14, 173–186.

Merzenich, M.M., Schreiner, C.E., Jenkins, W.M., & Wang, X. (1993). Neural mechanisms underlying temporal integration, segmentation, and input sequence representation: some implication for the origin of learning disabilities. In P. Tallal, A.M. Galaburda, R.R. Llinas, & C. von Euler (Eds.), Temporal information processing in the nervous system: special reference to dyslexia and disgraphia (Annals of the New York Academy of Sciences, 682, pp.1-22). New York: New York Academy of Sciences.

Milne, D.R., Hamm, J.P, Kirk, I.J., & Corballis, M.C. (2003). Anterior-posterior beta asymmetries in dyslexia during lexical decisions. Brain and Language, 84, 309-317.

Molfese, D. L. (2000). Predicting dyslexia at 8 years of age using neonatal brain responses. Brain and Language, 72, 238–245.

Molfese, D. L., & Molfese, V. J. (1997). Discrimination of language skills at five years of age using event-related potentials recorded at birth. Developmental Neuropsychology, 13, 135–156.

Molfese, V. J., Molfese, D. L., & Modglin, A. A. (2001). Newborn and preschool predictors of second-grade reading scores: An evaluation of categorical and continuous scores. Journal of Learning Disabilities, 34, 545–554.

Neville, H.J., Coffey, S.A., Holcomb, P.J., & Tallal, P. (1993). The neurobiology of sensory and language processing in language-impaired children. The Journal of Cognitive Neuroscience 5, 235–253.

Nicolson, R.I., & Fawcett, A.J. (1990). Automaticity: a framework for dyslexia research? Cognition, 35, 159-182.

Nicolson, R.I., Fawcett, A.J., & Dean, P. (2001). Developmental dyslexia: the cerebellar deficit hypothesis. Trends in Neurosciences, 24, 508–11.

Olson, R.K., (2002). Nature and nurture. Dyslexia, 8, 143-159.

Ortiz, T., Exposito, F.J., Miguel, F., Martin-Loeches, M., & Rubia, F.J. (1992). Brain mapping in dysphonemic dyslexia: in resting and phonemic discrimination conditions. Brain & Language, 42, 270-285.

Pantev, C., Makeig, S., Hoke, M., Galambos, R., Hampson, S., & Gallen, C. (1991). Human auditory evoked gamma-band magnetic fields. of the National Academy of Science of the United States of America 88, 8996-9000.

Paulesu, E., Démonet, J.F., Fazio, F., McCrory, E., Chanoine, V., Brunswick, N., Cappa, S.F., Cossu, G., Habib, M., Frith, C.D., & Frith, U.(2001). Dyslexia: cultural diversity and biological unity. Science, 291, 2165–67.

Paulesu E., Frith, U., Snowling, M., Gallagher, A., Morton, J., Frackoviak, R.S., & Frith, C.D. (1996). Is developmental dyslexia a disconnession syndrome? Evidence from PER scanning. Brain, 119, 143-157.

Pennington, B.F. (1997). Using genetics to dissect cognition. The American Journal of Human Genetics 60, 13.

Pennington, B.F., & Lefly, D.L. (2001). Early reading development in children at family risk for dyslexia. Child Development, 72, 816-833.

Penolazzi, B., Hauk, O., & Pulvermüller, F. (2007). Early semantic context integration and lexical access as revealed by event-related potentials. Biological Psychology, 74, 374-388.

Penolazzi, B., Spironelli, C., & Angrilli, A. (in press). EEG delta activity as index of linguistic impairment in dyslexic children (Psychophysiology).

Penolazzi, B., Spironelli, C., Vio C., & Angrilli, A. (2006). Altered hemispheric asymmetry during word processing in dyslexic children: an event related potential study. Neuroreport, 17, 429-433.

Peiffer, A.M., Rosen, G.D., & Fitch, R.H. (2002). Rapid auditory processing and MGN morphology inmicrogyric rats reared in varied acoustic environments. Developmental Brain Research, 138, 187–193.

Pihko, E., Leppänen, P.H.T., Eklund, K. M., Cheour, M., Guttorm, T. K., & Lyytinen, H. (1999). Cortical responses of infants with and without a genetic risk for dyslexia: I. Age effects. Neuroreport, 10, 901–905.

Pizzagalli, D.A. (2007). Electroencephalography and High-Density Electrophysiological Source Localization. In J. Cacioppo, L.G. Tassinary, G.G. Bernstom (Eds.), The handbook of psychophysiology (pp.56-84). Cambridge: Cambridge University Press.

Price, C.J., (1998). The functional anatomy of word comprehension and production. Trends in Cognitive Sciences, 2, 281-288.

Ramus, F. (2003). Developmental dyslexia: Specific phonological deficit or general sensorimotor dysfunction? Current Opinion in Neurobiology 13, 1-7.

Ramus, F. (2004). Neurobiology of dyslexia: A reinterpretation of the data. Trends in Neurosciences, 27, 720-726.

Ramus, F. (2006). A neurological model of dyslexia and other domain-specific developmental disorders with an associated sensorimotor syndrome. In G.D. Rosen (Ed.), The dyslexic brain: new pathways in neuroscience (pgg.75-101). Mahwah: Lawrence Erlbaum Associates.

Ramus, F., & Szenkovits, G. (2008). What phonological deficit? The Quarterly Journal of Experimental Psychology, 61, 129-141.

Ramus, F., Rosen, S., Dakin, S.C., Day, B.L., Castellote, J.M., White, S., & Frith, U., (2003). Theories of developmental dyslexia: Insights from a multiple case study of dyslexic adults. Brain 126, 841-865.

Rapin, I., & Allen, D.A. (1988). Syndromes in developmental dysphasia and adult aphasia. In F. Plum (Ed.), Language, comunication and brain (pgg. 57-75). New York: Raven Press.

Rippon, G., Brunswick, N. (1998). EEG correlates of phonological processing in dyslexic children. Journal of Psychophysiology 12, 261– 274.

Rippon, G., Brunswick, N. (2000). Trait and state EEG indices of information processing in developmental dyslexia. International Journal of Psychophysiology, 36, 251– 265.

Robichon, F., Besson, M., & Habib, M. (2002). An electrophysiological study of dyslexic and control adults in a sentence reading task. Biological Psychology, 59, 29-53.

Robichon, F., & Habib, M. (1998). Abnormal callosal morphology in male adult dyslexic: relationships to handedness and phonological abilities. Brain and Language, 62, 127-146.

Robichon, F., Lévrier, O., Farnarier, P., & Habib, M. (2000). Developmental dyslexia: atypical asymmetry of language areas and its functional significance. The European Journal of Neurology, 7, 35-46.

Rosen, G.D., Herman, A.E., & Galaburda, A.M. (1999). Sex differences in the effects of early neocortical injury on neuronal size distribution of the medial geniculate nucleus in the rat are mediated by perinatal gonadal steroids. Cerebral Cortex 9, 27–34.

Rosenthal, J. H., Boder, E., & Callaway, E. (1982). Typology of developmental dyslexia: Evidence for its construct validity. In R. N. Malastesha (Ed.), Reading disorders: Varieties and treatments (pp. 93–117). New York: Academic Press.

Sarnthein, J., Morel, A., von Stein, A., & Jeanmonod, D. (2003). Thalamic theta field potentials and EEG: High thalamocortical coherence in patients with neurogenic pain, epilepsy and movement disorders. Thalamus and Related Systems, 2, 231-238.

Sarnthein, J., Petsche, H., Rappelsberger P., Shaw, G.L., & von Stein, A. (1998). Synchronization between prefrontal and posterior association cortex during human working memory. Proceedings of the National Academy of Science of the United States of America, 95, 7092-7096.

Sauseng, P., Klimesch, W., Dopplemayr, M., Hanslmayr, S., Schabus, M., & Gruber, W.R. (2004). Theta coupling in the human electroencephalogram during a working memory task. Neuroscience Letters, 354, 123-126.

Sauseng, P., Klimesch, W., Schabus, M., & Dopplemayr, M. (2005). Fronto-parietal EEG coherence in theta and upper alpha reflect central executive functions of working memory. International Journal of Psychophysiology, 57, 97-103.

Schulte-Körne, G., Deimel, W., Bartling, J., & Remschmidt, H. (2001). Speech perception deficit in dyslexic adults as measured by mismatch negativity (MMN). International Journal of Psychophysiology, 40, 77–87.

Schulte-Körne, G., Deimel, W, Müller, K., Gutenbrunner, C., & Remschmidt, H. (1996). Familial aggregation of spelling disabilities. The Journal of Child Psychological Psychiatry, 37, 817-822.

Share, D.L., Jorm, A.F., MacLean, R., & Matthews. R. (2002). Temporal processing and reading disability. Reading and Writing, 15,151-178.

Shaywitz, S.E., (1998). Dyslexia. The New England Journal of Medicine, 338, 307-312.

Shaywitz, B.A., Shaywitz, S.E., Pugh, K.R., Mencl, W.E., Fulbright, R.K., Skudlarski, P., Constable, R.T., Marchione, K.E., Fletcher, J.M., Lyon, G.R., & Gore, J.C., (2002). Disruption of posterior brain systems for reading in children with developmental dyslexia. Biological Psychiatry, 52, 101-110.

Shaywitz, S.E., & Shaywitz, B.A., (2005). Dyslexia (Specific Reading Disability). Biological Psychiatry, 57, 1301-1309.

Shaywitz, S.E., Shaywitz, B.A., Fulbright, R.K., Skudlarski, P., Mencl, W.E., Constable, R.T., Pugh, K.R., Holahan, J.M., Marchione, K.E., Fletcher, J.M., Lyon, G.R., & Gore, J.C. (2003). Neural systems for compesation and persistence: Young adult outcome of childhood reading disability. Biological Psychiatry, 4, 25-33.

Simos, P.G., Breier, J.L., Fletcher, J.M., Bergman, E., & Papanicolaou, A.C., (2000). Cerebral mechanisms involved in word reading in dyslex children: A magnetic source imaging approach. Cerebral Cortex, 10, 809-816.

Snowling, M.J. (2001). From language to reading and dyslexia. Dyslexia, 7, 37-46.

Spironelli, C. & Angrilli, A. (2006). Language lateralization in Phonological, Semantic and Orthographic tasks: A slow evoked potential study. Behavioral Brain Research, 175, 296-304.

Spironelli, C., Penolazzi, B., & Angrilli, A. (2008). Dysfunctional hemispheric asymmetry of theta and beta EEG activity during linguistic tasks in developmental dyslexia. Biological Psychology, 77, 123-131.

Spironelli, C., Penolazzi, B., Vio, C., & Angrilli, A. (2006). Inverted EEG theta lateralization in dyslexic children during phonological processing. Neuropsychologia, 44, 2814-2821.

Sklar, B., Hanley, J., & Simmons, W.W. (1972). An EEG experiment aimed toward identifying dyslexic children. Nature, 240, 414-416.

Slotnick, S.D., Moo, L.R., Kraut, M.A., Lesser, R.P., & Hart, J.Jr. (2002). Interaction between thalamic and cortical rhythms during semantic memory recall in human. Proceedings of the National Academy of Science of the United States of America, 99, 6440-6443.

Smith, S.D., Gilger, J.W., & Pennington, B.F., (1996). Dyslexia and other specific learning disorders. In D.L. Rimoin, J.M. Connor, & R.E. Pyeritz, (Eds.), Principles and practice of medical genetics (pgg. 1767–89). New York: Churchill Livingstone.

Smith, S.D., Kelley, P.M., & Brower, A.M. (1998). Molecular approaches to the genetic analysis of specific reading disability. Human Biology, 70, 239-256.

Stein, J.F. (1993).Visuospatial perception in disabled readers. In D.M. Willows, & R.S. Kruk (Eds.), Visual processes in reading and reading disability (pp.331-346). Hillsdale: Lawrence Erlbaum Associates.

Stein, J. F. (2001). The magnocellular theory of developmental dyslexia. Dyslexia, 7,12-36.

Stein, J.F., & Talcott, J.B. (1999). Impaired neuronal timing in developmental dyslexia-The magnocellular hypothesis. Dyslexia, 5, 59-77.

Stein, J.F., & Walsh, V. (1997). To see but not to read: the magnocellular theory of dyslexia. Trends in Neurosciences, 20, 147-152.

Stelmack, R.M., Saxe, B.J., Noldy-Cullum, N., Campbell, K.B., & Armitage, R. (1988). Recognition memory for words and event-related potentials: A comparison of normal and disabled readers. The Journal of Clinical and Experimental Neuropsychology, 10, 185–200.

Stevenson, J., Graham, P., Fredman, G., & McLoughlin, V.A., (1987). Twin study of genetic influences on reading and spelling disability. The Journal of Child Psychology and Psychiatry, 229–47.

Tallal, P. (1980). Auditory temporal perception, phonics and reading disabilities in children. Brain and Language, 9, 182-198.

Tallal, P., & Piercy, M. (1973). Defects of non-verbal auditory perception in children with developmental aphasia. Nature, 241, 468-469.

Tallon-Baudry, C., & Bertrand, O. (1999). Oscillatory gamma activity in humans and its role in object representation. Trends in Cognitive Sciences 3, 151-162.

Taylor, M.J., & Keenan, N.K. (1990). Event –related potentials to visual and language stimuli in normal and dyslexic children. Psychophysiology, 27, 318-327.

Temple, E., Poldrack, R.A., Salidis, J., Deutsch, G.K., Tallal, P., Merzenich, M.M., & Gabrieli, J.D.E., (2001). Disrupted neural responses to phonological and orthographic processing in dyslex children: An fMRI study. Neuroreport 12, 299-307.

Tesche, C.D., & Karhu, J. (2000). Theta oscillations index human hippocampal activation during a working memory task. Proceedings of the National Academy of Science of the United States of America, 97, 919-924.

Valdois, S., Gèrard C., Vanault, P., & Dugas, M. (1995). Pheripheral developmental dyslexia: a visual attentional account? Cognitive Neuropsychology, 12, 31-67.

Vertes, R.P. (2005). Hippocampal theta rhythm: A tag for short-term memory. Hippocampus 15, 923-935.

Wadsworth, S.J., DeFries, J.C., Stevenson, J., Gilger, J.W., & Pennington, B.F. (1992). Gender ratios among reading-disabled children and their siblings as a function of parental impairment. The Journal of Child Psychology and Psychiatry, 33, 1229-39.

Wagner, R.K., & Torgesen, J.K., (1987). The nature of phonological processing and its causal role in the acquisition of reading skills. Psychological Bulletin, 101, 192-212.

Wienbruch, C., Moratti, S., Elbert, T., Vogel, U., Fehr, T., Kissler, J., Schiller, A., & Rockstroh, B. (2003). Source Distribution of Neuromagnetic Slow Wave Activity in Schizophrenic and Depressive Patients. Clinical Neurophysiology, 114, 2052-2060.

Wolf, M., Goldberg O'Rourke, A., Gidney, C., Lovett, M., Cirino, P., & Morris, R. (2002). The second deficit: an investigation of the independence of phonological and naming-speed deficits in developmental dyslexia. Reading and Writing, 15, 43-72.

World Health Organization (1993). The International Classification of Diseases, vol.10: Classification of Mental and Behavioural Disorders. Geneva: World Health Organization.

Yingling, C.D., Galin, D., Fein, G., Peltzman, D., & Davenport, L. (1986). Neurometrics does not detect "pure dyslexics". Electroencephalography and Clinical Neurophysiology, 63, 426-430.

Zoccolotti, P., De Luca, M., Di Pace, E., Judica, A., Orlandi, M., & Spinelli, D. (1999). Markers of developmental surface dyslexia in a language (Italian) with high grapheme–phoneme correspondence. Applied Psycholingusitics, 20, 191–216.

In: Children and Language: Development, Impairment … ISBN 978-1-60692-395-5
Editor: Michael A. Reed

Chapter 5

Interaction Between Flexible Cognition and Language Comprehension in Children with and Without Language Impairment

Klara Marton[1]
Brooklyn College, City University of New York
& Barczi Gusztav Faculty of Special Education,
Eotvos Lorand University, Budapest

Abstract

The focus of this chapter is on the impact of various cognitive functions on language acquisition and language processing in different groups of children. Empirical data are presented on individual variations of language and cognition in typically developing children, children with specific language impairment, and in young adults with dyslexia. The interaction between flexible cognition (attention switching, working memory, and inhibition control) and language comprehension was examined in English-speaking and Hungarian participants.

The findings suggest that working memory performance and language comprehension are strongly influenced by task complexity, age, and language structure. Working memory storage and processing are affected differently by stimulus complexity.

Children with specific language impairment and young adults with dyslexia showed deficits in flexible cognition and language comprehension (oral and written). Children with SLI performed more poorly than their age-matched and language-matched peers in tasks that measured working memory capacity and inhibition control. In addition to the group effects, participants with language impairment showed different errors and performance patterns than their peers.

[1] Correspondence: Klara Marton, Address: Brooklyn College, 2900 Bedford Ave., Brooklyn, NY 11210, Phone: (718) 951-4402, Fax: (718) 951-4167, Email: kmarton@brooklyn.cuny.edu

INTRODUCTION: INTERACTION BETWEEN LANGUAGE AND NON-LINGUISTIC COGNITIVE SKILLS

Language development and processing are entwined with non-linguistic cognitive skills in children and adults. The focus of this chapter is on the interaction between language acquisition and disorders and the development of higher level cognitive skills. Empirical results from typically developing school-age children, from children with specific language impairment (SLI), and from adolescents and young adults with dyslexia will be used to demonstrate the impact that working memory, inhibition control and other executive functions have on written and oral language performance.

The theoretical framework for this discussion is the neuroconstructivist account (Karmiloff-Smith, 1998). This theory suggests that cognitive development is closely linked to the changes in the underlying neurological structures. According to the neuroconstructivist approach, the adult modular information processing system is the result of development. Children are born with a less differentiated system that has domain-relevant capacities instead of domain-specific ones (Thomas, 2005). The infant's system shows more flexibility and different strengths and weaknesses than the adult structure (Paterson, Brown, Gsödl, Johnson, & Karmiloff-Smith, 1999). In accordance with the neuroconstructivist theory, there are constraints at each level from the genes to the social environment. Over the course of development, these structures interact with each other. Cognitive development cannot be understood without comprehending the constraints on neural development (Westermann, Mareschal, Johnson, Sirois, Spratling, & Thomas, 2007). There is continuous competition and collaboration among the different structures. The level of development will depend on the specific context in which the given structures compete and collaborate with each other.

The neuroconstructivist account has further implications for developmental disorders. In response to multiple constraints, the system goes through an adaptation process, similar to the one observed in typical development, but the constraints differ in atypical cases. Thus, this approach promotes a different view of atypical development from the more modular idea that assumes failures in isolated functions. Variations in the genes may change the course of development and their effects will differ across outcomes. They will have stronger impacts on certain functions and weaker influences on others. Because of the interactions across various levels in a dynamic context, one cannot separate intact and impaired modules. According to this view, there is a shift from dissociations to cross- syndrome associations (Karmiloff-Smith, 1998). Thus, the neuroconstructivist approach provides a more dynamic framework of developmental disorders than the traditional neuropsychological models.

Researchers studying neurocognitive disorders have argued that children diagnosed with different impairments show many overlapping characteristics in their cognitive and linguistic profiles. Although the groups of children with different neurocognitive disorders may vary in the rate of development (e.g., children with Down syndrome, with Williams syndrome, with specific language impairment, or with autistic spectrum disorder), they show many similarities in their performance profiles and errors (Bates, 2004). Thus, these impairments may lie on a continuum (e.g., Bishop, 2000).

During the first year of life, infants acquire numerous non-linguistic skills that promote the development of language. More complex language structures are established through associations between speech sounds and their meanings (Chiat, 2001). This mapping process is influenced by a number of non-linguistic cognitive skills, such as cross-modal perception and sensori-motor precision (Bates, 2004). Joint attention facilitates the mapping process during which children link the words and sentences with their corresponding objects and events (Baldwin, 1995). Infants are born with a higher level memory system that enables them to imitate actions even after a significant delay.

The first 18 months are characterized by a shift from experience-based mental representations to more hypothetical ones (Meltzoff, 1990). During this time, cross-modal integration develops and supports the emergence of various forms of imitation, which plays a central role in the development of motor control, speech-language-communication and social life (Tomasello, Kruger, & Ratner, 19993). The combination of joint reference and imitation facilitates the development of both the theory of mind and observational learning. Based on the assumption that language and cognition develop in interaction, if there is a deficit in any of the above mentioned cognitive functions, language learning will be altered. The rate of language development is also determined by more general cognitive factors, such as IQ and auditory memory (Tager-Flusberg, 2005).

During the preschool years, children's language level is highly correlated with their non-linguistic skills. For example, Marchman (1997) suggests that young children's production of suffixes is related to their rate of language acquisition. Children with more advanced phonological systems produce fewer errors in English past tense morphology than their peers.

Flexible cognition is an umbrella term for the cognitive system's ability to adapt to contextual and task-related changes by shifting attention, selecting relevant information, forming plans and monitoring performance (Deak, 2003). Flexible cognition has been found to influence language development to a great extent. In a conversation, children must remember the topic (topic maintenance), shift attention according to the progress of the dialogue, inhibit irrelevant thoughts, and consider their partner's perspective. To comprehend complex or potentially ambiguous sentences, children must recognize the words, selectively activate relevant meanings, inhibit irrelevant ideas, remember the words, and parse the sentence, keeping track of element order as well as long-distance grammatical relations (e.g., subject-verb agreement, tense, elements that have undergone movement and their traces, etc.). Sentences that can have more than one meaning (i.e., are initially ambiguous) also require suppression of one potential meaning. At a lexical level, in tasks like picture naming, children must selectively activate the correct word in a cohort of phonologically and semantically related words and inhibit related non-target items. They must selectively attend to segments and features that distinguish the target word from phonological neighbors.

The relationship between flexible cognition and language is bidirectional, but we do not know how much language development contributes to the advancement of cognition. Behavioral studies' results show that preschool-age children have problems in tasks that test flexible cognition. These children experience difficulty in inhibiting thoughts and responses that are not relevant anymore (Diamond, 1998), in flexible switching (Zelazo, Muller, Frye, & Marcovitch, 2003), and in selecting task cues (Deak, 2000). In the following parts of this chapter we will present data on the interaction between language and verbal working memory, inhibition control, and other executive functions.

Interaction Between Language and Verbal Working Memory: A Developmental Perspective

There is a clear relationship between working memory and language comprehension and production (e.g., Gathercole & Baddeley, 1993; Just & Carpenter, 2002; Marton, Schwartz, Farkas, & Katsnelson, 2006). Phonological working memory, which is a measure of short-term storage, is closely linked to vocabulary development, particularly during the first years of language acquisition. Young children with more limited phonological working memory capacity, as measured by nonword repetition, show slower vocabulary development than children with better nonword repetition skills. Nonwords do not activate the long-term lexical representations, therefore nonword repetition reflects the person's phonological storage capacity. As children become more advanced language learners, they rely more on their lexicon. They access their conceptual, semantic and phonological knowledge during vocabulary acquisition (Gathercole, 2006).

Language comprehension is also linked to verbal working memory. Various linguistic span tasks (reading span, listening span) have been shown to be great predictors of language comprehension (Daneman & Philip, 1996) because language processing has high computational and storage demands.

Participants' comprehension performance reflects individual differences in working memory capacity (e.g., Caplan & Waters, 1999; Just & Carpenter, 2002; King & Just, 1991). These differences, however, are not about the individual's phonological storage capacity, but imply more general executive functions (e.g., Conway & Engle, 1994; Engle & Cane, 2004). Working memory span is constrained by controlled attention (Engle, Kane, & Tuholski, 1999), by task-switching ability (Towse, Hitch, & Hutton, 1998), and by the inhibition of irrelevant information (Hasher & Zacks, 1988). According to Baddeley's working memory model (Baddeley, 2000), participants may demonstrate individual variations in processing and storage independently from a general executive capacity in complex working memory span tasks (Bayliss, Jarrold, Gunn, & Baddeley, 2003). The extent to which performance on complex working memory span tasks depends on processing and storage functions is still subject to debate (see more detailed conceptual reviews of working memory e.g., Baddeley, 2000; Engle & Kane, 2004; Miyake & Shah, 1999).

Developmental studies on working memory performance evidenced that executive functions develop gradually until adolescence (DeLuca, Wood, Anderson, Bucanan, Proffitt, Mahony, & Pantelis, 2003). Changes in working memory span reflect a combination of efficiency and speed of processing. Older children perform faster on the same tasks as younger children, therefore they need fewer resources to perform a particular activity (e.g., counting) and have more resources available for memory operations (Case, Kurland, & Goldberg, 1982). A different interpretation of age-related changes is provided by the task-switching model (Towse & Hitsch, 1995). In linguistic span tasks, participants may use the sentence context to help reconstruct the list of words that have to be remembered. If this reconstitution process is too difficult for the individual's system, then it may take so much time that some information could be lost. Younger children may make more errors because of difficulty in attention switching. In complex working memory tasks, span measures may reflect the ability to control/switch attention, whereas response times depend on retrieval speed (Hitsch, Towse, & Hutton, 2001; Kail & Salthouse, 1994). Increases in attentional capacity and advance in attention switching result in working memory span enhancement (Barrouillet & Camos, 2001).

In our own research, we examined the effects of age and sentence complexity on verbal working memory performance (Marton, Schwartz, & Braun, 2005). Previous studies that have investigated age-related changes in working memory structures used short and/or simple sentences in linguistic span tasks (Cain, Oakhill, & Bryant, 2004; Gathercole, Pickering, Ambridge, & Wearing, 2004). Although the findings of adult studies showed an effect of linguistic complexity on working memory performance, the relations between linguistic complexity and age in children's working memory production is an uncharted area. Our study extended previous work by exploring the effect of sentence length and complexity on working memory performance in groups of participants that differed in age. We examined whether stimulus length or complexity has a larger effect on working memory performance accuracy and language comprehension, and whether this relationship changes with age during childhood and adolescence. Further, this study tested the theory of working memory capacity and executive attention (Engle & Kane, 2004) from a developmental perspective.

Three groups of children and young adults participated in this experiment (n=75). There were 25 participants in each group; the groups differed in age (Group1: 7;0-8;6 years; Group 2: 9;6-11:00 years; Group 3: college students, 19-22 years). The rationale for choosing these age groups was based on previous findings that indicated immature executive functions, such as the maintenance of task goals, sustained attention, set shifting, and inhibition below 8-8;6 years of age. Although memory span improves between age 10 and adulthood, resistance to interference matures around 10 years of age (DeLuca, Wood, Anderson, Buchanan, Proffitt, Mahony, & Pantelis, 2003; Hale, Bronik, & Fry, 1997).

To measure the relations between working memory and language comprehension, we developed a Modified Listening Span task (MLS). The task included 90 sentences (30 syntactically simple short sentences, 30 syntactically complex short sentences, and 30 syntactically complex long sentences) with a question for each sentence. Sentence-length was determined by the number of syllables (M = 7.91, SD = 1.64 for the short sentences; M = 17.64, SD = 3.47 for the long sentences). The complex sentences included relative clauses. The last word in each sentence was replaced with a nonword (2-, 3-, 4-syllable). The nonwords were part of the syntactic structure of the sentences. The task required that

participants listen to a sentence, repeat the sentence-final nonword and answer a question about the content of the sentence. Thus, the task required simultaneous processing and attention switching. The traditional linguistic span task (TLS) consisted of 9 sets of sentences with 5 sentences in each set (3 sets with syntactically simple short sentences, 3 sets with syntactically complex short sentences, and 3 sets with syntactically complex long sentences). Participants were asked to listen to the sentences and repeat the 5 sentence-final words in the order of presentation. The words were real words with similar phonotactic patterns, syllable length, and frequency of occurrence. Following sentence presentation, yes/no questions were randomly asked. In addition to the listening span tasks, a single nonword repetition task was used as a baseline measure of phonological working memory. The task consisted of 24 nonwords (2-3-4 syllables).

The results in each working memory task showed an age effect; younger children made more errors than the older participants. Performance accuracy also differed between Groups 2 and 3, particularly with more complex items.

Age-related changes were further observed in different error types and performance patterns, especially with an increase in stimulus complexity.

In addition to an age effect, the results of the linguistic span tasks showed an effect of sentence complexity on working memory performance. Participants in each group showed higher working memory performance accuracy following the simple sentences than the complex sentences. Sentence length differences did not impact performance accuracy in this study. This finding is similar to the results of Willis & Gathercole (2001). The authors reported that increased length of stimulus items did not affect sentence comprehension.

In contrast to sentence length, syntactic complexity did have a significant effect on working memory performance. The two dependent measures of the MLS task reflected the contribution of storage and processing efficiency separately. Sentence complexity affected the answers to the questions, but not nonword repetition. Nonword repetition accuracy was influenced by word length, but not by syntactic complexity. The idea of separate contributions of storage and processing efficiency in the MLS task was further supported by the high correlation between single nonword repetition and nonword repetition in the MLS task, and by the high correlation between the answers to the questions in the MLS and the TLS tasks.

These findings are in line with the results of Bayliss and colleagues (2003). The authors suggested that processing efficiency and storage capacity constrain complex span performance independently. The results of the linguistic span tasks (MLS, TLS) in our study were also in agreement with the findings of Gathercole, Pickering, Ambridge, and Wearing (2004), and showed the effect of age on executive functions. In linguistic span tasks, executive functions are used to integrate phonological, lexical, syntactic, and semantic representations.

Younger children rely more on their storage resources and show more difficulty in attention switching and flexible adaptation to changing task requirements. In our study, this was evidenced not only by these children's lower scores, but also by the age-related differences in performance pattern. In contrast to the results of the older participants, younger children (Group 1) produced more interference errors than omissions with each sentence type. They showed more difficulty in blocking the effects of prior sentence information. The children in Group 2 produced a higher number of interference errors only with increased sentence complexity. Most of their errors were omissions with the simple sentences. Performance accuracy in young adults (Group 3) was also influenced by sentence complexity, but they made significantly fewer interference errors than the children in Groups 1 and 2, even with the complex sentences. Young adults showed better monitoring of previously recalled items. These data are similar to the results of McCormack, Brown, & Vousden (2000); the authors reported an age-related decrease in interference errors in short-term memory tasks.

A similar age-related pattern emerged when performance on the TLS task was scored with 2 different methods: free recall versus recall with order. There was no difference between the scores using the 2 scoring methods for the participants in Group 3. Children in Group 2, received similar scores with the two methods for the simple sentences, but not for the complex sentences. In complex sentences, children's recall scores were higher with the free scoring method than with the one that included order scoring. The youngest children (Group 1) showed score differences with each sentence type, even with the simple sentences. The finding that children in Group 1 received higher scores with the free scoring method following each sentence type shows that they were able to remember the words but not the order of presentation. This finding supports the idea that younger children may rely more on storage resources than on general processing. Remembering both the items and their order of presentation requires the ability to maintain goal-relevant information and continuous attention switching.

Although processing efficiency was influenced by sentence complexity, but not by sentence length, nonword repetition performance -that reflects the storage function rather than processing- showed a word-length effect. Performance on both tasks, single nonword repetition and nonword repetition with sentence context, decreased with the increase of syllable length. In the MLS task, there was an interaction between word length and age. The younger children performed more poorly than the older participants at each syllable length; performance accuracy between Groups 2 and 3 did not differ for the 2-syllable nonwords,

only with the longer nonwords. Working memory span continues to improve between 10-11 years of age and adulthood.

Taken these results together with the findings on the linguistic span measures, the two functions of working memory, storage and processing efficiency were differently affected by the structure and complexity of the stimuli. Nonword repetition, the measure of the storage function, was influenced by stimulus length, but not by the sentence type, whereas the answers to the questions and listening span, that reflect processing efficiency, were affected by sentence complexity, but not sentence length. The results of the two listening span tasks support the theory of working memory capacity and executive attention (Engle & Kane, 2004). Performance accuracy increased and the proportion of interference errors decreased with age. These age-related differences reflect better attention switching and executive control. Participants needed to switch attention continuously during the processing of complex linguistic structures in the listening span tasks. There was a gradual

increase in performance accuracy across groups: the listening span tasks were most demanding on working memory for the youngest children (Group 1), who performed more poorly than groups 2 and 3 with each sentence type. Group 2 differed from Group 3 only with the complex sentences.

The development of executive functions and their effect on working memory performance were also reflected in children's errors. Younger children showed more difficulty in blocking previously presented information. This problem resulted in a high number of interference errors. Monitoring previously recalled items requires executive functions that develop with age. In conclusion, both age and language structure influence working memory performance. There is an interaction between these two factors that has an additional impact on individual performance variations in working memory tasks. The

findings indicate that different working memory tasks do not involve the same processes and that both factors, language and age, may influence them differently.

INTERACTION BETWEEN LANGUAGE AND VERBAL WORKING MEMORY IN CHILDREN WITH SLI

Phonological Storage and Processing

Children with SLI have significant limitations in their language abilities in the absence of hearing impairment and frank neurological damage. These children show typical interaction with people and objects and they show no signs of pervasive developmental disorders, such as autism. Their language scores on standardized tests are at least 1.25 SD lower than the average (<81 IQ) and/or their language-age is at least 12 months below their chronological age. These children's non-verbal intelligence is within the typical range (Leonard, 1998).

Children with specific language impairment perform more poorly than their age-matched or language-matched peers in verbal working memory tasks (Edwards & Lahey, 1998, Hoffmann & Gillam, 2004, Marton & Schwartz, 2003, Montgomery, 2000). These children show a deficit in repetition of single nonwords and nonword lists that are reflecting the function of phonological storage (Gathercole & Baddeley, 1990). Several explanations have been offered for their poor performance. One of them was that these children have difficulty in phonological encoding. Phonological encoding has been measured by the comparison of repetition accuracy of phonologically similar and dissimilar word lists (Gathercole & Baddeley, 1990; Montgomery, 1995; van der Lely & Howard, 1993). These authors found that poor nonword repetition in children with SLI was not a consequence of an encoding deficit because, like typically developing children, children with SLI showed greater difficulty repeating phonologically similar lists (e.g., bat, cap, cat) than dissimilar words (phonological similarity effect). Further, children with SLI showed a word-length effect similar to that of controls (Gathercole & Baddeley, 1990; Montgomery, 1995). All children showed more difficulty in repeating single nonwords as their length increased.

A deficit in verbal rehearsal has also been suspected to underlie poor nonword repetition in this population. Rehearsal is the ability to maintain stimulus items that have been encoded. Children with better rehearsal rates are able to keep more items in an active state than persons with lower rehearsal rates. Children with SLI did not show poor rehearsal; they did not differ from typically developing peers in word retrieval tasks. Their rate of articulation was comparable to the typically developing children's rate (Gathercole & Baddeley, 1990; Gillam, Cowan, & Day; 1995; Montgomery, 1995; van der Lely & Howard, 1993).

A further component that was controlled in some working memory studies using children with SLI was planning and executing the speech motor program. Edwards and Lahey (1998) suggested that errors on consonant clusters are related to difficulties with motor execution. In our own study (Marton & Schwartz, 2003), the planning and execution requirements were equally demanding across tasks; it was only the memory load that differed in the tasks that included word or nonword repetition. The error analysis data showed that children with SLI did not make many cluster reduction and/or cluster deletion errors. The ratio of the consonant cluster errors compared to the total number of errors was similar in the groups of children with and without SLI.

The last candidate for causing a deficit in nonword repetition was phonological discrimination. The discrimination data in the literature are mixed. Montgomery (1995) found significant differences in discrimination accuracy in nonword pairs that differed in one phoneme, but only with four-syllable nonwords. Gathercole and Baddeley (1990) found that children with SLI demonstrated accurate discrimination of nonwords and real words. The stimuli in their study were all monosyllabic words. Further support for no discrimination problems in children with SLI comes from the study by Edwards and Lahey (1998). The authors considered the production of unstressed syllables and stop consonants to signal auditory discrimination difficulties. Children with SLI did not show significantly more errors with unstressed syllables and stop consonants than their typically developing peers. These findings are similar to our own data that suggest no perceptual classification problems in children with SLI (Marton & Schwartz, 2003). These children performed as well as their peers in discriminating nonwords of varying lengths. These nonwords were minimal pairs that differed in their stress patterns only. Although the children in our study may have used multiple phonetic parameters (e.g., duration, intensity, pitch, etc.) to enhance discrimination, differentiating words that differ only in the suprasegmentals is always more difficult than discriminating minimal pairs that differ in one or two segments. One explanation for the difference between Montgomery's data and our results is related to the variation in methods. Montgomery presented each nonword pair twice successively to decrease the memory load of the task. In contrast, we presented our nonword pairs only once. Montgomery's dual presentation may have caused item interference. For example, the second presentation of word 1 might have interfered with the preceding presentation of word 2 (e.g., 1. zopanishful–topanishful, 2. zopanishful–topanishful).

Why is nonword repetition then so difficult for children with SLI? Our alternative hypothesis suggests that the nonword repetition errors in children with SLI are related to their difficulties in simultaneous processing of information (Marton, 2006). Evidence for this argument comes from our error analysis data and from findings on nonword repetition with stimuli that included meaningful parts (mono-syllabic real words). According to an account of phonological encoding in word retrieval, the phonemes of a word and the word's metrical frame are processed separately. The metrical frame includes the number of syllables and information on the words' stress pattern; the segmental part consists of information on the phonemes (consonants, vowels, clusters). The "segment-to-frame-association" theory (Biran & Friedmann, 2004; Levelt, 1992) proposes that segments/phonemes are inserted into the metrical frame of a word during phonological encoding. In word retrieval, these 2 types of information are integrated by the mechanism of "segment-to-frame-association". Evidence for this account comes from speech errors in different populations, e.g., stress exchange, anticipatory and perseveratory phoneme substitutions, and changes in syllabification (Biran & Friedmann, 2004; Meyer, 1992).

Detailed analyses of nonword repetition errors in children with SLI indicated that the majority of the errors were segment substitutions with notable assimilation errors (when the production of one part of the nonword influenced the production of another part of the same nonword). In contrast to the many segmental errors, the metrical frames of these nonwords were produced correctly; the number of syllables and the stress patterns were correct.

Further support for the argument that nonword repetition requires simultaneous processing and therefore it is highly demanding on language impaired children's working memory comes from our experiments where we compared nonword repetition accuracy of stimuli with no meaningful syllables to nonwords that consisted of 1 mono-syllabic real word and 2-3 syllables that had no meaning. Previous research showed that children's nonword repetition accuracy improves if the nonwords include meaningful syllables (Dollaghan, Biber,

& Campbell, 1995). Our results showed a similar pattern for the age-matched and the language-matched groups. The children with SLI, however, did not show a difference in performance accuracy across the nonword lists. Their performance did not improve, even when we ensured that they knew the words that were inserted in the nonwords. The children with TLD did benefit from their lexical knowledge, whereas the children with SLI did not take advantage of their long-term knowledge (see more information on this topic in the section "Interaction between working memory and the long-term lexicon in children with SLI" below).

One explanation for these findings is that simultaneously processing and integrating the different phonological structures (metrical frame and segments) is so demanding for the children with SLI that they do not have more resources to process the semantic information of the inserted mono-syllabic words. There are various functions that influence simultaneous processing and integration of information; one candidate for the difficulties observed in children with SLI is a weakness in attention switching (see further discussion on attention switching in children with SLI later in this chapter). Complex tasks that involve the concurrent processing of information require continuous attention switching. Children with SLI have extreme difficulty in these tasks and they are often not able to use even their existing knowledge to support their working memory performance.

Functional Working Memory and Language Comprehension

The interaction between language comprehension and working memory in children with SLI has not been investigated to the same extent than phonological storage and processing. The few studies that have studied sentence comprehension and working memory in children with SLI (e.g., Ellis-Weismer, Evans, & Hesketh, 1999; Montgomery, 1995, 2000) used stimuli with limited syntactic complexity: either short simple sentences or sentences varying in length without a variation in syntactic complexity. Consequently, in our studies we examined the effect of variations in sentence length and syntactic complexity on working memory performance in children with SLI (Marton & Schwartz, 2003; Marton et al., 2006). The comprehension of sentences with increasing length and complexity requires simultaneous processing. Simultaneous processing in these tasks involves continuous attention switching between encoding and rehearsal. Thus, tasks targeting simultaneous processing are highly demanding not only on working memory resources but also on attentional capacity.

A storage and processing trade-off was used to explain the performance of children with SLI in tasks that focused on functional working memory capacity (Montgomery 2000). The children were asked to recall as many words as possible under three conditions: no load (simple span), single load (storage and one mental operation) and dual load (storage and two mental operations). The children with SLI had a storage capacity similar to their peers' when the processing requirements were low. As the processing requirements increased (dual load), the children with SLI exhibited a trade-off between storage and processing. These children comprehended fewer redundant (long) sentences than the age-matched and the vocabulary-matched younger children. The findings were interpreted as further support for a processing deficit in children with SLI.

Our own research on working memory and language comprehension in children with SLI included several studies using similar experimental paradigms, but different languages and populations. In our first study, we had 13 children with SLI and 13 age-matched peers (ages 7-10 years). All children with SLI were enrolled in speech-language treatment and their language performance was at least 1.5 SD below the age-appropriate language performance level as measured by a standardized language test (Clinical Evaluation of Language Fundamentals–Revised; Semel, Wiig, & Secord, 1987). All children with SLI fell within the normal range of Performance IQ (i.e., between 90 and 120, with a mean of 102 on the Wechsler Intelligence Scale for Children–Revised; Wechsler, 1974). To test the interaction between working memory and language comprehension, we used our own traditional listening span task and modified listening span task (see their description in section "Interaction between language and verbal working memory: a developmental perspective above).

The findings in English-speaking children with SLI revealed a larger effect of syntactic complexity than sentence length on performance accuracy. Both children with SLI and their age-matched peers showed great difficulty in the MLS task, where they listened to sentences that varied in lengths and in syntactic complexity. As described earlier in this chapter, in the MLS task, a non-word was embedded in the sentence and children were asked to repeat that nonword. Following the recall of the nonword, children answered a question that targeted sentence content. The task required from the participants to pay close attention to sentence content while storing the words to-be-remembered. Most children with SLI were not able to process simultaneously the nonwords and the semantic and syntactic information of the sentences. These children performed more poorly than their age-matched peers. The results in the TLS task were similar to the findings in the MLS task. In the TLS task, children with SLI performed more poorly than their peers and made frequent interference errors. They repeated items from previous lists and from the middle of the sentences. Their recall pattern reflected diminished primacy and recency effects. Children with SLI showed difficulty in switching attentional focus according to the test requirements. They were not able to switch their attention from encoding to rehearsal and vice versa. The interference errors may have resulted from poor attention switching or from a deficit in inhibition control (see data on inhibition in children with SLI later in this chapter).

The effects of syntactic complexity on language comprehension were consistent with adults' performance on traditional listening span tasks. In adults, increased syntactic complexity resulted in increased reaction time and decreased repetition accuracy of real words (MacDonald, Just, & Carpenter, 1992). The authors' explanation for their findings was that processing more complex sentences requires more working memory capacity than processing simple sentences. They interpreted their data within the framework of the processing capacity theory (Just and Carpenter 1992).

An alternative hypothesis is that the retrieval of words to-be-remembered in complex sentence contexts may result in prolonging the recall process for a longer time period than in simple sentential contexts. This prolongation may be long enough for some information to be lost (Cowan et al. 2003). The efficiency of sentence processing is strongly related to the demands that sentence structure variations place on memory resources (McElree, Foraker, & Dyer 2003).

In a second study on language comprehension and working memory, we performed a cross-linguistic comparison. We examined how the variations of the linguistic structures in different languages influence verbal working memory performance and language comprehension. This research was based on the assumption that verbal working memory is not a language-independent system (Thorn and Gathercole 1999). There is evidence that SLI manifests differently cross-linguistically, because it reflects the features of a given language (Leonard 1998). Thus, we expected that verbal working memory deficits would reflect an interaction of the core deficits associated with SLI and language-specific features. English and Hungarian languages were used to examine this effect. In contrast to English, Hungarian is a language with relatively free word order and a rich agglutinative morphology.

In the first experiment of this cross-linguistic comparison, we used adaptations of our MLS and TLS tasks to compare working memory performance of Hungarian children with SLI with our previous findings in English-speaking children. The question was the same as in our previous study; whether the effect of syntactic complexity or of sentence length has a larger impact on working memory performance. Another question was whether Hungarian children with SLI show a similar deficit to English-speaking children in language comprehension with syntactically complex sentences if the memory load is high. Seventeen children with SLI and 17 age-matched typically developing children (ages 7;6-10;5 years) participated in this experiment.

Similarly to the English data, there was a group effect; children with SLI performed more poorly than their age-matched peers. Unlike the English results, the data from both listening span tasks showed that children answered more questions correctly following the simple short and complex short sentences than they did with the complex long sentences. Their performance decreased with the increase of sentence length. This finding was in contrast to our previous data from English-speaking children because in that population sentence complexity had a larger effect on working memory performance than sentence length. One explanation for these contradictory findings was related to the morphological differences between the languages. Hungarian is an agglutinative language with a rich morphological system, whereas English has relatively sparse morphology. The increase in sentence length did not change the morphological complexity in English, but it did in Hungarian. The results showed the impact of language-specific structures on working memory performance and language comprehension.

In addition to the group difference in performance accuracy - children with SLI performed more poorly than the control participants in both listening span tasks - the groups showed different error patterns. The error analysis data from the listening span tasks were similar to the data from the English-speaking children (Marton and Schwartz 2003). Typically developing children usually make three types of errors in serial recall: intrusion, omission, and movement. Preschool-age children produce many intrusions (items outside of the list). With an increase in age and the development of executive functions, the number of intrusions decreases; 10 year old children produce more omissions and movement errors than intrusions. Adults still make movement errors, but the number of omissions decreases to a great extent (McCormack, et al., 2000). The main error category for the control children in our study was in agreement with the literature. The typically developing children produced omissions in both listening span tasks. This was not surprising because executive functions are not fully developed at this age. Thus, 10-year-old children exhibit slower memory search and retrieval processes than adults (McCormack et al. 2000). Another common error among the typically developing children was semantic substitutions. The use of synonyms and words with similar meanings within the same grammatical category indicate large and flexible vocabularies in these children. In contrast, the majority of the errors produced by the children with SLI were interference errors in both tasks. Their answers were often words from previous lists or items that were presented in the middle of one of the preceding sentences, but were not sentence-final items that had to-be-remembered. Children with SLI had difficulty inhibiting previously activated items (see more details on inhibition in the next section of this chapter). Inhibitory processes allow only those items to enter working memory that are consistent with the goals of the listener. Inhibitory mechanisms also suppress the activation of irrelevant information (Lorsbach and Reiner, 1997).

Based on the findings of Experiment 1, in the second experiment of this study we examined whether an increase in sentence length or an increase in the sentences' morphological complexity has a larger effect on working memory performance and on language comprehension. Previous findings in English-speaking adults evidenced that working memory performance depends more on the ability to control attention, to suppress irrelevant information and to focus on task-relevant goals than on the ability to store more items (Engle et al. 1999; Lustig, May, & Hasher, 2001; Miyake 2001). Thus, the simple increase of the number of words in a sentence, without an increase in grammatical complexity, should not influence performance accuracy to the same extent as the increase in morphological complexity. The agglutinative nature of Hungarian enabled us to examine working memory performance and language comprehension using sentences that differed in their morphological structures: short sentences with simple morphological structures, long sentences with simple morphology, and long sentences with complex morphological structures. We hypothesized that sentences with complex morphological structures are more demanding on working memory than sentences with simple morphological structures, even when the sentence length is the same. A group effect was expected with each sentence type. This experiment included 25 children with SLI and 25 control participants (ages: 8-11 years).

The results revealed that morphological complexity has a greater impact on working memory performance and language comprehension than sentence length. An increase in morphological complexity caused a significant decrease in performance accuracy in children with SLI. There was no difference in performance accuracy between the short and long sentences, when morphology was simple. Thus, similar to our findings in English-speaking children, Hungarian children showed more difficulty as stimulus complexity increased, but complexity affected working memory performance differently across languages. In English, it was the increase in syntactic complexity that resulted in a decrease in working memory performance and language comprehension accuracy. In Hungarian, a language with a rich morphological system, it was the increase in morphology that resulted in decreased performance accuracy.

These findings raise issues regarding the interaction between working memory and language comprehension. Different working memory models provide various descriptions of storage that can be devoted to language operations, such as processing words, syntax, and morphosyntax (e.g. Just and Carpenter 1992). Although the complexity effects manifested differently across languages, there was consistency in their impact on working memory performance and language comprehension. These results suggest that the interaction between working memory and language comprehension may best be described by those models that posit a workspace with limited capacity rather than a more traditional capacity-limited storage for material.

Regardless of the particular language, the error analysis data were similar across our studies. As the demands on working memory increased, typically developing children forgot some information or substituted a synonym for the target word. In contrast, the children with

SLI produced a high number of interference / inhibition errors. These observations motivated our next study.

WORKING MEMORY AND INHIBITION IN CHILDREN WITH SLI

Based on our previous error analysis data, we examined the "inefficient inhibition" hypothesis by Bjorklund and Harnishfeger (1990) in children with and without SLI. According to this account, individuals with better inhibition skills have more processing capacity than people who are less efficient in inhibition control. Thus, individuals with efficient inhibition skills perform better on various working memory tasks because they are able to keep out irrelevant information from working memory. This mechanism helps people to stay focused and to be goal-relevant (Hasher, Lustig, & Zacks, 2007). Hasher and colleagues proposed 3 functions of inhibition: controlling attentional focus, deleting irrelevant information from working memory, and suppressing inappropriate responses. In behavioral tests, these inhibitory functions interact with each other and are often difficult to separate.

Our previous findings showed that the majority of errors in children with SLI, across various listening span tasks, indicated a weakness in inhibition control. These children's working memory difficulties were not simply related to limitations in storage. Children with SLI showed a deficit in repeating words in interfering contexts. In the MLS task, the answers to the questions prior word repetition interfered with the words to-be-remembered. Gillam and colleagues (1995) also reported problems with suppressing irrelevant information in children with SLI. In their study, children with SLI showed larger suffix effects than their peers. The suffix is an item that is added after the list-final item, therefore it diminishes the recency effect. Children with SLI produced more interference errors with the suffix than the control group because they did not suppress the irrelevant information.

The results of various attention tasks showed similar problems in children with SLI. These children experienced difficulty in focusing on the relevant information, particularly in tasks that were more demanding on working memory (Noterdaeme, Amorosa, Mildenberger, Sitter, & Minow, 2001). Children with SLI showed comparable performance to their peers' results on simple vigilance tasks and on other attention tasks with low working memory load. In tasks with higher working memory demands (e.g., test of sustained visual attention), the children with SLI made more errors than did the children in the control group. The findings revealed that children with SLI experience difficulty with both selective and sustained attention when the tasks have high working memory demands.

In our inhibition study we examined the contribution of inhibition control to working memory performance and language comprehension in children with SLI, in their age-matched and language-matched peers (Marton, Kelmenson, & Pinkhasova, 2007). Each group consisted of 15 children (ages: 8-10 years). A listening span task with 2 lists (84 sentences) was used to study inhibition control across groups. All sentences in this task were short (10 or fewer syllables). The lists included sets of sentences that increased in the number of items (3 sets of 2 sentences per set, 3 sets of 3 sentences per set, 3 sets of 4 sentences per set, and 3 sets of 5 sentences per set in each list).Error analysis was performed as follows. All answers that were a target of a previous list or a non sentence-final word were considered as an inhibition error. These errors could occur immediately following stimulus presentation or with a delay. We considered errors from the current set as immediate, from a previous set, as delayed. Another categorization of errors consisted of contextual distractions and perseverations. Contextual distractions were errors where the child recalled a non-target word from the middle of the sentence or from the question, whereas perseverations included errors where the child repeated either a previously recalled sentence-final word or the answer to the question.

Children with SLI produced a significantly higher number of immediate inhibition errors than the controls. These children produced words that were previously relevant, but then had to be suppressed. There was no group difference in delayed inhibition. It was more difficult for everyone to suppress relatively recent items than items from earlier sets.

Many errors made by the children with SLI reflected contextual distraction. These words had to be encoded during sentence processing, but they were not target items. Children in both control groups performed better than the children with SLI. Even the younger, language-matched children performed with much fewer inhibition errors than the children with SLI. The children with SLI showed difficulty with expelling previously activated information from working memory when that information was not relevant anymore. This was further evidenced by the high number of perseverations in children with SLI. Most of the perseverations were repetitions of the answer to the questions. These findings are similar to the results of Cornoldi et al. (2001) in children with attention deficit disorders. Those children performed poorly on working memory tasks and showed significant interference between relevant information and information that first had to be processed, and subsequently excluded from memory.

Although we found an association between inhibition control and working memory capacity, the direction of causality is not clear. Inhibition control is not limited to the suppression of irrelevant information. The evaluation of resistance to interference in children with SLI may help to clarify the relations between inhibition and working memory capacity. If resistance to interference works efficiently, irrelevant items are not encoded into working memory. Our study was limited to the analysis of items that had been encoded previously. Thus, these data show that children with SLI have difficulty with suppressing information that is not relevant anymore; they show problems with expelling unnecessary material from working memory. These findings support the "inefficient inhibition" account, but more research is needed to understand SLI children's inhibition functions and their impact on working memory performance.

Interaction Between Working Memory and the Long-Term Lexicon in Children with SLI

Working memory does not operate in isolation; permanent knowledge has an impact on it (Gathercole, 2006). Long-term knowledge and processing capacity are interrelated (Mainela-Arnold & Evans, 2005). This is evidenced by data showing higher accuracy for sentence-recall than for word lists (Jefferies, Lambon Ralph, & Baddeley, 2004). The lexical characteristics of stimulus items for immediate recall influence working memory performance to a great extent. Moreover, sublexical and super-lexical knowledge contribute to immediate recall. Children's phonological working memory performance improves if the nonwords include meaningful syllables because of the interaction between the long-term lexicon and working memory (Dollaghan et al., 1995). Memory span is larger for words than for nonwords, particularly for high frequency words and for concrete words (Hulme, Maughan, & Brown, 1991; Hulme, Roodenrys, Schweickert, Brown, Martin, & Stuart, 1997; Walker & Hulme, 1999). All these processes have been related to redintegration; a process that is responsible for reconstructing the decaying traces in short-term memory with the support of long-term lexical and semantic knowledge (Roodenrys, Hulme, Alban, & Ellis, 1994).

Our data on nonword repetition with stimuli that included a meaningful syllable showed that unlike typically developing children, children with SLI do not support their working memory performance with their long-term knowledge. It is also known from the literature that children with SLI have more limited vocabularies and show more difficulties with accessing the information in their long-term lexicon than typically developing children. These findings motivated our next study in which we developed a specific listening span task to examine the interaction between working memory and the long-term lexicon in this population. In this new task (Active Listening Span task, ALS), children were first required to complete the sentences with their own words. Afterwards, the children were presented with these sentences as the stimuli of a listening span task. Each child was told that the sentences were exactly the same as they had completed them. The data from this task were compared with the results of our TLS task (described in the "Working memory and inhibition in children with SLI" section above). Three groups of 8-10 years old children participated in this study (children with SLI, age-matched, and language-matched controls).

The typically developing children performed significantly better in the ALS task than in the TLS task. In the former task, participants recalled words that they had previously activated. Thus, all words were familiar to the children and had a relatively high activation level. In contrast to the age-matched and language-matched groups, the children with SLI showed no difference in recall accuracy across the listening span tasks (ALS versus TLS). These children did not benefit from their long-term knowledge and from the previous activation of the stimuli. These findings reveal problems in the interaction between working memory and the long-term lexicon in children with SLI. Further, they contradict the hypothesis that these children's working memory difficulties are caused by weak word representations. Typically developing children's data suggest that repeated items become stronger, thus they are more likely to be produced correctly and remembered more accurately (Gershkoff-Stowe, 2002). In the ALS task, children completed the sentences with familiar words. They activated these words as they performed the task. Despite the familiarity and higher activation level of these words, children with SLI did not perform better than in the TLS task, where the words have not been active previously. One reason for this finding is that the task required continuous attention switching and simultaneous processing (listening to the new incoming items and rehearsing the already presented words), which was too demanding for the children with SLI. It is important for future research to examine the contribution of the long-term lexicon to working memory performance at various levels (sublexical, lexical, super-lexical) in children with SLI. If we enhance the contribution of the long-term lexicon in maintaining words, then the attentional requirements for retaining these words in working memory decreases. Thus, more attention can be focused on the recall processes.

WORKING MEMORY IN ADOLESCENTS AND YOUNG ADULTS WITH DYSLEXIA

In this section of the present chapter we explore the interaction between cognition and language comprehension in young individuals with a diagnosis of dyslexia. Individuals with a history of childhood dyslexia often experience difficulty with written language even as adults. In most cases, these problems are not limited to reading. Young individuals with reading difficulties also show a deficit in word recognition and in working memory. The literature is mixed regarding the relationship between word recognition and reading comprehension. In some participants, performance on word recognition tasks showed an association with their reading level, but many young people's results indicated dissociation between word recognition and reading comprehension (Lefly & Pennington, 1991). Thus, the ability to recognize and identify single words is not always a good predictor of reading.

Young individuals (ages 17-23 years) with dyslexia performed more poorly than the controls in tasks on phonological processing, naming speed, general knowledge, vocabulary, listening comprehension, and working memory (Ransby & Swanson, 2003). Based on a hierarchical regression model, the authors concluded that both higher order and lower order processes mediate reading comprehension. In predicting reading comprehension fluency, working memory and listening comprehension were the most important factors. Working memory capacity and lexical processing were the functions that had the most influence on individual differences within groups. Engle and colleagues also suggest that individuals with greater working memory capacity are able to comprehend more complex discourse than people with low working memory span. Better working memory skills enhance the retention of story details and facilitate the integration of separated propositions (Engle, Cantor, & Carullo, 1992).

The results of an fMRI study revealed that individuals with dyslexia use similar brain areas in verbal working memory tasks than the controls, but the groups differ in the degree and extent of activation, particularly, with an increase in cognitive demands (Vasic, Lohr, Steinbrink, Martin, & Wolf, 2007). The overall data from of the above study suggest that individuals with dyslexia are not limited in storage capacity, but have a deficit in executive functions that prevent them from efficient manipulations of verbal material according to task demands.

Two groups of adults with a childhood diagnosis of dyslexia were compared with non-impaired readers in another fMRI study by Shaywitz and her colleagues (Shaywitz et al., 2003). The authors examined whether young individuals with persistent reading difficulties differ form people with a compensated reading profile. The documents from participants' childhood revealed that all individuals began school with comparable reading skills and similar socioeconomic status. The 2 groups differed, however, in their cognitive skills. The second group showed higher cognitive scores than the first group. It was their better cognitive ability that allowed participants in the second group to compensate for their phonological deficit, so that as adults these individuals performed similarly to the controls in reading comprehension. The results of the study demonstrate that cognitive ability is an important factor in predicting reading comprehension in adults.

Based on the above literature, we examined the cognitive and reading profiles of 44 adolescents and young adults (ages: 13-22 years) with persistent difficulties in written language (Jaszberenyi & Marton, in press). Similar to children, young individuals with dyslexia showed a discrepancy between their verbal and performance IQs on the Wechsler intelligence test (Kun & Szegedi, 1972, Hungarian version of the Wechsler Adult Intelligence Scale). Participants with dyslexia showed significantly better Performance IQs than Verbal IQs. The multiple regression analysis data revealed that the best predictors for the overall IQ were scores on information, arithmetic, and digit span tasks. These findings and the following data suggest that individuals with dyslexia show a weakness in their language skills even in adulthood.

There was a negative correlation between verbal IQ and the number of reading errors (individuals with lower verbal IQ performed with more errors on the reading task). Further analyses revealed that the number of reading errors was closely linked to these individuals' working memory and executive functions skills. Participants with a deficit in working memory performed with more errors on the reading task and on the Raven Advanced Matrices (Raven, 1962) test. This finding is in line with previous research that indicated a strong relationship between performance on the Raven test and working memory capacity (Verguts & De Boeck, 2002). Typically, individuals with good working memory skills perform better in applying rules, particularly, if those rules were used earlier in the test. Individuals with good working memory skills profit from rules that occur repeatedly. The results in our study did not show this advantage for the young individuals with dyslexia. Our participants showed an overall deficit in applying rules. This was reflected in their performance on the Raven test and in their writing samples. Most of their writing errors were rule-based problems. These errors were related to these individuals' difficulty with simultaneous processing, to their limitations in processing capacity.

This was further evidenced by the comparison of participants' short-term memory and working memory data. These individuals showed much better performance on the verbal short-term memory tests than on the verbal working memory tasks. Moreover, the written language errors (both reading and writing) did not correlate with the short-term memory scores. In contrast to short-term memory, written language errors highly correlated with working memory performance in young adults with dyslexia. These young people did not show any difficulty in remembering a larger amount of information, but they experienced severe problems with application of rules and knowledge. They were not sure how and when to manipulate information in order to solve a problem efficiently.

SUMMARY

This chapter focused on the interaction between cognition and language in different populations. Data from typically developing school-age children, children with SLI, and adolescents and young individuals with dyslexia have been analyzed to demonstrate the impact of various cognitive functions on language acquisition and language processing. The data confirmed the role of flexible cognition in language comprehension.

According to the neuroconstructivist account (Karmiloff-Smith, 1998), children's cognitive-linguistic system changes from a less detailed, domain-relevant structure to a more specified, domain-specific one during development. Certain non-linguistic cognitive functions, such as imitation, cross-modal integration, attention and memory serve as prerequisites for language acquisition (Bates, 2004). Thus, language development is not isolated from changes in cognitive skills. In this chapter, we examined the contribution of flexible cognition, particularly of working memory, inhibition, and attention switching to the development of language comprehension. Language comprehension is a multifaceted skill that includes various cognitive-linguistic processes, such as the perception of speech sounds, the connection of the processed phonemes to the mental lexicon, the interpretation of grammatical structures, and the use of semantic, syntactic, and social context to decipher the speaker's intended meaning (Bishop, 1997). This complex process is strongly influenced by flexible cognition. To comprehend a sentence, one must recognize the words and continuously update his/her working memory, selectively activate relevant meanings, inhibit irrelevant thoughts and responses, remember the words, and parse the sentence, keeping track of element order as well as long-distance grammatical relations, process the pragmatic context of the sentence.

The findings from numerous working memory studies revealed an interaction between task complexity and age. Younger children (6-8 years of age) performed less accurately than older children at each complexity level. These children made different errors than the older children and the adults. The majority of their errors reflected a weakness in those cognitive skills that set up flexible cognition. These errors included distractions from task context and perseverations. Young children's errors demonstrate the age-related weakness in task switching and in blocking previously relevant items. The executive functions that support task switching show substantial improvement with age during school age (Cepeda, Kramer, Gonzalez de Shalter, 2001). Older children (10-11 years of age) made not only fewer errors than their younger peers, but older children produced errors that were similar to the ones observed in adults. Most of their errors were omissions. As the working memory load of the tasks increased, older children and young adults omitted some information. In simple tasks with low working memory demands, older children performed comparable to young adults. In addition to the observed developmental changes, the results confirmed that working memory storage and processing were affected differently by the complexity of the stimuli.

Children with SLI and young adults with dyslexia showed deficits in working memory and executive functions. Both groups' performance showed a strong interaction between language comprehension and production, and working memory, task switching, and inhibition. The findings described in this chapter do not support the notion of SLI as a deficit in linguistic knowledge (e.g., van der Lely, 1998, 2001) because these children showed extreme difficulties in flexible cognition as well. These children produced many interference and perseverative errors across tasks that reflected their difficulty in attention switching, inhibition, and in working memory. Their performance differed from their age-matched and younger, language-matched peers. Their recall patterns did not show the typical U shape. Most children with language impairment performed with diminished primacy and recency effects. These problems are related to difficulty in simultaneous processing. One must encode the new information concurrently with the rehearsal of the old material. Both English-speaking and Hungarian children showed diminished effects. Although children with SLI performed similarly across languages, the cross-linguistic comparison revealed the effects of language structure on working memory performance. Researchers studying working memory in different populations across languages are encouraged to consider the effect of language structure on working memory.

The findings strengthen the concept that children with SLI not only perform more poorly on tasks of inhibition control and working memory than their peers, but also mobilize different functions during task performance. This was reflected in the group differences in error types and performance patterns. Further research is needed to analyze in more details these qualitative group differences including the examination of strategy use across populations. It is essential for future studies to examine perseveration in children with language impairment. Although we observed a very high number of perseveration errors in children with SLI, we do not know what exactly causes this problem. It may be related to deficits in attention switching, inhibition, and / or working memory or to a combination of these functions. As suggested by the neuroconstructivist perspective, it is crucial to seek more subtle effects beyond the unique ones (Karmiloff-Smith, 1998).

ACKNOWLEDGMENTS

The studies described in this chapter were supported by the following grants and awards:

1. "The impact of inhibition control on working memory performance in children with SLI", 1R15DC009040-01, NIH-NIDCD; 2007-2010,
2. "Inhibition control in children with specific language impairment", PSC-CUNY grant 2007-2008;
3. Brooklyn College, sabbatical fellowship, 2006-2007;
4. "Working memory capacity in children with SLI", R03DC41449, NIH-NIDCD; 2002-2005;
5. "Reading comprehension and working memory in children with specific language impairment", PSC-CUNY grant, 2003-2004;
6. Szent-Györgyi Albert fellowship from the Hungarian Ministry of Education, 2003-2004;
7. "Lexical influence on working memory performance in children with specific language impairment", PSC-CUNY grant, 2002-2003;
8. "Working Memory for Structural-Linguistic Information in Adults and Children", CUNY Collaborative Incentive Grants Program, 2001-2003;
9. "Developmental changes in phonological working memory performance in school-age children", PSC-CUNY grant, 2001-2002.

REFERENCES

Baddeley, A. D. (2000). The episodic buffer: A new component of working memory? *Trends in Cognitive Sciences, 4*, 417–422.

Baldwin, D. A. (1995). Understanding the link between joint attention and language. In. C, Moore & P. J. Dunham (Eds.), *Joint attention. Its origin and role in development.* Lawrence Erlbaum Associates, 131-158.

Barrouillet, P., & Camos, V. (2001). Developmental increase in working memory span: Resource sharing or temporal decay? *Journal of Memory and Language, 45*, 1-20.

Bates, E. (2004). Explaining & interpreting deficits in language development across clinical groups: Where do we go from here? *Brain & Language, 88*, 248-253.

Bayliss, D. M., Jarrold, C., Gunn, D. M., & Baddeley, A. D. (2003). The complexities of complex span: Explaining individual differences in working memory in children and adults. *Journal of Experimental Psychology: General, 132*, 71-92.

Biran, M, & Friedmann, N. (2005). From phonological paraphasias to the structure of the phonological output lexicon. *Language and Cognitive Processes, 20*, 589-616.

Bishop, D. V. M. (2000). Pragmatic language impairment: A correlate of SLI, a distinct subgroup, or part of the autistic continuum? In: D. V. M. Bishop & L. B. Leonard (Eds.). Speech and language impairment in children. Causes, characteristics, intervention and outcome. Taylor and Francis: Psychology Press.

Bjorklund, D. F., & Harnishfeger, K. K. (1990). The resources construct in cognitive development: Diverse sources of evidence and a theory of inefficient inhibition. *Developmental Review, 10*, 48-71.

Cain, K., Oakhill, J., & Bryant, P. (2004). Children's reading comprehension ability: Concurrent prediction by working memory, verbal ability, and component skills. *Journal of Educational Psychology, 96*, 31-42.

Caplan, D. & Waters, G. S. (1999). Verbal working memory and sentence comprehension. *Behavioral and Brain Sciences, 22*, 77-94.

Case, R., Kurland, D. M., & Goldberg, J. (1982). Operational efficiency and the growth of short-term memory span. *Journal of Experimental Child Psychology, 33*, 386–404.

Cepeda, N. J., Kramer, A. F., & Gonzalez de Sather, J. C. (2001). Changes in executive control across the life span: Examination of task-switching performance. *Developmental Psychology, 37*, 715–730.

Chiat, S. (2001). Mapping theories of developmental language impairment: Premises, predictions and evidence. *Language and Cognitive Processes, 16*, 113–142.

Conway, A. R. A., & Engle, R. W. (1994). Working memory and retrieval: A resource-dependent inhibition model. *Journal of Experimental Psychology: General, 123*, 354-373.

Cowan, N., Towse, J. N., Hamilton, Z., Saults, J. S., Elliott, E. M., Lacey, J. F., Moreno, M. V., & Hitsch, G. J. (2003). Children's working memory processes: A response-timing analysis. *Journal of Experimental Psychology: General, 132*, 113–132.

Daneman, M. & Philip, M. M. (1996). Working memory and language comprehension: A meta-analysis. *Psychonomic Bulletin & Review, 3 (4)*, 422-433.

Deák, G. O. (2000). The growth of flexible problem solving: Preschool children use changing verbal cues to infer multiple word meanings. *Journal of Cognition and Development, 1*, 157–192.

Deák, O. G. (2003). The development of cognitive flexibility and language abilities. *Advances in Child Development and Behavior, 31*, 271-327.

DeLuca, C. R., Wood, S. J., Anderson, V., Bucanan, J., Proffitt, T. M., Mahony, K., & Pantelis, C. (2003). Normative data from the Cantab: I. Development of executive function over the lifespan. *Journal of Clinical & Experimental Neuropsychology, 25*, 242-254.

Diamond, A. (1998). Evidence of the importance of dopamine for prefrontal cortex functions early in life. In: A. Roberts, T. Robbins, & L. Weiskrantz (Eds.), *The prefrontal cortex*. Oxford: University Press, 144-164.

Dollaghan, C. A., Biber, M. E., & Campbell, T. F. (1995). Lexical influences on nonword repetition. *Applied Psycholinguistics, 16*, 211-222.

Edwards, J., & Lahey, M. (1998). Nonword repetitions of children with specific language impairment: Exploration of some explanations for their inaccuracies. *Applied Psycholinguistics, 19*, 279–309.

Engle, R. W., Cantor, J., & Carullo, J. J. (1992). Individual differences in working memory and comprehension: A test of four hypotheses. *Journal of Experimental Psychology: Learning, Memory, and Cognition, 18*, 972–992.

Engle, R. W. & Kane, M. J. (2004). Executive attention, working memory capacity, and two-factor theory of cognitive control. *The Psychology of Learning and Motivation, 44*, 145-199.

Engle, R. W., Kane, M. J., & Tuholski, S. W. (1999). Individual differences in working memory capacity and what they tell us about controlled attention, general fluid intelligence and functions of the prefrontal cortex. In: Miyake, A. & Shah, P. (Eds.), *Models of WM: Mechanisms of active maintenance and executive control*. London: Cambridge Press, 102-134.

Gathercole, S. E. (2006). Nonword repetition and word learning: The nature of the relationship. *Applied Psycholinguistics, 27*, 513-543.

Gathercole, S. E., & Baddeley, A. D. (1990). Phonological memory deficits in language disordered children: Is there a causal connection? *Journal of Memory and Language, 29*, 336–360.

Gathercole, S. E., Pickering, S. J., Ambridge, B., & Wearing, H. (2004). The structure of working memory from 4 to 15 years of age. Developmental Psychology, 40, 177-190.

Gershkoff-Stowe, L. (2002). Object naming, vocabulary growth, and the development of word retrieval abilities. *Journal of Memory and Language, 46 (4)*, 665-687.

Gillam, R. B., Cowan, N., & Day, L. S. (1995). Sequential memory in children with and without language impairment. *Journal of Speech and Hearing Research, 38*, 393–402.

Hale, S., Bronik, M. D., & Fry, A. F. (1997). Verbal and spatial working memory in school-age children: Developmental differences in susceptibility to interference. *Developmental Psychology, 33 (2)*, 364-371.

Hasher, L., Lustig, C., & Zacks, R. T. (2007). Inhibitory mechanisms and the control of attention. In: A. Conway, C. Jarrold, M. Kane, A. Miyake, & J. Towse (Eds.), *Variation in working memory*. Oxford University Press, 227-249.

Hasher, L., & Zacks, R. T. (1988). Working memory, comprehension, and aging: A review and a new view. In: G. H. Bower (Ed.) *The psychology of learning and motivation, 22*, New York, NY: Academic Press, 193-225.

Hoffmann, L. V. M. & Gillam, R. B. (2004). Verbal and spatial information processing constraints in children with specific language impairment. *Journal of Speech, Language, and Hearing Research, 47*, 114-125.

Hulme, C., Maughan, S., & Brown, G. D. A. (1991). Memory for familiar and unfamiliar words: Evidence for a long-term memory contribution to short-term memory span. *Journal of Memory and Language, 30*, 685-701.

Hulme, C., Roodenrys, S., Schweickert, R., Brown, G. D. A., Martin, S., & Stuart, G. (1997). Word frequency effects on short-term memory tasks: Evidence for a redintegration process in immediate serial recall. *Journal of Experimental Psychology: Learning, Memory, and Cognition, 23*, 1217-1232.

Jaszberenyi, M. & Marton, K. (in press). Clinical examination of young adults with reading difficulties in light of Evidence Based Practice. In: K. Marton (Ed.), Diagnostics and therapy of neurocognitive developmental disorders: On the way to Evidence Based Practice. Budapest, Eotvos Kiado (in Hungarian).

Just, M. A. & Carpenter, P. A. (1992). A capacity theory of comprehension: individual differences in working memory. *Psychological Review, 99*, 122–149.

Just, M. A. & Carpenter, P. A. (2002). A capacity theory of comprehension: Individual differences in working memory. In: T. A. Polk & C. M. Seifert (Eds.), *Cognitive modeling*. Cambridge, MA: The MIT Press, 131-178.

Kail, R & Salthouse, T. A. (1994). Processing speed as a mental capacity. *Acta Psychologica, 86*, 199-255.

Karmiloff-Smith, A. (1998). Development itself is the key to understanding developmental disorders. *Trends in Cognitive Sciences, 2 (10)*, 389-398.

King, J., & Just, M. A. (1991). Individual differences in syntactic processing: The role of working memory. *Journal of Memory and Language, 30*, 580–602.

Kun, M. & Szegedi, M. (1972). Measurement of intelligence. Budapest: Akademia Kiado (in Hungarian).

Lefly, D. L., & Pennington, B. F. (1991). Spelling errors and reading fluency incompensated adult dyslexics. *Annals of Dyslexia, 41*, 143–162.

Leonard, L. B. (1998). *Children with specific language impairment*. Bradford Books.

Levelt, W. J. M. (1992). Accessing words in speech production: stages, processes and representations. *Cognition, 42*, 1-22.

Lorsbach, T.C. & Reiner, J. F. (1997). Developmental changes in the inhibition of previously relevant information. *Journal of Experimental Child Psychology, 64*, 317–342.

Lustig, C., May, C. P., & Hasher, L. (2001). Working memory span and the role of proactive interference. *Journal of Experimental Psychology, 130*, 199–207.

MacDonald, M. C., Just, M. A., & Carpenter, P. A. (1992). Working memory constraints on the processing of syntactic ambiguity. *Cognitive Psychology, 24*, 56–98.

Mainela-Arnold, E. & Evans, J. L. (2005). Beyond capacity limitations: Determinants of word recall performance on verbal working memory span tasks in children with SLI. *Journal of Speech, Language, and Hearing Research, 48*, 897-909.

Marchman, V.A. (1997). Children's productivity in the English past tense: The role of frequency, phonology, and neighborhood structure. *Cognitive Science: A Multidisciplinary Journal, 21 (3)*, 283-304.

Marton, K. (2006). Do nonword repetition errors in children with specific language impairment (SLI) reflect a weakness in an unidentified skill specific to nonword repetition or a deficit in simultaneous processing? *Applied Psycholinguistics, 27(4)*, 569-573.

Marton, K., Kelmenson, L., & Pinkhasova, L. (2007). Inhibition control and working memory capacity in children with SLI. *Psychologia, 50*, 110-121.

Marton, K. & Schwartz, R. G. (2003). Working memory capacity limitations and language processes in children with specific language impairment. *Journal of Speech, Language, and Hearing Research, 46*, 1138-1153.

Marton, K., Schwartz, R. G., & Braun, A. (2005). The effect of age and language structure in working memory performance. In Bara, B. G., Barsalou, L., & Bucciarelli, M. (Eds.).

Proceedings of the XXVII. Annual Meeting of the Cognitive Science Society. Mahwah, NJ: Lawrence Erlbaum Associates, Inc., 1413-1418.

Marton, K., Schwartz, R. G., Farkas, L., & Katsnelson, V. (2006). Effect of sentence length and complexity on working memory performance in Hungarian children with specific language impairment (SLI): a cross-linguistic comparison. *International Journal of Language & Communication Disorders, 41 (6),* 653-673.

McCormack, T., Brown, G. D. A., & Vousden, J. I. (2000). Children's serial recall errors: Implications for theories of short-term memory development. *Journal of Experimental Child Psychology, 76*, 222–252.

McElree, B., Foraker, S., & Dyer, L. (2003). Memory structures that subserve sentence comprehension. *Journal of Memory and Language, 48*, 67–91.

Meltzoff, A. N. (1990). Towards a developmental cognitive science. The implications of cross-modal matching and imitation for the development of representation and memory in infancy. *Annals of the New York Academy of Sciences, 608*, 1-31.

Meyer, A. S. (1992). Investigation of phonological encoding through speech error analyses: Achievements, limitations, and alternatives. *Cognition, 42*, 181-211.

Miyake, A. (2001). Individual differences in working memory. Introduction to the special section. *Journal of Experimental Psychology, 130*, 163–168.

Miyake, A. & Shah, P. (1999). *Models of working memory: Mechanisms of active maintenance and executive control*. London: Cambridge Press.

Montgomery, J. W. (1995). Examination of phonological working memory in specifically language impaired children. *Applied Psycholinguistics, 16*, 335–378.

Montgomery, J. W. (2000). Verbal working memory and sentence comprehension in children with specific language impairment. *Journal of Speech, Language, and Hearing Research, 43*, 293–308.

Noterdaeme, M., Amorosa, H., Mildenberger, K., Sitter, S., & Minow, F. (2001). Evaluation of attention problems in children with autism and in children with specific language disorder. *European Child & Adolescent Psychiatry, 10*, 58-66.

Paterson, S. J., Brown, J. H., Gsödl, M. K., Johnson, M. H., & Karmiloff-Smith, A. (1999). Cognitive modularity and genetic disorders. *Science, 286*, 2355–2358.

Ransby, M. J. & Swanson, H. L. (2003). Reading comprehension skills of young adults with childhood diagnoses of dyslexia. *Journal of Learning Disabilities, 36 (6)*, 538-555.

Raven, J. C. (1962). *Advanced progressive matrices, set II*. London, UK: H. K. Lewis.

Roodenrys, S. Hulme, C., Alban, J., & Ellis, A. W. (1994). Effects of word frequency and age of acquisition on short-term memory span. *Memory and Cognition, 22*, 695-701.

Semel, E., Wiig, E. H., & Secord, W. A. (1987). *Clinical Evaluation of Language Fundamentals–Revised*. San Antonio, TX: The Psychological Corporation.

Tager-Flusberg, H. (2005). Designing studies to investigate the relationships between genes, environments, and developmental language disorders. *Applied Psycholinguistics, 26*, 29-39.

Thomas, M. S. C. (2005). Constraints on language development: Insights from developmental disorders. In: P. Fletcher & J. Miller (Eds.) Language Disorders and Developmental Theory. John Benjamins, 11-34.

Thorn, A. S. C. & Gathercole, S. E. (1999). Language-specific knowledge and short-term memory in bilingual and non-bilingual children. *Quarterly Journal of Experimental Psychology, 52A*, 303–324.

Tomasello, M., Kruger, A, & Ratner, H. (1993). Cultural learning. *Behavioral and Brain Sciences, 16*, 495-552.

Towse, J. N., & Hitch, G. J. (1995). Is there a relationship between task demand and storage space in tests of working memory capacity? *Quarterly Journal of Experimental Psychology: Human Experimental Psychology, 48A*, 108–124.

Towse J. N., Hitch, G. J., & Hutton, U. (1998). A reevaluation of working memory capacity in children. *Journal of Memory and Language, 39*, 195-217.

van der Lely, H. K. J. (1998). SLI in Children: Movement, Economy, and Deficits in the Computational-Syntactic System. *Language Acquisition, 7 (2-4)*, 161-192.

van der Lely, H. K. J. (2001). Past tense morphology in specifically language impaired and normally developing children. *Language and Cognitive Processes, 16 (2 & 3)*, 177–217.

van der Lely, H., & Howard, D. (1993). Children with specific language impairment: Linguistic impairment or short-term memory deficit? *Journal of Speech and Hearing Research, 36*, 1193–1207.

Vasic, N., Lohr, C., Steinbrink, C., Martin, C., & Wolf, R. C. (2007). Neural correlates of working memory performance in adolescents and young adults with dyslexia. *Neuropsychologia, 46 (2)*, 640-648.

Verguts, T. & De Boeck, P. (2002). On the correlation between working memory capacity and performance on intelligence tests. *Learning and Individual Differences 13*, 37–55.

Walker, I. & Hulme, C. (1999). Concrete words are easier to recall than abstract words: Evidence for a semantic contribution to short-term serial recall. Journal of Experimental Psychology: Learning, Memory, and Cognition, 25, 1256- 1271.

Wechsler, D. (1974). *Wechsler Intelligence Scale for Children–Revised.* San Antonio, TX: The Psychological Corporation.

Westermann, G., Mareschal, D., Johnson, M. H., Sirois, S., Spratling, M. W., & Thomas, M. S. C. (2007). Neuroconstructivism. *Developmental Science, 10 (1)*, 75-83.

Willis, C. S., & Gathercole, S. E. (2001). Phonological short-term memory contributions to sentence processing in young children. *Memory, 9*, 349–364.

Zelazzo, P. D., Muller, U., Frye, D., & Marcovitch, S. (2003). *The development of executive function in early childhood. Monographs of the Society for Research in Child Language Development*, 68.

In: Children and Language: Development, Impairment … ISBN 978-1-60692-395-5
Editor: Michael A. Reed

Chapter 6

READY FOR TOMORROW'S INTERNATIONAL WORLD: CONTENT AND LANGUAGE INTEGRATED LEARNING (CLIL) PROVIDING CHILDREN WITH GOOD FIRST AND FOREIGN LANGUAGE SKILLS

Tuula Merisuo-Storm
Department of Teacher Education, University of Turku, Finland

ABSTRACT

The study described in the article investigated the effects of bilingual teaching (Content and Language Integrated Learning, CLIL) on the development of children's literacy skills during their first six school years. In the CLIL classes 20–25 per cent of the instruction was given in a foreign language. The results of the study showed that the children in the CLIL classes learned to read and write their first language equally well than their peers in monolingual classes. In addition, bilingual teaching did not have a negative effect on the development of those children who started school with poor learning readiness either. After the two first study years the children in the CLIL classes were more fluent readers and had better reading comprehension and spelling skills than their peers in the other classes.

After four school years it was obvious that the children's creative writing skills had also benefited from bilingual teaching. The students in the CLIL classes had learned to pay attention to languages, as well to their mother tongue as to other languages. Moreover, they had more positive attitudes towards reading, writing and foreign language learning. Especially the boys' attitudes proved to be more positive in the CLIL classes than in the other classes.

After six study years the students in the CLIL classes had achieved significantly better first language spelling skills than the students in the other classes. They made significantly less spelling errors and understood significantly better different texts. Furthermore, they showed more proficiency in deriving the meaning of new words from the written context than the other students. Likewise, they succeeded significantly better in finding the most important facts of the non-fiction text and summarising the text than their peers in the other classes. It is worth mentioning that in the other classes the girls' skills were significantly better than the boys' skills but in CLIL classes the difference was not significant. The students in the CLIL classes enjoyed studying the foreign language and also studying through it. Consequently, their foreign language skills developed very well.

INTRODUCTION

A good command of the mother tongue is considered the basis of all learning. There is not an area in curriculum that does not demand an ability to read and write. Reading skills, including being capable of discovering the meaning and of finding information in written texts, and learning to remember this information and to relate it to previous knowledge, are the necessary tools for the study of any school subject. The older the students get the more they need reading skills to acquire new information and the more complex texts they have to be able to comprehend. In addition, students have to achieve good foreign language skills to be able to manage in today's international world. The use of a foreign language as the medium of instruction has proved to be an effective method of developing versatile language skills. The results of the study described in this article showed that also students' first language skills benefit from bilingual education.

CONTENT AND LANGUAGE INTEGRATED LEARNING (CLIL)

The acronym *CLIL (Content and Language Integrated Learning)* is the platform for a methodological approach of far broader scope than language teaching. It seeks to develop proficiency as well in a non-language subject as in the language through which it is taught. In addition, achieving this dual aim demands a special approach to teaching. In CLIL education the non-language subject is not taught in a foreign language but with and through a foreign language. This involves a more integrated approach to teaching and learning. Consequently, the teachers should not only consider how languages should be taught but also give special thought to the educational process in general. (Content and Language Integrated Learning at School in Europe 2005, p. 7.)

The goal in CLIL education is to ensure that students acquire knowledge of subject matter and simultaneously develop their competence in a foreign language. In Finland the important aims related to CLIL education are:

- providing students facilities for life in an internationalised society
- enabling students to develop effective foreign language communication skills and motivating them to learn languages by using them for genuine practical purposes
- enabling students to extend subject-related knowledge and learning skills and enhancing the assimilation of subject matter by use of a different and innovative approach (Content and Language Integrated Learning at School in Europe 2005, p. 22.)

Language learning becomes meaningful and efficient when the student receives new information through the medium of a foreign language and can practise language in real communicative situations and discussions. He or she has extensive opportunities to hear language used by others and use it himself of herself in purposeful ways. In addition, content-based language teaching provides more time for students in contact with a foreign language while only minimally decreasing the amount of time assigned for non-language subjects. CLIL can also provide opportunities for students to gain cultural understanding and skills in knowing how to communicate with people from foreign countries. (Met 2004, p. 217; Richards & Rodgers 2001, p. 207.)

In the Action plan 2004–2006 of the Commission of the European Communities for promoting language learning and linguistic diversity it is stated: "CLIL has a major contribution to make to the Union's language learning goals. It can provide effective opportunities for students to use their language skills now rather than learn them now for later use." Therefore the schools that wish to introduce a content and language integrated learning approach should receive increased support. (Commission of the European Communities 2003.) Largely due to the language policy of the European Commission, CLIL has increased its popularity during the last ten years.

The study reported below was conducted in Finland, a country in Northern Europe with approximately five million inhabitants. Finnish language is a Finno-Ugric language, which is very different from the major languages spoken by hundreds of millions of people in the world. Therefore, the Finns need ability to use foreign languages in communication with people from other countries. Already since the 1970s more than 90 per cent of schoolchildren in Finland have studied English as a foreign language, and at the beginning of the 1990s a national decision was made to allow instruction through a language other than the official languages of the country (Finnish, Swedish or Sami) in general education. In recent years there has been a vast increase, at all levels of education, from kindergarten to higher education to use English, Swedish, French, German and Russian as a language of instruction. However, English is by far the most popular one. (Järvinen 2005, pp. 437–438; Nikula 2007, p. 206; Nikula 2005, pp. 27–28.)

In many Finnish schools development of CLIL has started as an experiment of individual teachers who have had interest in this form of teaching. Consequently, CLIL is not an elite school phenomenon in Finland. Forms of CLIL have been offered in schools across the country, as well in rural as in urban areas. In addition, parents encourage schools to start bilingual teaching, as they wish their children to obtain a good basis for language proficiency and courage to communicate in a foreign language. In most cases students' participation in CLIL education is voluntary, especially if a large part of the teaching takes place through a foreign language. Therefore, students participating in it are generally interested in language learning. (Merisuo-Storm 2007a, p. 228; Nikula 2005, p. 31.)

CLIL provides for the students opportunities to hear and use foreign language in a meaningful context. When teaching a subject through a foreign language the teacher should use illustrative and concrete teaching methods in order to make understanding and learning process easier. Language that is used to convey subject matter needs to be highlighted in a manner that makes certain features more salient to learners. Although the teaching is lucid and concise, occasionally it is necessary to use students' mother tongue to clarify the contents. Especially for young children some contents can be taught first in their first language and afterwards in a foreign language. (Nikula & Marsh 1997, pp. 52–54.) It is also necessary to repeat same concepts several times in various ways. Sometimes it may be difficult for a struggling or a young learner to understand teaching, which is given through a foreign language, but if the teacher uses familiar, repetitious routines and structures of instruction, he or she can predict what will happen next. Important components of teaching for instance, phrases and expressions related to the school day, are repeated day after day. Games, songs, stories and nursery rhymes are excellent means for learning new words and phrases. (Merisuo-Storm 2007a, pp. 227–228; Merisuo-Storm 2002, p. 31.)

According to a study conducted by Nikula and Marsh (1997, pp. 110–111) students in CLIL classes *learn contents of non-language subjects* equally well as their peers who study them in their mother tongue. Furthermore, they found out that for some students their interest in language learning has motivated them to put more effort also in subject matter learning. Nevertheless, some educators are concerned that teaching through a foreign language can effect negatively the development of children's first language reading and writing skills. Good reading skills are the necessary tools for studying almost any school subject. Furthermore, writing skills are necessary for learning, thinking and communication. For a student writing is a learning tool of various school subjects and skills. Therefore, a student's writing problems can hinder his or her learning of other essential skills and lead to more widespread learning disabilities. (Mäki 2002, p. 11.)

2. Reading comprehension

Three key issues related to the growth of a student's reading skills are developing fluency, expanding comprehension, and broadening vocabulary. These components overlap and each supports the others. Reading fluency involves the ability to read text accurately and quickly, and one of the primary advances in literacy development is made when a young reader is able to proceed from slowly sounding out every word to reading words rapidly and accurately. Fluent reading includes decoding with facility, automatic word identification, and expressiveness in reading. When a student is capable of reading most of a text fluently he or she can focus on comprehension rather than on deciphering individual words. (Barone, Mallette & Xu 2005, p. 114.)

Comprehension is a *multidimensional thinking process*: the reader has to construct meaning by interacting with text using his or her previous knowledge and experience and the information that can be found in the text. The understanding of the text may vary greatly because interpretation is unique to the reader. While reading a text a reader activates his or her previous knowledge about the topic. The more background information connected to the text a reader has, the more easily he or she will comprehend the text. Meaning constructed from the same text may differ greatly among readers. It is possible that a reader does not have knowledge enough about the topic or he or she is not able to use his or her experiential backgrounds. In addition, he or she may not be able to use the clues the text offers. Other factors that influence a reader's interaction are, for example, how well the text is written, how easy it is to read, how closely it follows the conventions of its genre or structure, the language it is written in, and even the type and the size of font. (Blair-Larsen & Vallance 2004, p. 37.)

Reading is thinking based on the cues that a text provides. Skilful readers are able to find essential information from the text. Accurate comprehension is necessary when reading non-fiction but also when reading fiction. In non-fiction, a reader needs to understand the topic, learn new facts, and be able to locate and keep in mind important information. (Scharer, Pinnell, Lyons & Fountas 2005, p. 25.) Different types of texts have a different kind of structure. Expository texts can involve several patterns for instance, description, sequence, compare–contrast, cause–effect, and problem solution. Narrative texts usually follow a general structural pattern called story grammar. Children develop already before school age sensitivity to narrative structure and they use it to understand simple stories. They pay attention on the setting (time, place, and characters), problems or conflicts (actions and reactions of the characters), and the story resolution when reading. However, skilful comprehension involves generalisation beyond the characters and the events of the story to the people and the events in real life. Furthermore, expository texts are usually more difficult to understand because they contain many different structures and they more often involve unfamiliar content. In addition, most parents read more often stories than non-fiction to young children. (Williams 2005, p. 7.) Reutzel, Smith and Fawson (2005, pp. 277–278) argue that research has clearly shown that young children do not get many opportunities of reading and writing information texts in school either. However, integrating the instruction of comprehension strategies to learning information in content areas could be an effective manner of proceeding.

Skilful readers use *comprehension strategies* to make the construction of meaning easier. These strategies can provide access to knowledge that is beyond a reader's personal experience. Students that preview, activate their prior knowledge, predict, make connections, monitor, organise, summarise, ask questions, and visualise, are likely to understand the text. Researchers suggest that using such strategies helps students to become meta-cognitive readers. To become a skilful comprehender, a reader needs to learn to choose appropriate strategies depending on the content of the text and its level of difficulty. When reading a difficult text, the reader needs to consciously direct the process of meaning construction. (Bimmel & van Schooten 2004, p. 86; McLaughlin 2006, p. 6.)

Van der Schoot, Vasbinder, Horseley and van Lieshout (2008, p. 220) found out in their study that more and less skilful 10–12-year-old comprehenders differ in their use of reading strategies. More successful comprehenders spent more time in processing important than unimportant text elements but the less successful comprehenders used equally long time processing important and unimportant elements of text. They suggest that this shows that skilful comprehenders construct meaning actively and less skilful comprehenders are more passive readers. In addition, the more skilful comprehenders constructed an integrated and coherent text model and had no difficulties in tracing back the referent of a referring expression.

Skilled comprehenders are *fluent readers*. Non-fluent reading demands mental capacity that would be needed for comprehension process. However, students can have difficulties in comprehending a text despite being able to read single words correctly. This is due to difficulties located in particular in the higher order skills of making conclusions, forming a logical meaning of a text and monitoring their comprehension. (Hurry & Doctor 2007, p. 44.) In addition, for skilful comprehension the reader needs *extensive vocabulary*, for comprehension does not occur if he or she does not understand the individual words. However, good readers' comprehension processes involve comprehension above the word level. (Pressley 2002, p. 297; Snow, Sweet, Alvermann, Kamil & Stricland 2002, pp. 95, 98.) Increasing vocabulary acquisition has a positive influence in reading comprehension, but also increasing reading practice can increase vocabulary and comprehension. Research has shown that often children with reading disabilities have lower-than-average vocabularies. This is due to the effects of language problems as well as limited exposure to print. It appears that parents have an important role in children's vocabulary growth, especially before third school year. (Biemiller 2003, p. 326.)

Written language is lexically richer than spoken language, and when children become more fluent readers they start reading texts that include many words that are not part of their oral vocabulary. It is a demanding task for a young reader to *derive the meaning of an unknown word* from the written context. If the word is related to a familiar concept it may be a simple synonym. However, the word can refer to unknown concepts. Furthermore, contexts do not always reveal the full meaning of a word, even when explicit clues are present. Sometimes the context is even misleading. It is necessary that the reader also analyses the text to distinguish the relevant clues from the irrelevant ones. Sometimes children produce incorrect definitions of words because they select irrelevant information or only part of the relevant context from the text. (Cain 2007, pp. 348–349.) Additionally, the difficulty of deriving the meaning of a word from the context is connected to the concreteness of the unfamiliar concept. (Fukkink 2005, p. 24.) In the study conducted by Fukkink, Blok, and de Glopper (2001, p. 409) the effect of concreteness proved to be especially strong for the young students.

In non-fiction texts, a reader often has to put together information from several idea units, which can be found in different places throughout a passage. The longer the distance between the pieces of information the more difficult it is to integrate them. A student's small memory capacity makes the process even more demanding. (Cain, Oakhill & Lemmon 2004, p. 672.) It is also necessary to understand that students cannot be expected to give dictionary-like definitions of the unfamiliar words that the text includes.

Summarising is a very demanding comprehension strategy. Many students have great difficulties in determining which are the main ideas and themes in a text as well as in integrating similar ideas, and synthesising them into a coherent whole. Therefore, they often repeat most of the text or give a very vague statement. Nevertheless, a good summary should give a complete picture of the text but include only the important parts. When the students become older they have to use more and more often comprehension skills to acquire new information. After reading a text they are expected to remember the main ideas and concepts of it. (Swanson & De La Paz 1998.)

WRITING

During the first six grades students spend plenty of time in rehearsing spelling, handwriting, and composing stories and other texts. They learn to use writing as a tool of communication. When spelling, a child has to be able to connect a phoneme with a corresponding grapheme and to use language-specific spelling rules. In addition, adequate visual-motor coordination is needed for handwriting. A student may have difficulties in manipulating and guiding the pen. Poor spelling is often combined with untidy handwriting. When letter formation is difficult, a student has to focus on the motor requisites for writing. As a result, less capacity is left for spelling. (Mäki 2002, pp. 11, 19; Pollock & Waller 1997, p. 81.)

Writing in Finnish Language

In Finnish language there is a close correspondence between sounds and letters. Therefore, children learn a spelling strategy that enables them to write any word needed. However, in Finnish words there are many double consonants and vowels and often a word can be distinguished from another word with the difference between short and long sounds (e.g. *'uni'* – *'uuni'* [dream – oven]; *'kisa'* – *'kissa'* [sports event – cat]; *'liina'* – *'linna'* [scarf – castle]; *'siili'* – *'silli'* [hedgehog – herring]). (Mäki 2002, p. 12.) There are also several groups of words that are almost the same but have very different meanings (e.g. *'muta'* – *'mutta'* – *'muuta'* – *'muuttaa'* [mud – but – something else – move]). If a child has difficulties in auditory discrimination this can be quite confusing and cause spelling errors.

In addition, in Finnish language there is a large number of very long words and compound words that are written as one word and often children have difficulties in writing them correctly (e.g. *'omenamehu'* [apple juice], *'urheilutapahtuma'* [sports event], *'talviurheilutapahtuma'* [winter sports event], and *'kevättalviurheilutapahtuma'* [late winter sports event]). The meaning of a word can change if its parts are written separate (e.g. *'äidinkieli'* [mother tongue] – *'äidin kieli'* [mother's tongue], *'kirkonkello'* [church bell] – *'kirkon kello'* [clock in a church], and *'isoisä'* [grandfather] – *'iso isä'* [a big father]. (Merisuo-Storm 2007b, p. 376.)

Creative Writing

The process of writing includes planning, translating and reviewing. Planning consists of idea generating, translating of text generating and transcription, and reviewing of evaluating and revising. Good writers should be able to construct meaningful sentences that express their ideas, emotions and views appropriately and in a creative and mature style. In addition, they should be able to use grammatically accurate language and adequate syntactic, morphological and semantic elements in their texts. (Berninger, Abbot, Whitaker, Sylvester & Nolen 1995, p. 295; Hurry & Doctor 2007, p. 40.)

More than twenty years ago Heikkilä and Kantola (1983, pp. 124–131) described Yamamoto's assessment system of children's stories from the nineteen sixties. Yamamoto's main criteria of assessment included individual style and interesting contents. The positive characteristics of a fictional text that Kantola herself listed were: it is imaginative, illustrative, it includes surprises and different ideas, it has an original but clear structure, it has rhythm – and also changes of rhythm – and the language is rich and colourful. In addition, the story has different layers and it shows that the author has a sensitive and inquiring mind, a personal view, individual writing style, a sense of humour, and he or she skilfully connects and compares different ideas. (Heikkilä & Kantola 1983, pp. 157–158.)

Nelson, Bahr and Van Meter (2004) suggest that when beginning the assessment of a student's narrative one should pay attention to the story structure; how the elements are combined and do they create a clear, logical, and interesting story. In addition, one should consider how well the text conveys meaning to a reader. The assessment can be guided with e.g. following questions: Is the story interesting? Does it make sense? Has the writer met his or her intended goals successfully? Is the story congruent with the given instructions. After that one should focus on the productivity and fluency, discourse structure and maternity, and cohesion. In addition, one should bear in mind that a long story is not always a better story than a short one. However, the length of a story can indicate that the writer creates text with facility. Students who have difficulties in composing a story use often short and simple sentences. (Nelson et al. 2004, pp. 379–382.)

Most seven-year-old children are capable of inventing stories with a plot. Their stories include a beginning, characters with a problem to solve or injustice to redress, and a description of how the characters try to solve the problems and how they succeed in that. By the time the children reach nine years they are usually able to describe several characters' observations and feelings in their narratives. The combination of structural elements produces a story structure that is familiar and predictable. In Western European cultures, the most common story type includes seven story grammar elements: 1) setting (time, place, and characters), 2) problem or conflict that sets events of the story in motion, 3) character's feelings in response of the problem, 4) statement of ideas or plans to address the problem, 5) action taken to solve the problem, 6) resolution or outcome, and 7) story closing and ending. (Nelson et al. 2004, pp. 379–385.)

THE STUDY

The goal of the study was to find out if bilingual education affects the development of students' first language literacy skills negatively or if children in CLIL education achieve the same level of literacy as their peers who study exclusively in Finnish. The development of the students' reading and writing skills in three bilingual CLIL classes and in three monolingual classes were observed from the beginning of first grade to the end of sixth grade. At the beginning of the first school year in these classes there were 138 students, 78 of them studied in the CLIL classes and 58 in the other classes. In the CLIL classes 20–25 per cent of the teaching was in English. All students came from Finnish-speaking families.

The study included five measurements during six years. The students' starting level was measured at the beginning of first grade, when they were six or seven years old. *The initial test* was used to measure the students' general level of school readiness, auditory and visual perception, mathematic skills and memory. The results showed that the students studying in the CLIL classes had, as a group, better initial skills than the other students. This was due to the entrance procedures for the CLIL classes. However, it should also be pointed out that although the students studying in the bilingual classes showed, as a group, a higher starting level, there were on one hand also in the control group students who showed excellent performance in the initial test and on the other hand in the CLIL classes students who had poor initial skills.

Three reading tests were used to measure the students' reading skills at the end of the first, the second, and the sixth school year. *The first and the second grade reading tests* included reading aloud and reading comprehension tasks and *the sixth grade reading test* measured the students ability to comprehend different kinds of texts. The students' spelling skills were measured with *the first, the second, and the sixth grade writing from dictation tests*. When the children were in fourth grade the focus was on their *creative writing skills*. All the measurements were performed in class, and on average no more than one lesson (45 minutes) was used during the same day for measurements. The test results were analysed using an SPPS program. The results may have been somewhat effected by the loss in the number of the students. In the end of the sixth school year only 60 per cent of the students (n=134) were the same as in the beginning of the first school year. However, it is worth mentioning that in the CLIL classes the wastage rate of the students was notably smaller than in the other classes. The families were in most cases so happy to have their children in a CLIL class that they did not want to move them to another school.

Spelling

After the first school year there was no great difference between the bilingual group and the monolingual group in regard to the number of errors in the writing from dictation test. However, after two study years the students in the CLIL classes made significantly fewer spelling errors than the students in the other classes (t= 4.83, p= .000). Furthermore, in the last weeks of the sixth school year the students in CLIL classes had significantly better spelling skills than their peers in monolingual classes (t= 4.22, p= .000). There was a strong correlation between the results of the sixth grade spelling test and the spelling tests of first and second grade (r= .44, p= .000; r= .65, p= .000). Figure 1 shows the results of the sixth grade spelling test (10= no mistakes,..., 4= plenty of mistakes). In the CLIL classes 22 per cent of the students and only 10 per cent of the students in the other classes had excellent marks (9 or 10). In the other classes 10 per cent of the students had made so many errors in the writing from dictation task that their marks were very poor (4). No one in the CLIL classes had performed equally poorly in the task.

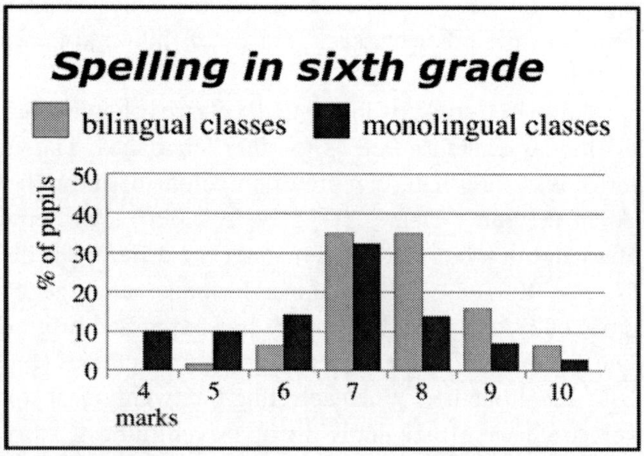

Figure 1. The percentage distribution of the students' marks of the writing from dictation test in the bilingual (CLIL) classes and the monolingual classes (10 = no mistakes .... 4 = plenty of mistakes).

In monolingual classes the girls' marks were significantly better than the boys' marks but this was not the case in the CLIL classes. Moreover, the boys' marks in the CLIL classes were significantly better than the boys' marks in the other classes but there was no significant difference in the marks of the girls of the two groups.

In sixth grade the most common errors in the students' papers were compound word mistakes and capital letter mistakes. It seems, however, that the different ways of writing compound words and using capital letters in Finnish and English had not increased the number of these errors in the CLIL classes. On the contrary, the students in the monolingual classes made them significantly more often ($t= -3.37$, $p= .001$; $t= -4.46$, $p= .000$) than the students in the CLIL classes.

Creative Writing

In fourth grade the focus of the study was on the students' creative writing. The students were asked to write a story about someone's journey to a destination that was very different from where he or she lived. The instructions for the task were as follows: The writer should invent the title of the story himself or herself. The main character of the story could be the writer himself or herself, another person, an animal, or an imaginary character. The destination of the journey could be either an existing location or an imaginary place. The inhabitants there spoke a foreign language. Moreover, the writers were encouraged to use colourful and rich language, and invent interesting and amusing events. The students wrote the stories in class and the time for the task was not limited.

The most apparent differences between the stories composed by the students in the CLIL classes and in the other classes were related to the writers' consciousness of the existence of different languages. It was obvious that languages played a more important role in the lives of the children studying in the CLIL classes than for their peers in the other classes. For instance, 60 per cent of them mentioned the different language of the new place in their stories, but in the other classes only 21 per cent did this. In addition, in 41 per cent of their stories the inhabitants of the new place used in the dialogues language that the authors themselves had invented. In the other classes, phrases of this kind appeared only in six per cent of the stories.

The stories composed by the students in the CLIL classes showed that they had learned to pay attention to their first language as well as to other languages. The Finnish language that they used in their stories was significantly more often colourful and rich than the language in the stories composed in the other classes ($t= 5.19$, $p= .000$). Furthermore, they described significantly more often and in a more detailed manner the differences between home and the new place ($t= -5.17$, $p= .000$), as well as the appearance and the characteristics of the characters ($t= -3.15$, $p= .002$), and in addition, they had expressed original thoughts or clever remarks significantly more often than the students in the other classes ($t= 3.94$, $p= .000$).

There were 138 stories altogether. When selecting the twenty best stories out of them, the main criteria that were used were their individuality, eventfulness, story structure, rich and colourful language, and fluency of narration. The attention was also paid to the fashion in which the author sketched the difference between home and the new place and described the characters of the story, and whether he or she had shown original thinking or made clever remarks. Each of these features were scored from 0 to 2. For instance, assessing the description of the story characters: 0 = no description, 1 = description of the persons' physical appearance or personality, 2 = description of both of the qualities of the persons. When describing the new place the writer could sketch the environment and the different language spoken there. Score 2 was given if both were found in the text. The other criteria were assessed from 0 to 2 according to the quality or the degree of the aspect assessed. Of the twenty stories that best met these criteria, seventeen came from the CLIL classes and only three from the other classes.

Reading

After the first and the second school year the students in the CLIL classes read with greater accuracy and speed than the students in the other classes. After two years in school especially the reading comprehension skills were significantly better in the CLIL classes than in the other classes (t= 7.10, p= .000). When observing the students who started school with a poor level of school readiness or the students who started school with an excellent level of school readiness, there was no significant difference in regard to the development of literacy skills between the bilingual and the monolingual group.

During the last weeks of the sixth school year the students' reading comprehension skills were measured with a test that consisted of three different texts. In addition, the focus was on the students' ability to derive the meaning of a word from the written context and to summarise a text. The first text was a story written by H.C. Andersen, the second a newspaper article about H.C. Andersen, and the third a non-fiction text about orang-utans and their living conditions in today's world.

H.C. Andersen's story was called *"What the old man does is always right"*. After reading the story the students answered 20 questions. To some questions it was easy to find answers in the text. However, there were several more demanding questions, such as *"What were the main characters like?"* The most difficult questions to answer were those in which the students had to put together more than one peace of information from the text. The question about the title, *"What is the title based on?"* was very difficult. Although most students understood that the man in the story did many very foolish things, they accepted the title as a fact. Only 30 per cent of them mentioned that it was only an expression that his wife used or that it was her opinion about the matter. In this section of the test the difference between the two groups was not significant (t= 2.21, p= .029, Figure 2). However, the students in the CLIL classes proved to have heard or read more Andersen's stories than their peers in the other classes. They could significantly more often produce a title of another story by Andersen. The difference between the two groups was significant (t= 4.11, p= .000).

The second text in the reading comprehension test was *a newspaper article about H.C. Andersen*. The title of the article was "In the large footsteps of H.C. Andersen". After reading the article the students' task was to answer ten questions and explain the meaning of ten words picked from the text. In these tasks the students in the CLIL classes performed significantly better than the students in the other classes (t= 3.16, p= .002, Figure 3). Their scores varied from 20 to 8 and the scores of the students in the other classes from 19 to 3.

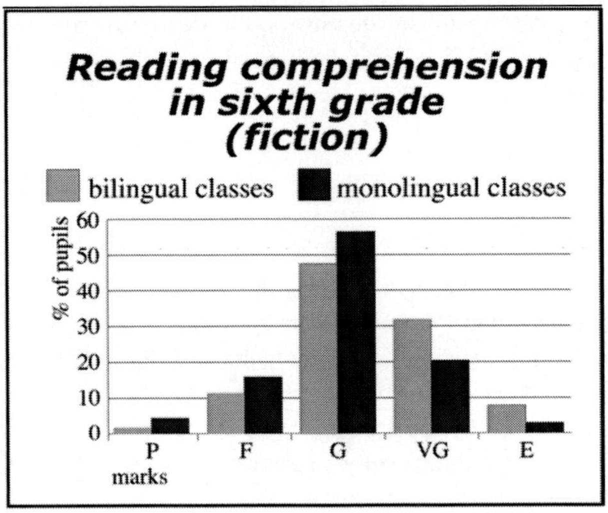

Figure 2. The percentage distribution of the students' marks in the fiction section of the reading comprehension test in the bilingual and the monolingual classes in sixth grade (p= poor, f= fair, g= good, vg= very good, e= excellent)

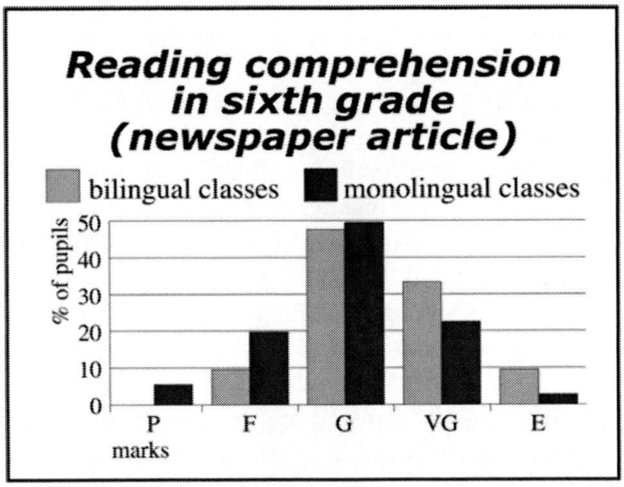

Figure 3. The percentage distribution of the students' marks in the newspaper text section of the reading comprehension test in the bilingual and the monolingual classes in sixth grade (p= poor, f= fair, g= good, vg= very good, e= excellent)

Also in this section the most difficult questions to answer were those in which the students had to integrate more than one peace of information from the text. The last question *"Which two things does the expression 'in the large footsteps' in the title of the article refer to?"* was most demanding. It was mentioned in the text that Andersen's shoe size was 47. In addition, the students had to understand that the phrase in question could also refer to the fact that Andersen was a great author, who is famous all over the world. Only 28 per cent of the students (33% in the CLIL classes and 24 % in the other classes) produced the right answer.

The ten words that the students had to explain could be found in the article. The students were asked to write what the words meant in this particular text. As was mentioned above, deriving the meaning of an unknown word from the written context is a demanding task. Some words proved to be especially difficult. In addition, it was obvious that all students were not capable to take the advantage of the clues in the text. Consequently, several students gave an explanation that the word has in some other context. The most difficult word appeared to be *'välähdys'* ['a glimpse'] in a sentence "Ne näyttävät vierailijalle *välähdyksiä* kirjailijan elämän arkisistakin puolista". ["They show the visitor *glimpses* of the author's everyday life."] In this context the word 'välähdys' means 'a glimpse of something' but in a different context the same word means 'a flash' or 'a gleam'. Some students did not pay attention to the context and gave a false explanation. This was the case significantly more often in the monolingual classes than in the CLIL classes (t= 3.57, p= .000).

The students in the CLIL classes succeeded also significantly better than the other students in explaining the word *'kohde'* (t= 4.00, p= .000). In many occasions it could be translated into English as 'a target' but in this context it meant a place where visitors could see or hear something connected to Andersen's life or work. On the whole, the students in the CLIL classes produced significantly more often a correct explanation for the ten words (t= 4.11, p= .000).

The third section of the test proved to be the most difficult. The students were asked to read *a non-fiction text* about orang-outans and their living conditions in today's world and then write a five-sentence summary of it. It was stressed that the summary should include the most essential aspects of the text. In the CLIL classes there was no difference in the results of the three sections of the test. However, in the other classes finding the most important facts in the text and summing them up into five sentences appeared to be significantly more difficult than answering the questions in the two previous sections. In the CLIL classes almost half of the students (48 %) and in the other classes only 11 per cent of the students achieved excellent or very good marks in this section. In contrast, in the monolingual classes almost half of the students' marks (46 %) were poor or fair but only 13 per cent of the students in the bilingual classes succeeded as poorly in summarising the text. The difference between the marks of the two groups was significant (t= 5.80, p= .000, Figure 4).

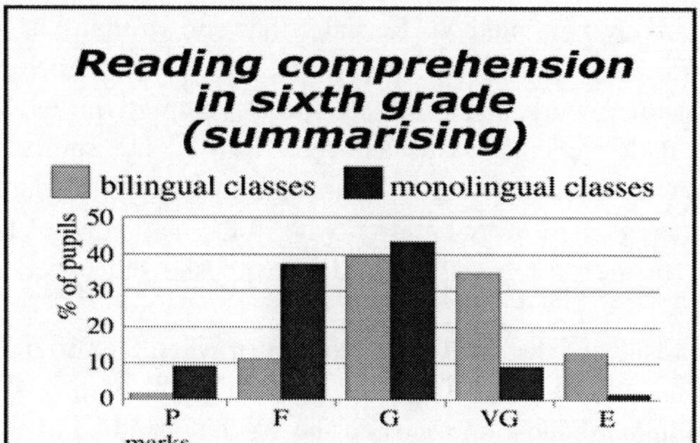

Figure 4. The percentage distribution of the students' marks in the non-fiction and summarising section of the reading comprehension test in the bilingual and the monolingual classes in sixth grade (p= poor, f= fair, g= good, vg= very good, e= excellent)

Conclusion

The results of the study showed that bilingual education had not effected the development of the students' literacy skills negatively. After six study years the students in the CLIL classes had achieved significantly better spelling skills than the students in the other classes. Furthermore, the dissimilarities in spelling English and Finnish language did not seem to cause errors in writing Finnish. For instance, the different ways of writing compound words and using capital letters in the two languages had not increased the number of these errors in the CLIL classes. On the contrary, the students in the CLIL classes made them significantly less than the students in the other classes.

The students in the CLIL classes had learned to pay attention to languages, as well to their mother tongue as to other languages. They were aware of several similarities and dissimilarities in the languages. For instance, in fourth grade the most distinguishable differences between the stories composed in the CLIL classes and in the other classes were related to the writers' consciousness of the existence of different languages. It was obvious that languages played a more important role in the lives of the students studying in the CLIL classes than for the students in the other classes.

In addition, in sixth grade the students in the CLIL classes understood different texts better than their peers in the other classes. They succeeded equally well in comprehending non-fiction, fiction and newspaper texts while the students in the other classes had much more difficulties in understanding the non-fiction text and the newspaper article than the narrative text. The students in the CLIL classes showed also more proficiency in deriving the meaning of new words from the written context than the other students. In addition, they succeeded significantly better in finding the most important facts of the non-fiction text and summarising the text than their peers in the other classes.

Still, when assessing the results of the study it is necessary to keep in mind certain facts: Firstly, most parents whose children studied in the CLIL classes were interested in their children's studies and sought to help them to succeed in them. They attended parent–teacher meetings more often than parents on average. Furthermore, it is possible that they encouraged their children to read and write also outside school more often than other parents. All this has had a positive effect on the children's development. Secondly, teaching through two languages is a relatively new method. Research has shown that when teachers start using a new teaching method they put more effort to their work. The teachers in the CLIL classes were interested in their work and motivated to develop it further. This may have had a positive effect in their students' skills as well. Thirdly, the students in the CLIL classes showed, as a group, a higher starting level in the initial test six years earlier. Nevertheless, also in the CLIL classes there were children who in the beginning of first grade showed poor starting level and in the other classes children who showed excellent performance in the initial test.

However, the results of the study show that even when the different starting levels of the two groups were taken in account the pupils' reading and writing skills developed at least equally well in bilingual education as when the students studied exclusively in their mother tongue. Furthermore, studying through one or two languages did not appear to have any significant effect on the development of a student's literacy skills when his or her starting level at the beginning of the first school year had been poor of excellent. The results showed that when most of the teaching is carried out in the students' first language, CLIL education does not affect the development of first language skills negatively. Children are able to keep the two languages separate.

When the students were in fourth grade they took part also in a study that aimed to find out what kind of attitudes they had towards reading, writing, and foreign language learning (Merisuo-Storm 2007a). The results of the study revealed that in the CLIL classes the students' attitudes towards language learning were more positive than the attitudes of their peers in the monolingual classes. Although the boys, at the age of ten, did not appear to be as interested in reading and writing as the girls, the difference between the attitudes of the two genders was not as apparent in the CLIL classes as in the other classes. Moreover, in the monolingual classes there was a significant difference between the boys' and the girls' attitudes towards language learning, whereas this was not the case in the CLIL classes.

After having used the English language in an everyday context for four years the students in the CLIL classes found speaking and writing in English and hearing and reading it natural. Moreover, they did not feel uncomfortable studying through it. Consequently, their attitudes towards foreign language learning were more positive than the pupils' attitudes in the other classes and therefore also their foreign language skills developed very well. The results of the study showed that especially boys benefited of bilingual education. In the CLIL classes boys' attitudes towards reading, writing and language learning were more positive than the attitudes of the boys in the other classes.

In Finland students move after six school years to secondary school. There they need versatile reading and writing skills to be able to acquire effectively new information, to understand and to summarise more and more complex texts, and to perform various writing tasks. It seemed that the students in the CLIL classes were well prepared for successful studies also in secondary school.

References

Barone, D.M., Mallette, M.H. & Xu, S.H. (2005). *Teaching Early Literacy: Development, Assessment, and Instruction.* New York, NY: The Guilford Press.

Berninger, V.W., Abbott, R.D., Whitaker, D., Sylvester, L. & Nolen, S.B. (1995). Integrating low- and high-level skills in instructional protocols for writing disabilities. *Learning Disability Quarterly 18* (4), 293–309.

Biemiller, A. (2003). Vocabulary: Needed if more children are to read well. *Reading Psychology 24* (3/4), 323–335.

Bimmel, P. & van Schooten, E. (2004). The relationship between strategic reading activities and reading comprehension. *L1 – Educational Studies in Language and Literature 4* (1), 85–102.

Blair-Larsen, S.M. & Vallance, K.M. (2004). Comprehension Instruction in a Balanced Reading Classroom. In S.M. Blair-Larsen & K.A. Williams (Eds.) *The Balanced Reading Program: Helping All Students Achieve Success* (pp. 37–52) Newark, DE: International Reading Association.

Cain, K. (2007). Deriving word meanings from context: does explanation facilitate contextual analysis? *Journal of Research in Reading 30* (4), 347–359.

Cain, K., Oakhill, J. & Lemmon, K. (2004). Individual Differences in the Inference of Word Meanings From Context: The Influence of Reading Comprehension, Vocabulary Knowledge, and Memory Capacity. *Journal of Educational Psychology 96* (4), 671–681.

Commission of the European Communities (2003). *Promoting language learning and linguistic diversity: An action plan 2004–2006. Communication from the Commission to the Council, the European Parliament, the Economic and Social Committee and the Committee of the regions* (COM 449 final). <http://ec.europa.eu/education/doc/official/keydoc/actlang/act_lang_en.pdf>

Content and Language Integrated Learning (CLIL) at School in Europe 2005. Brussels, Belgium: Eurydice.

Fukkink, R.G. (2005). Deriving word meaning from written context: a process analysis. *Learning and Instruction 44* (1), 23–43.

Fukkink, R.G., Blok, H. & de Glopper, K. (2001). Deriving word meaning from written context: A multicomponitial skill. *Language Learning 51* (3), 477–496.

Hannon, P. (1997). *Literacy, Home and School: Research and Practice in Teaching Literacy with Parents.* London, UK: The Falmer Press.

Heikkilä, J. & Kantola, K. (1983). *Luova kirjoittaminen [Creative writing].* Juva, Finland: WSOY.

Hurry, J. & Doctor, E. (2007). Assessing Literacy in Children and Adolescents. *Child and Adolescent Mental Health 12* (1), 38–45.

Järvinen, H-M. (2005). Language learning in content-based instruction. In A. Housen & M. Pierrard (Eds.) *Investigations in Instructed Second Language Acquisition* (pp. 433–456). Berlin, Germany: Mouton de Gruyter.

McLaughlin, M. (2006). *Guided Comprehension in the Primary Grades.* Newark, DE: International Reading Association.

Merisuo-Storm, T. (2007a). Pupils' attitudes towards foreign language learning and the development of literacy skills in bilingual education. *Teaching and Teacher Education 23* (2), 226–235.

Merisuo-Storm, T. (2007b). The development of writing skills of boys and girls during six school years. *Nordisk Pedagogik 27* (4), 373–385.

Merisuo-Storm, T. (2002). *Oppilaan äidinkielen lukemisen ja kirjoittamisen taitojen kehittyminen kaksikielisessä alkuopetuksessa. [The development of pupils' first language literacy skills in bilingual education in first and second grades of the Finnish comprehensive school].* Turku, Finland: University of Turku.

Met, M. (2004). Improving Students' Capacity in Foreign Languages. *Phi Delta Kappan 86* (3), 214–218.

Mäki, H. (2002). *Elements of Spelling and Composition. Studies on Predicting and Supporting Writing Skills in Primary Grades.* Turku, Finland: University of Turku.

Nelson, N.W., Bahr, C.M. & Van Meter, A.M. (2004). *The Writing Lab Approach to Language Instruction and Intervention.* Baltimore, MD: Paul H. Brooks.

Nikula, T. (2007). Speaking English in Finnish content-based classrooms. *World Englishes 26* (2), 206–223.

Nikula, T. (2005). English as an object of study in classrooms: Interactional effects and pragmatic implications. *Linguistics and Education 16* (1), 27–58.

Nikula, T. & Marsh, D. (1997). *Vieraskielisen opetuksen tavoitteet ja toteuttaminen. [Goals and realization of bilingual teaching].* Helsinki, Finland: Opetushallitus.

Pollock, J. & Waller, E. (1997). *Day-to Day Dyslexia in the Classroom.* Revised edition. London, UK: Routledge.

Pressley. M. (2002). Metacognition and Self-Regulated Comprehension. In A.E. Farstrup & S.J. Samuels (Eds.) *What Research Has to Say About Reading Instruction.* (third edition, pp. 291–309) Newark, DE: International Reading Association.

Reutzel, D.R., Smith, J.A. & Fawson, P.C. (2005). An evaluation of two approaches for teaching reading comprehension strategies in the primary years using science information texts. *Early Childhood Research Quarterly 20*, 276–305.

Richards, J.C. & Rodgers, T.S. (2001). *Approaches and methods in language teaching* (second edition). Cambridge, UK: Cambridge University.

Scharer, P.L., Pinnell, G.S., Lyons, C. & Fountas, I. (2005). Becoming an Engaged Reader. *Educational Leadership 63* (2), 24–26.

van der Schoot, M., Vasbinder, A.L., Horsley, T.M. & van Lieshout, E.C.D.M. (2008). The role of two reading strategies in text comprehension: An eye fixation study in primary school children. *Journal of Research in Reading 31* (2), 203–223.

Snow,C. , Sweet, A.P., Alvermann, D.E., Kamil, M.L., & Stricland, D.S. (2002). Formulating a Research Agenda About Reading for Understanding. In A.M. Roller (Ed.) *Comprehensive Reading Instruction Across the Grade Levels. A collection of papers from the Reading Research 2001 Conference* (pp. 88–110). Newark, DE: International Reading Association.

Swanson, P.N. & De La Paz, S. (1998). Teaching effective comprehension strategies to students with learning and reading disabilities. *Intervention in School & Clinic 33* (4), 209–218.

Whitehead, M. (1999). *Supporting Language and Literacy Development in the Early Years.* Buckingham, UK: Open University Press.

Williams, J.P. (2005). Instruction in Reading Comprehension for Primary-Grade Students: A Focus on Text Structure. *The Journal of Special Education 39* (1), 6–18.

In: Children and Language: Development, Impairment ... ISBN 978-1-60692-395-5
Editor: Michael A. Reed

Chapter 7

LANGUAGE DEVELOPMENT IN SPECIAL POPULATIONS: THE CASE OF SELECTIVE MUTISM

Matilda E. Nowakowski*[1]*, Louis A. Schmidt*[1] [1]*,
***Charles E. Cunningham*[2]*, and Angela E. McHolm*[3]**

[1]Department of Psychology, Neuroscience & Behaviour, McMaster University, Hamilton, ON
[2] Department of Psychiatry & Behavioural Neurosciences, McMaster University, Hamilton, ON
[3]Department of Psychology, University of Guelph, Guelph, ON

INTRODUCTION

Selective mutism is a disorder that is characterized by a lack of speech in specific unfamiliar situations or in the presence of unfamiliar individuals despite speaking normally in other situations (APA, 2000). Although the disorder usually first appears in the preschool years (Black & Uhde, 1995; Cunningham, McHolm, Boyle, & Patel, 2004; Dummit, Klein, Tancer, Asche, Martin, & Fairbanks, 1997; Steinhausen & Juzi, 1996), it is typically not diagnosed until the child is between 6.5 to 9 years of age (Ford, Sladesczek, Carlson, & Krochwell, 1998; Kumpulainen, Rasenen, Raaska, & Somppi, 1998; Remschmidt, Poller, Herpertz-Dahlmann, Hennighausen, & Gutenbrunner, 2001; Standart & Le Couteur, 2003). Given that the disorder manifests itself early in development, the child' limited speaking in select situations and its impact on language development warrants careful consideration.

The purpose of the present chapter is to review the literature on language performance in children with selective mutism. The chapter is divided among three sections. In the first section, we provide an overview of selective mutism, including its definition, prevalence, diagnosis, classification, etiology and functional impairment. In section two, we review the

---

[1] Correspondence should be addressed to Dr. Louis A. Schmidt, Department of Psychology, Neuroscience & Behaviour, McMaster University, Hamilton, Ontario, L8S 4K1 Canada; fax: 905-529-6225; email: schmidtl@mcmaster.ca

research that has been conducted to date on language performance in children with selective mutism. We conclude the chapter in section three with a review of possible developmental pathways for the association between selective mutism and language performance as well as implications for future research.

SELECTIVE MUTISM

Definition

The constellation of symptoms presently identified as selective mutism date back to the 19th century (Dummit et al., 1997; Kopp & Gillberg, 1997). In 1877, the German physician Kussmaul first described a disorder in which children failed to speak in certain situations despite having the ability to speak. He termed this disorder 'aphasia voluntaria', emphasizing the belief that these children were voluntarily making the decision to not speak (Dow, Sonies, Scheib, Moss, & Leonard, 1995). Moritz Tramer (1934), a Swiss child psychiatrist, developed the term 'elective mutism' to describe the same constellation of symptoms, again emphasizing the belief that these children were electing not to speak (Dow et al., 1995). Although the International Classification of Diseases and Related Health Problems (ICD; World Health Organization, 1994) has retained the term elective mutism, the 4th Edition of the Diagnostic and Statistical Manual of the American Psychiatric Association (DSM-IV; APA, 1994) has changed the term elective mutism to selective mutism, placing greater focus on the fact that these children fail to speak in specific situations or in the presence of specific individuals and emphasizing that the lack of speech is context-specific.

The hallmark diagnostic characteristic of selective mutism is a persistent lack of speaking in specific social situations (e.g., the school setting), despite speaking normally in other situations (APA, 2000). This lack of speech results in significant functional and educational impairment and is not better explained by a lack of knowledge of the language, a communication disorder, or a pervasive developmental disorder. The lack of speech must persist for a minimum of 1 month, excluding the first month of school, as this is a time when children are often apprehensive, shy, and hesitant to communicate because they are adjusting to new surroundings and expectations (APA, 2000). As well, in immigrant children, it has been suggested that selective mutism should last a minimum of 6 months and be present in both the native and non-native language in order to ensure that the lack of speech is not due to a lack of knowledge of language or a transient reaction to adapting to the new environment (Toppelberg, Tabors, Coggins, Lum, & Burger, 2005).

Selective mutism first appears during the preschool years (Black & Uhde, 1995; Cunningham et al., 2004; Dummit et al., 1997; Steinhausen & Juzi, 1996). It is usually not diagnosed, however, until around 6.5 to 9 years of age (Ford et al., 1998; Kumpulainen et al., 1998; Remschmidt et al., 2001; Standart & Le Couteur, 2003), when the child has been consistently identified as not meeting the expectations for speech and verbal participation in the school setting.

PREVALENCE

The prevalence of selective mutism has been estimated at between 0.7% and 2% (Bergman, Piacentini, & McCracken, 2002; Kopp & Gillberg, 1997; Kumpulainen et al., 1998; Elizur & Perednik, 2003). The differing rates of the disorder across studies are most likely due to the use of differing diagnostic criteria, samples, and ages. For instance, it was not until the DSM-IV that interference with functioning was included as one of the criteria that needed to be met for a diagnosis of selective mutism (Bergman et al., 2002; Cohan, Price, & Stein, 2006; Elizur & Perednik, 2003; Kumpulainen et al., 1998). As well, the age range included in these studies results in different prevalence rates. Studies that use older children will report lower prevalence rates than studies that use younger children, due to the fact that selective mutism is most commonly diagnosed during the early school (Kopp & Gillberg, 1997; Kumpulainen et al., 1998). Studies using clinical samples have also reported lower prevalence rates than studies using school samples, again probably due to the fact that selective mutism presents itself most commonly in the school setting (Standart & Le Couteur, 2003). Most studies have found that selective mutism is slightly more common in females than in males with ratios varying from 1.2-to-1 to 2.6-to-1 (Black & Uhde, 1995; Dummit et al., 1997; Kristensen, 2000; Steinhausen & Juzi, 1996, but not Bergman et al., 2002; Elizur & Perednik, 2003; Cunningham et al., 2006) and has a higher rate among immigrant children (Elizur & Perednik, 2003).

COMORBIDITY AND CLASSIFICATION

Selective mutism is often comorbid with other disorders, including anxiety disorders (Bergman et al., 2002; Cunningham et al., 2004; Cunnigham, McHolm, & Boyle, 2006; Dummit et al., 1997; Manassis, Tannock, Garland, Minde, McInnes, & Clark, 2007; Steinhausen & Juzi, 1996; Vecchio & Kearney, 2005; Yeganeh, Beidel, & Turner, 2006; Yeganeh, Beidel, Turner, Pina, & Silverman, 2003), communication disorders (Dummit et al., 1997), developmental delay (Elizur & Perednik, 2003; Kristensen, 2000; Steinhausen & Juzi, 1996), oppositional defiant disorder (Steinhausen & Juzi, 1996; Yeganeh et al., 2006), and elimination disorders (Kristensen, 2000; Steinhausen & Juzi, 1996). Selective mutism is currently classified under the other disorders of infancy, childhood and adolescence in the Fourth Revised Edition of the Diagnostic and Statistical Manual (DSM-IV-R; APA, 2000). There is, however, much debate in the literature as to the accuracy of this classification with many researchers suggesting that selective mutism should be classified as an anxiety disorder (Andstendig, 1999; Sharp, Sherman, & Gross, 2007; Vecchio & Kearney, 2005), or, even more specifically, as a variant of social phobia (Yeganeh et al., 2006). These arguments are based on studies that have found high rates of comorbidity between selective mutism and anxiety disorders, especially social phobia (Black & Uhde, 1995; Dummit et al., 1997; Vecchio & Kearney, 2005), higher rates of family histories of social phobia in children with selective mutism (Black & Uhde, 1995; Kumpulainen, 2002; Schwartz, Freedy, & Sheridan, 2006), and higher rates of anxiety disorders in adolescents and adults with a childhood history of selective mutism (Joseph, 1999).

Using clinical samples, researchers have found high rates of comorbid anxiety disorders in children with selective mutism (Black & Uhde, 1995; Dummit et al., 1997; Vecchio & Kearney, 2005). For instance, in a large clinical sample of 50 children, Dummit and colleagues (1997) found that, of the children with selective mutism, 100% had a comorbid diagnosis of social phobia while approximately 50% had a diagnosis of a second anxiety disorder. Similarly, Black and Uhde (1995) found that in a sample of thirty children with selective mutism, 97% had a comorbid diagnosis of social phobia. Furthermore, longitudinal research has shown that adults and adolescents with a history of selective mutism experience higher rates of social phobia, shyness, and social difficulties even when they overcome the selective mutism (Joseph, 1999; Remschmidt et al., 2001). Family studies have also found that the parents of children with selective mutism have higher rates of anxiety disorders, especially social phobia (Black & Uhde, 1995; Schwartz, Freedy, & Sheridan, 2006; Steinhausen, & Adamek, 1997), compared to parents of control children (Kumpulainen, 2002).

Behavioral studies have highlighted the similarities between selective mutism and behavioral inhibition (Black & Uhde, 1995; Dummit et al., 1997), which is considered a developmental risk factor for social phobia (Oberklaid, Sanson, Pedlow, & Prior, 1993). Behavioral inhibition, as first defined by Kagan and his Harvard research group, is characterized by behaviors such as clinging to the mother, long latencies to approach and communicate, withdrawal, and expressions of distress in novel social and non-social situations (Garcia-Coll, Kagan, & Reznick, 1984). According to Kagan and colleagues (1987), a lack of speech is one of the cardinal characteristics of behavioral inhibition. Given that many parents whose children are diagnosed with selective mutism retrospectively report that their children were always shy and withdrawn (Garcia, Freeman, Francis, Miller, & Leonard, 2004), and that there are a number of behavioral similarities between children with selective mutism and children with behavioral inhibition, many researchers have suggested that selective mutism and social phobia may be on a developmental continuum with behavioral inhibition.

Given the early labels of 'aphasia voluntaria' and 'elective mutism', which implied that the children were making the decision to not speak in order to be defiant or manipulate individuals or their environment (Manassis, Fung, Tannock, Sloman, Fiksenbaum, & McInnes, 2003), it is not surprising that researchers have also suggested that selective mutism may be associated with oppositional behaviors (Kumpulainen et al., 1998; Kristensen & Torgersen, 2001; Steinhausen & Juzi, 1996; Yeganeh et al., 2006 but not Cunningham et al., 2004; Cunningham et al., 2006). Compared to the conceptualization of selective mutism as an anxiety disorder, however, there have been few studies that have shown strong evidence for oppositional behaviours among children with selective mutism. For instance, Steinhausen and Juzi (1996) found that 66% of their sample of children with selective mutism had a comorbid anxiety disorder, while only 20% met the criteria for oppositional behaviours. Furthermore, of the 50 children studied by Dummit and colleagues (1997), all of them met the diagnostic criteria for social phobia or avoidant disorder, while only one child met the criteria for oppositional-defiant disorder. Current studies suggest that only a small sample of children with selective mutism are oppositional (Yeganeh et al., 2006) and most studies appear to support the conceptualization of selective mutism as an anxiety disorder.

Etiology

The etiology of selective mutism is poorly understood due the relative rarity and heterogeneous presentation of the disorder. The little research that has been done on the topic suggests that the developmental pathways to selective mutism are complex and determined by a number of interacting factors, including, genetics, temperament, social factors and attainment of developmental milestones (Cohan et al., 2006). Researchers have also found a number of factors that are present in children with selective mutism at higher rates than in typically developing children that may provide preliminary insights into possible etiological factors, including, immigration and learning a new language (Elizir & Perednik, 2003; Steinhausen & Juzi, 1996; Steinhausen, Wachter, Laimbock, & Metzke, 2006), a family history of a reticent personality (Steinhausen et al., 2006), reduced auditory capacity (Arie et al., 2007), and histories of language and communication difficulties (Dummit et al., 1997; Kristensen, 2000; Steinhausen & Juzi, 1996).

In fact, with regards to immigration, researchers have suggested that there may be two different pathways to the development of selective mutism depending on whether the selective mutism appears in children who are native speakers of the language or in children who are immigrants. Selective mutism in children who are native speakers of the language is associated with higher rates of developmental disorder or delay, while selective mutism in immigrants is associated with higher rates of social phobia(Elizir & Perednik, 2003).

Functional Impairment and Prognosis

A limited number of studies have investigated the functional impairment caused by selective mutism. Using the Children's Global Assessment Scale (Shaffer et al., 1983), clinicians have rated children with selective mutism as moderately impaired, defined as exhibiting moderate levels of functional impairment in all areas of life or exhibiting a severe level of functional impairment in one specific area (Dummit et al., 1997; Manassis et al., 2003). Similar results were found in a prospective study in which teachers rated the children with selective mutism on the Children's Global Assessment Scale (Shaffer et al., 1983) at two time-points 6 months apart. Although children with selective mutism were rated lower in functional impairment at the 6-month follow-up, they still remained functionally impaired compared to the controls (Bergman et al., 2002). In a study of 33 children with selective mutism, teachers rated 51% of the children as having "serious school and social problems (Schwartz et al., 2006). Similarly, teachers and parents rated children with selective mutism as having significant deficits in verbal and nonverbal social skills compared to a community control group (Cunningham et al., 2006; Cunningham et al., 2004). Despite the lack of demonstrated social skills, however, children with selective mutism did not experience an increased rate of peer victimization (Cunningham et al., 2004). In a follow-up study of patients with selective mutism, all 25 patients who were interviewed at a mean follow-up period of 12 years revealed that they viewed their selective mutism as a serious disorder and that they experienced high levels of suffering (Remschmidt et al., 2001).

Selective mutism is a serious disorder that results in significant functional impairment. One area of functional impairment that has been investigated is language development and performance. The most common context in which children with selective mutism fail to speak is the school setting (Steinhausen & Juzi, 1996). Given that school-age children spend more than half of their day in school, children with selective mutism miss out on many opportunities to practice and develop their language and social communication skills. Therefore, a natural question is, how does selective mutism impact language performance and development?

Selective Mutism and Language Development

Extant Studies

Studies of speech and language disorders in children with selective mutism have estimated that between 20% and 50% of children with selective mutism present with co-occurring speech and/or language disorders (Andersson & Thomas, 1998; Black & Uhde, 1995; Kristensen, 2000; Kolvin & Fundudis, 1981; Kumpulainen et al., 1998; Remschmidt et al., 2001; Steinhausen & Juzi, 1996; Wilkins, 1985; Wright, 1968). Kolvin and Fundudis (1981) found that in a sample of 24 children identified retrospectively based on hospital records as having elective mutism, 50% had delayed speech development or some other type of speech difficulties. In a more recent study, Kristensen (2000) found that in a sample of 54 children with selective mutism with a mean age of 9 years and 108 matched controls, 50% of the children with selective mutism had a communication disorder compared to only 11.5% of the controls. Kristensen (2000) found a significantly higher rate of mixed receptive-expressive language disorders (17.3% vs. 1%), expressive language disorders (6% vs. 1%), and phonological disorders (42.6% vs. 10.2%) in children with selective mutism compared to the controls.

These studies are limited by a number of methodological difficulties, including: 1) inconsistencies in the definitions of selective mutism and inclusion criteria; and 2) lack of specificity, and possibly consistency, in how children's speech and language abilities were determined. Although the study by Kristensen (2000) used well-defined standardized assessments to determine the presence of disorders, many other studies have used case notes (e.g., Wilkins, 1986), teacher reports (e.g., Kumpulainen et al., 1998), parent reports (e.g., Black & Uhde, 1995) or audio-tapes of the child's speech in the home setting (e.g., Kolvin & Fundus, 1981). Overall, there is a lack of detail in the manner in which speech and language disorders were assessed in these studies. As suggested by Cleator and Hand (2001), in many cases it appears that there was no systematic assessment but rather speech and language disorders were identified based on observation. This creates a bias as it raises the possibility of a large amount of heterogeneity across participants in the manner in which the diagnosis of a language or speech disorder was established.

More recent studies on speech and language development in children with selective mutism have focused increasingly on the development and use of standardized assessment techniques, thus creating more consistency across participants. Admittedly, the assessment of speech and language abilities in children with selective mutism presents a number of unique challenges. First, it is difficult to determine what exactly is being measured when children with selective mutism are given tests of expressive and receptive language performance. Given that these children fail to speak in unfamiliar situations and towards unfamiliar individuals (APA, 2000) and often become withdrawn in such situations, their decreased scores may not be a measure of decreased speech and/or language abilities but rather of inhibition in the unfamiliar testing situation and towards the unfamiliar examiner.

Second, although receptive language performance can be assessed through the use of testing methods that allow for nonverbal responses such as pointing (Cleator & Hand, 2001; Dow et al., 1995), assessment of expressive language performance is much more difficult. While one method is to rely on anecdotal reports from the parents, some research has found that parents often overestimate the expressive language abilities of their children (Stein, Rapin, & Yapko, 2001, but not Chaffee, Cunningham, Secord-Gilbert, Elbard, & Richards, 1991). Another approach is to have parents unobtrusively record their children's speech in the home setting in interactions with them and then to conduct the assessment based on this sample of the child's speech. The challenge with this approach, however, is that such unstructured interactions with their parents in the home setting may not access the type of speech that would be elicited in a formal assessment setting (McInnes, Fung, Manassis, Fiksenbaum, & Tannock, 2004).

Much of the recent research on speech and language development in children with selective mutism has been conducted by Manassis and her research group (Manassis et al., 2003; Manassis et al., 2007; McInnes et al., 2004). The researchers have been successful in developing innovative methods through which to attain adequate measures of receptive and expressive language performance from children with selective mutism.

In a study of 14 children with selective mutism (*M* age = 10.07 years) and 9 children with social phobia (*M* age = 11.33 years), Manassis and colleagues (2004) found that children with selective mutism performed significantly lower on discrimination of speech sounds compared to children with social phobia. There were no significant differences between the groups in their performance on perceiving the number and order of sounds in spoken syllables, or in their ability to follow directions of varying complexity and length. There was a trend for receptive language performance, with the selective mutism group performing lower than the social phobia group (Manassis et al., 2003). In an analysis of expressive language performance, McInnes and colleagues (2004) used the same sample as Manassis and colleagues (2003) and audio-recorded the children's retelling of stories to their mothers in both the home and a quiet room in the laboratory. Children with selective mutism (n = 7, *M* age = 9.7) had significantly shorter, less complex, and less content-rich linguistic narratives compared to children with social phobia (n =7, *M* age = 11.1), controlling for age differences and despite no differences between the two groups in cognitive and receptive language performance.

Although both of the above studies are limited by their small sample sizes and the lack of a normal control group, they make significant contributions to the study of speech and language in children with selective mutism. They present methodology that enables the collection of adequate speech samples from children with selective mutism across two different contexts as well as successful administration of standardized assessments of language performance. The results provide preliminary evidence that children with selective mutism have lower speech and language performance compared to children with social phobia, and that this lower performance may span across both receptive and expressive language. This finding is consistent with that of Cleator and Hand (2001) who found that, in a sample of 5 children with selective mutism ranging in age from 3 to 8 years, there was no consistency in the type of language and/or speech disorder identified. Rather, there was a range of language and speech disorders such that some children only had speech difficulties, others only language difficulties, and still others a combination of both language and speech difficulties.

In the most recent study conducted to date, Manassis and colleagues (2007) addressed some of the limitations mentioned above by including a normal control group and increasing the sample size. Using standardized measures, the authors found that children with selective mutism ($n = 44$, M age = 7.87 year) were distinguished from children with anxiety disorders ($n = 28$, M age = 9.09 years) and normal controls ($n = 19$, M age = 9.07 years) by their performance on standardized tests of receptive language and reception of grammar. The selective mutism group performed significantly lower on both of these measures compared to the other two groups. Although the differences may be statistically significant, their clinical significance is uncertain.

First, as mentioned above, it is impossible to separate the effects of inhibition in the test situation from actual language difficulties, thus bringing into question whether the significant differences are due to a true language difficulty or a reflection of the child's inhibition in the situation. Second, the scores for both the PPVT-III (Dunn & Dunn, 1997) and the Test of Reception of Grammar (TROG; Bishop, 2003) are standardized on a mean of 100 and a standard deviation of 15. For the TROG (Bishop, 2003), the mean score for the selective mutism group was 89.86 while the mean scores for the anxiety and control groups were 100.86 and 102.26, respectively. Similarly, the mean score for the children with selective mutism on the PPVT-III (Dunn & Dunn, 1997) was 97.35, while the mean scores for the children with anxiety disorders and the community controls were 111, and 110.95, respectively. Given that the mean scores for the children with selective mutism were within 1 standard deviation, this brings into question the clinical significance of the differences between groups. Although the authors did not provide effect sizes, calculations of Cohen's d (Cohen, 1992) based on the provided means and standard deviations reveal that the differences between groups on the PPVT-III reflect large effect sizes while the differences on the TROG reflect medium to large effect sizes. This indicates that the statistically significant differences between the groups on both receptive language and reception of grammar are of practical concern and should be viewed as an area of importance in children with selective mutism.

The interpretation of the scores for the PPVT-III is further complicated by the fact that there is a tendency for score inflation on the PPVT-III (Ukrainetz & Duncan, 2000). Williams (1998) found that when she tested the same group of children on the PPVT-R (Dunn & Dunn, 1981) and the PPVT-III (Dunn & Dunn, 1997), the standardized scores were significantly higher on the PPVT-III than the PPVT-R. This score inflation was especially seen in children between the ages of 4 and 10 years. This age group had a score inflation of about 10 points (Williams, 1998). Thus, although the mean score of the children with selective mutism in the study by Manassis and colleagues (2007) appears to be average when we consider the mean on which the PPVT-III (Dunn & Dunn, 1997) is standardized, it is not clear whether the score is in fact average or whether it is a reflection of the score inflation that has been reported on the PPVT-III (Dunn & Dunn, 1997). If we were to consider a score inflation of 10 points, without this inflation the score would be around 87.35. Although this is still within 1 standard deviation of the mean, as evidenced above through the calculation of effect sizes, it is still a difference that is of practical concern and should not be ignored.

One of the challenges with the results that we have discussed thus far is that they are all focused on average scores. Given that selective mutism is a heterogenous disorder, it is important to not only analyze group averages but to also look at individual scores and the distribution of scores. Manassis and colleagues (2007) recognized the importance of this and found that a significantly higher rate of children with selective mutism had scores in the clinical range, thus bringing forth the question of what factors differentiate this group of children from those whose scores may be lower but not in the clinical range.

Kristensen and Torgersen (2002) have attempted to answer this question through a cross-sectional study evaluating differences in child and parent temperament between children with selective mutism with (n = 26, M age = 9 years) and without (n = 26, M age = 8.6 years) communication disorders. The parents of children with selective mutism and a communication disorder did not differ significantly from the parents of the control children on any measure of temperament while the parents of children with selective mutism and no communication disorder had significantly higher levels of distress and fear and significantly lower levels of activity compared to the parents of control children. Kristensen and Torgersen (2002) have proposed that this pattern of temperamental differences may suggest different developmental pathways for children with selective mutism with or without communication disorders such that the lack of speech in children with communication disorders is due to self-consciousness while in children without a communication disorder, the lack of speech is due to a genetically transmitted predisposition to show higher levels of distress and withdrawal. The results found by Kristensen and Torgersen (2002) are preliminary and need to be viewed as such. Further research is needed with larger sample sizes and looking at temperament longitudinally to ascertain the findings and developmental pathways suggested. However, the study does highlight the need for researchers to consider individual differences in their attempts to identify developmental pathways for selective mutism and speech and language development.

In combination, the findings by Manassis and group indicate that it is possible to attain adequate assessments of receptive and expressive language performance in children with selective mutism and that these assessments should be included as part of the protocol used for the diagnosis of selective mutism. Children with selective mutism performed significantly lower compared to children with social phobia and community controls on a number of standardized and non-standardized measures of speech and language performance that spanned across both receptive and expressive language.

It is interesting that the studies discussed above did not find any significant gender differences in language performance, given that females tend to have higher rates of language development compared to males (Bornstein, Hahn, & Haynes, 2004). In a study we recently conducted (Nowakowski et al., in press), we found a significant group by gender interaction on language performance as measured by the PPVT-III (Dunn & Dunn, 1997). Girls in the selective mutism (n = 16, M age = 7.9 years) and mixed anxiety (n = 22, M age = 9.4 years) groups attained significantly lower scores on receptive language performance compared to girls in the community control group (n = 15, M age = 7.9 years). In contrast, there were no significant differences on receptive language performance among the groups for boys. These results suggest that the picture may be more complicated such that girls with selective mutism may be more likely to have lower receptive language performance compared to boys. Much like Manassis and colleagues (2007), we found that although the mean standardized score on the PPVT-III for girls with selective mutism was within 1 standard deviation of the mean, the effect size was large, indicating that the difference was of clinical concern.

Taken together, although limited, the research on language performance in children with selective mutism suggests that selective mutism is associated with higher rates of difficulties in both receptive and expressive language. The large effect sizes for these differences suggest that, although all of the standardized scores for the children with selective mutism are within 1 standard deviation of the mean, the differences are still of practical concern and require attention. Furthermore, they highlight the need to not only investigate group means but also individual scores when considering language performance, given the heterogeneity that is present in selective mutism. It is important to note, however, that it is not clear whether the differences seen between groups are true differences in language ability or reflect the inhibition of the child in the unfamiliar testing situation.

Developmental Pathways

As discussed by Manassis and colleagues (2003), there are a number of potential developmental pathways the development of speech and language difficulties in children with selective mutism. First, it is possible that speech and language difficulties appear developmentally before selective mutism. This would suggest that the lack of speaking in children with selective mutism may be a result of the labour-intensive process and frustration they experience due to their speech and language impairments. A number of empirical findings have provided preliminary support for this line of thought. Arie and colleagues (2007) found that some children with selective mutism have reduced auditory processing, whereby they fail to sensitize to the sound of their own voices. Consequently, these children focus extensively on the sound of their own voices and are unable to focus on what is spoken around them. Manassis and colleagues (2007) also found that a combination of grammatical ability and maternal report of the child's level of social phobiawere the best predictors of the severity of selective mutism, accounting for 38% of the variance. Lastly, adopting the view that selective mutism is an anxiety disorder closely linked to social phobia (and possibly a predictor of later social phobia), Beitchman and colleagues (2001) found that language impairments in early childhood significantly predicted adolescent social phobia.

A second possible developmental pathway is that speech and language difficulties develop after selective mutism. This would suggest that the speech and language difficulties are a result of the children's tendency to be mute in various situations, especially the school setting, and are thus not using incidental learning opportunities to practice and develop their speech and language abilities.

A third possibility may be that there is some third factor that has not yet been identified that interacts with speech and language and results in selective mutism or that interacts with selective mutism and leads to speech and language problems. Thus, it is clear that there is a strong need for longitudinal studies to start to delineate the association between selective mutism and speech and language performance.

CONCLUSIONS AND FUTURE DIRECTIONS

Although selective mutism was first identified in 1977, the disorder has undergone much reconceptualization and only in the last 10 to 15 years have we seen research on selective mutism move away from clinical case studies and towards more systematic empirical studies of larger samples of children. With regards to the relation between selective mutism and speech and language, the research to date suggests that, overall, individuals with selective mutism have higher rates of both receptive and expressive language difficulties compared to community controls and possibly children with anxiety disorders, especially social phobia. It is unclear, however, the extent to which these differences reflect true speech and language difficulties or are a reflection of children's inhibition in the testing situation.

The research to date on speech and language performance in children with selective mutism has utilized primarily retrospective and cross-sectional approaches as well as a variety of language assessment methods, including case reports, teacher-reports, parent-reports, audiotapes of children's speech, and standardized measures. In order to further delineate the different possible developmental pathways discussed above, there is a great need for longitudinal and laboratory-based studies of children with selective mutism. Such studies would not only inform speech and language development but would also provide insight into other etiological factors in the development of selective mutism.

Longitudinal studies are essential to enabling researchers and clinicians to attain a stronger understanding of various aspects of speech and language development and performance in children with selective mutism, including: 1) Do children show an improvement in speech and language performance when selective mutism is successfully treated, defined as the elimination of the core symptoms? 2) How does selective mutism affect speech and language development in later years given that the studies to date have focused on children ages 10 years and younger? 3) Does speech and language performance in children with selective mutism become more clinically impaired as children become older? 4) What factors determine whether children with selective mutism experience speech and language performance difficulties? and 5) Do children who have difficulties in expressive and receptive language experience greater functional impairment and more severe selective mutism?

In summary, although not all children with selective mutism experience low performance on expressive and receptive language tests, a higher rate than would be expected by chance do. Accordingly, there is a high rate of co-occurrence of receptive and expressive language difficulties in children with selective mutism. What remains unclear, however, is the developmental pathway through which this co-occurrence develops. It is essential that future longitudinal research encourages collaboration amongst developmental and child clinical psychologists and speech-language pathologists in order to provide greater insight into the association between speech and language difficulties and selective mutism.

ACKNOWLEDGEMENTS

The writing of this chapter was supported by a Predoctoral Scholarship from the Social Sciences and Humanities Research Council (SSHRC) of Canada awarded to the first author under the direction of the second author and Operating Grants from SSHRC and the Natural Sciences and Engineering Research Council (NSERC) of Canada awarded to the second author and the Ontario Mental Health Foundation (OMHF) awarded to the third author.

References

American Psychiatric Association. (1994). *Diagnsotic and statistical manual of mental disorders (4th ed.)*. Washington, DC: Author.

American Psychiatric Association. (2000). Diagnostic and statistical manual of mental disorders (4th ed., Text Revision (DSM-IV-TR). Washington, DC: American Psychiatric Press.

Andersson, C.B., & Thomsen, P.H. (1998). Electively mute children: An analysis of 37 Danish cases. *Nordic Journal of Psychiatry, 52*, 231-238.

Anstendig, K.D. (1999). Is selective mutism and anxiety disorder? Rethinking its DSM-IV classification. *Journal of Anxiety Disorder, 13*, 417-434.

Arie, M., Henkin, Y., Lamy, D., Tetin-Schneider, S., Apter, A., Sadeh, A., & Bar-Haim, Y. (2007). Reduced auditory processing capacity during vocalization in children with selective mutism. *Biological Psychiatry, 61*, 419-421.

Beitchman, J.H., Wilson, B., Johnson, C., Aitkinson, L., Young, A., Adlaf, E., Escobar, M., & Douglas, L. (2001). Fourteen year follow-up of speech/language-impaired and control children: Psychiatric outcome. *Journal of the American Academy of Child and Adolescent Psychiatry, 40*, 75-82.

Bergman, L.R., Piacentini, J., & McCracken, J.T. (2002). Prevalence and description of selective mutism in a school-based sample. *Journal of the American Academy of Child and Adolescent Psychiatry, 41*, 938-946.

Bishop, D.V.M. (2003). *Test for Reception of Grammar (Version 2): TROG-2 Manual.* London: Psychological Corporation.

Black, B., & Uhde, T.W. (1995). Psychiatric characteristics of children with selective mutism: A pilot study. *Journal of the American Academy of Child and Adolescent Psychiatry, 34*, 847-856.

Bornstein, M.H., Hahn, C., & Haynes, M.O. (2004). Specific and general language performance across early childhood: Stability and gender considerations. *First Language, 24*, 267-304.

Chaffee, C.A., Cunningham, C.E., Secord-Gilbert, M., Elbard, H., & Richards, J. (1991). The influence of parenting stress and children behavior problems on parental estimates of expressive and receptive language development. Journal of Abnormal Child Psychology, 19, 65-74.

Cleator, H., & Hand, L. (2001). Selective mutism: How a successful speech and language assessment really is possible. *International Journal of Language and Communication Disorders, 36*(Suppl.), 126-131.

Cohan, S.L., Price, J.M., & Stein, M.B. (2006). Suffering in silence: Why a developmental psychopathology perspective on selective mutism is needed. *Developmental and Behavioral Pediatrics, 27*, 341-355.

Cohen, J. (1992). A power primer. *Psychological Bulletin, 112*, 155-159.

Cunningham, C.E., McHolm, A.E., & Boyle, M.H. (2006). Social phobia, anxiety, oppositional behavior, social skills, and self-concept in children with specific selective mutism, generalized selective mutism, and community controls. *European Journal of Child Adolescent Psychiatry, 15*, 245-255.

Cunningham, C.E., McHolm, A., Boyle, M.H., & Patel, S. (2004). Behavioral and emotional adjustment, family functioning, academic performance, and social relationships in children with selective mutism. *Journal of Child Psychology and Psychiatry, 45*, 1363-1372.

Dow, S.P., Sonies, B.C., Scheib, D., Moss, S.E, & Leonard, H.L. (1995). Practical guidelines for the assessment and treatment of selective mutism. *Journal of the American Academy of Child and Adolescent Psychiatry, 34*, 836-845.

Dummit, S.E., Klein, R.G., Tancer, N.K., Asche, B., Martin, J., & Fairbanks, J.A. (1997). Systematic assessment of 50 children with selective mutism. *Journal of the American Academy of Child and Adolescent Psychiatry, 36*, 653-660.

Dunn, L.M., & Dunn, L.M. (1981). *Peabody Picture Vocabulary Test – Revised.* Circle Pines, MN: American Guidance Service.

Dunn, L.M. & Dunn, L.M. (1997). *Peabody Picture Vocabulary Test – Third Edition.* American Guidance Service: MN.

Elizur, Y, & Perednik, R. (2003). Prevalence and description of selective mutism in immigrant and native families: A controlled study. *Journal of the American Academy of Child and Adolescent Psychiatry, 42*, 1451-1459.

Ford, M.A., Sladesczek, I.E., Carlson, J., & Krochwell, T.R. (1998). Selective mutism: Phenomenological characteristics. *School Psychology Quarterly, 13*, 192-227.

Garcia, A., Freeman, J., Francis, G., Miller, L.M., & Leonard, H.L. (2004). Selective mutism. In T. Ollendick (Ed.), *Phobic and anxiety disorders in children and adolescents: A clinician's guide to effective psychosocial and pharmacological interventions.* London: Oxford University Press.

Garcia-Coll, C., Kagan, J., & Reznick, S. (1984). Behavioral inhibition in young children. *Child Development, 55*, 1005-1019.

Joseph, P.R. (1999). Selective mutism: The child who doesn't speak at school. *Pediatrics, 104*, 308-310.

Kagan, J., Reznick, J.S., & Snidman, N. (1987). The physiology and psychology of behavioral inhibition in children. *Child Development, 58*, 1459-1473.

Kolvin, I., & Fundudis, T. (1981). Elective mute children: Psychological development and background factors. *Journal of Child Psychology and Psychiatry, 22*, 219-232.

Kopp, S., & Gillberg, C. (1997). Selective mutism: A population based study: A research note. *Journal of Child Psychology and Psychiatry, 38*, 257-262.

Kristensen, H. (2000). Selective mutism and comorbidity with developmental disorder/delay, anxiety disorder, and elimination disorder. *Journal of the American Academy of Child and Adolescent Psychiatry, 39*, 249-256.

Kristensen, H., & Torgersen, S. (2001). MCMI-II personality traits and symptom traits in parents of children with selective mutism: A case-control study. *Journal of Abnormal Psychology, 110*, 648-652.

Kristensen, H., & Torgersen, S. (2002). A case-control study of EAS child and parental temperaments in selectively mute children with and without a co-morbid communication disorder. *Nordic Journal of Psychiatry, 56*, 347-353.

Kumpulainen, K. (2002). Phenomenology and treatment of selective mutism. *CNS Drugs, 16*, 175-180.

Kumpulainen, K., Rasenen, E., Rasska, H., & Somppi, V. (1998). Selective mutism among second graders in elementary school. *European Child and Adolescent Psychiatry, 11*, 71-78.

Manassis, K., Fung, D., Tannock, R., Sloman, L., Fiksenbaum, L., & McInnes, A. (2003). Characterizing selective mutism: Is it more than social anxiety? *Depression and Anxiety, 18*, 153-161.

Manassis, K., Tannock, R., Garland, J.E., Minde, K., McInnes, A., & Clark, S. (2007). The sounds of silence: Language, cognition, and anxiety in selective mutism. *Journal of the American Academy of Child and Adolescent Psychiatry, 46*, 1187-1195.

McInnes, A., Fung, D., Manassis, K., Fiksenbaum, L., & Tannock, R. (2004). Narrative skills in children with selective mutism: An exploratory study. *American Journal of Speech-Language Pathology, 13*, 304-315.

Nowakowski, M.E., Cunningham, C.E., McHolm, A.E., Evan, M.A., Edison, S., St. Pierre, J., Boyle, M.H., & Schmidt, L.A. (In press). Language and academic abilities in children with selective mutism. *Infant and Child Development.*

Oberklaid, F., Sanson, A., Pedlow, R., & Prior, M. (1993). Predicting preschool behavior problems from temperament and other variables in infancy. *Pediatrics, 91*, 113-120.

Remschmidt, H., Poller, M., Herpertz-Dahlmann, B., Hennighausen, K., & Gutenbrunner, C. (2001). A follow-up study of 45 patients with elective mutism. *European Archives of Psychiatry and Clinical Neuroscience, 251*, 284-296.

Schwartz, R.H., Freedy, A.S., & Sheridan, M.J. (2006). Selective mutism: Are primary care physicians missing the silence? *Clinical Pediatrics, 45*, 43-48.

Shaffer, D., Grould, M.S., Brasic, J., Ambrosini, P., Fisher, P., Bird, H., Aluwahlia, S. (1983). A global assessment scale (CGAS). *Archives of General Psychiatry, 40*, 1228-1231.

Sharp, W.G., Sherman, C., & Gross, A.M. (2007). Selective mutism and anxiety: A review of the current conceptualization of the disorder. *Journal of Anxiety Disorders, 21*, 568-579.

Standart, S., & Le Couteur, A. (2003). The quiet child: A literature review of selective mutism. *Child & Adolescent Mental Health, 8*, 154-160.

Stein, M.T., Rapin, I., & Yapko, D. (2001). Selective mutism. *Journal of Developmental and Behavioral Pediatrics, 22*(Suppl. 2), S123-S126.

Steinhausen, H.C., & Adamek, R. (1997). The family history of children with elective mutism: A research report. *European Journal of Child and Adolescent Psychiatry, 6*, 107-111.

Steinhausen, H.C., & Juzi, C. (1996). Elective mutism: An analysis of 100 cases. *Journal of the American Academy of Child and Adolescent Psychiatry, 35*, 606-614.

Steinhausen, C.H., Wachter, M., Laimbock, K., & Metzke, C.W. (2006). A long-term outcome study of selective mutism in childhood. *Journal of Child Psychology and Psychiatry, 47*, 751-756.

Toppelberg, C.O., Tabors, P., Coggins, A., Lum, K., & Burger, C. (2005). Differential diagnosis of selective mutism in bilingual children. *Journal of the American Academy of Child and Adolescent Psychiatry, 44*, 592-595.

Ukrainetz, T.A., & Duncan, D.S. (2000). From old to new: Examining score increases on the Peabody Picture Vocabulary Test – III. *Language, Speech, and Hearing Services in Schools, 31*, 336-339.

Vecchio, J.L., & Kearney, C.A. (2005). Selective mutism in children: Comparison to youths with and without anxiety disorders. *Journal of Psychopathology and Behavioral Assessment, 27*, 31-37.

Wilkins (1985). A comparison of elective mutism and emotional disorders in children. *British Journal of Psychiatry, 146*, 198-203.

Williams, K.T. (1998). Peabody Picture Vocabulary Test – III: What is new and different? *Clinical Connection, 11*, 6-8.

World Health Organization. (1994). *International statistical classification of diseases and related health problems* (10th rev.). Geneva, Switzerland: Author.

Wright, H.L. (1968). A clinical study of children who refuse to talk in school. *Journal of the American Academy of Child Psychiatry, 7*, 603-617.

Yeganeh, R., Beidel, D.C., & Turner, S.M. (2006). Selective mutism: More than social anxiety? *Depression and anxiety, 23*, 117-123.

Yeganeh, R., Beidel, D.C., Turner, S.M., Pina, A.A., & Silverman, W.K. (2003). Clinical distinction between selective mutism and social phobia: An investigation of childhood psychopathology. *Journal of the American Academy of Child and Adolescent Psychiatry, 42*, 1069-1075.

In: Children and Language: Development, Impairment … ISBN 978-60692-395-5
Editor: Michael A. Reed

Chapter 8

EARLY COMMUNICATIVE CHANNEL IN CHILDHOOD: DEVELOPMENT AND IMPAIRMENT

Gianluca Esposito and Paola Venuti
Department of Cognitive Science, University of Trento, Italy

ABSTRACT

Crying, which represents the very first communicative channel infants can use to communicate with their environment, plays an important role in child development. Crying is a biological signal that alerts those in the caregiving environment about the needs and wants of the infant and motivates them to respond. Cries act to release specific and appropriate patterns of caregiving actions, thereby ensuring the infant's survival. The aim of this chapter is to review studies that have investigated expressions of distress, specifically crying, during early stages of development in infancy. Emphasized is the importance of cry evaluation in specific psychopathology, particularly Autism Spectrum Disorders (ASD). First the neurobiological activation that takes place during an episode of crying, both in the caregiver and the infant brain, is described. A description of the function of crying episodes and their evolution, starting from the fetal stage through childhood, follows. Finally, how anomalies in the expression of cry can bias the caregiver's perception of them, and how parents' reactions to pathological crying can be qualitatively different from their reactions to typical crying of same-aged children, is described. Such differences can confound parental attempts to share feelings and develop inter-subjectivity with their children.

Key words: crying, responses to young infant's cries, early communication, developmental disorders

Introduction

Crying represents the very first communicative channel infants can use to express their needs and communicate with their environment. These social behaviors, which are driven by genetically predetermined factors, elicit a series of physiological reactions in adults, such as increases in heart rate (Huffman, Bryan, del Carmen, Pedersen, Doussard-Roosevelt, & Porges, 1998) and endocrine responses (Fleming, Corter, Stallings, & Steiner, 2002). These reactions are greater in parents than in non-parents; for example, while hearing episodes of crying, higher levels of testosterone were found in fathers than non-fathers (Fleming et al., 2002). Such physiological reactions activate those listening to cries to take measures to eliminate the cause of the uneasiness that is shared both by newborn and adult (Gustafson, Wood, & Green, 2000; LaGasse, Neal, Lester, & 2005). Starting from these considerations, the aim of this chapter is to describe expressions of distress, specifically crying, during early stages of development in infancy. In the next pages we describe:

1. Physiology of human crying
2. Evolutionary trajectory of crying
3. Parental reaction to human cries
4. Cries in children with atypical development
5. How cries are perceived in children with atypical development: The case of Autism Spectrum Disorder

1. Physiology Of Human Crying

An episode of crying activates the central nervous system (CNS) of both the infant (the producer) and the caregiver (the listener), and this activation creates a state of reciprocal attention. For this reason crying has been considered a complex behavioral mechanism that regulates the infant-caregiver relationship. This complex behavioral mechanism guarantees the building of a specific tie, and this tie assures infant survival. In particular, infant survival is guaranteed primarily because the caregiver hearing the infant crying is alerted and can attend to the infant's primary needs (Murray, 1979) and affective, social, and cognitive needs as well.

In a typically developing infant, an episode of crying is a response to an external or internal negative stimulus and results from the coordination of several brain regions, such as cranial nerves, brainstem, and limbic system. The limbic system, which is the central core of socio-emotional life, is linked to the lower part of the brainstem, which controls the muscles of the larynx, pharynx, and thorax. From a physiological perspective, infant crying comprises a rhythmic alternation of utterances (the cry sounds) and inspiration. Crying is part of the expiratory phase of respiration with phonation (or sound) produced by the larynx. The larynx contains the vocal cords and the *glottis vocalis* (or simply glottis) that is the opening between the vocal cords. The larynx is the major source of sound during a crying episode and it generates sound through the rhythmic opening and closing of the vocal folds. The production of sound during an episode of crying is the same as every other vocalization (such as speech or song). In particular, in order to oscillate, the vocal folds are brought near enough together so that air pressure builds up beneath the larynx. The cords are pushed apart by this increased subglottal pressure. The elasticity of the cords brings them back together. Under typical conditions, this oscillation pattern sustains itself. In essence, sound is generated in the larynx by cutting the flow of air into little whiffs. This vibration is the fundamental frequency (f0) and is heard as the pitch of the cry (La Gasse et al., 2005). Damage in the vagal cranial nerve complex has been related to atypical patterns of fundamental frequency. Extremely rapid shifts in the fundamental frequency are often related to some degree of instability in the neural control system, especially at the level of the brainstem.

Mainly, three different cry modes, related to different vocal fold vibrations, have been identified. Each modality is related to a different infant need (Wolff, 1969, Golub, 1989; La Gasse et al., 2005).

1. basic cry or phonation, characterized by rhythmic vocalizations with cycles of opening and closing of the vocal cord (approximately 250 to 450 Hz or cycles per second in normal, healthy newborns).
2. high pitch cry or hyperphonation (1000–2000 Hz or cycles per second). The high frequencies of this mode express a high level of distress; for this reason it is often refereed to as a pain cry. Typically after an initial high frequency pitch the child tends to hold his breath.
3. turbulent cry or dysphonation, characterized by no harmonic vibration of the vocal folds. It is often refereed to as a cry of frustration.

These cry modes are present in all typically developing children, and also children from different cultures (Wolf, 1969; Barr, Konner, Bakeman, & Adamson, 1991).

In a recent study, Esposito and Venuti (2007) described the shape of the "narrative structure" of a crying cycle. In typically developing infants, some degree of h*omogeneity* across cultures exists (Barr et al., 1991). In particular the general shape of such cycles seems stable (see fig. 1). The general shape or *narrative* of each crying cycle is composed of 4 phases: (i) an initial phase, when the fundamental frequency starts to increase from a baseline level (usually silence). Soon after this initial phase there is a second phase, called (ii) *plateau*, when the fundamental frequency reaches its highest level. The plateau phase is then followed by (iii) the *aspiration/expiration* phase, during which the cry sound follows the breathing rhythm. The last or final phase (iv) concludes the cycle. During this last phase the fundamental frequency decreases to its baseline level. A crying episode can be composed of several cycles, and the proportion of time spent in each phase can differ from cycle to cycle.

For example pain cry, which usually require an immediate response from caregivers in order to assure the infant's safety (and, in extreme cases, survival), tend to have a higher and longer plateau phase and a shorter initial, aspiration/expiration and final phase than other cries. In this way the perceptual system of the caregiver, which, for neurophisiological reasons, is typically more activated by higher pitch stimuli, will be activated sooner. On the other hand, hunger cry, which do not always require an immediate response from the caregiver (the child will survive if the response is not immediate), tend to have a longer initial and aspiration/expiration phase and shorter plateau and final phases.

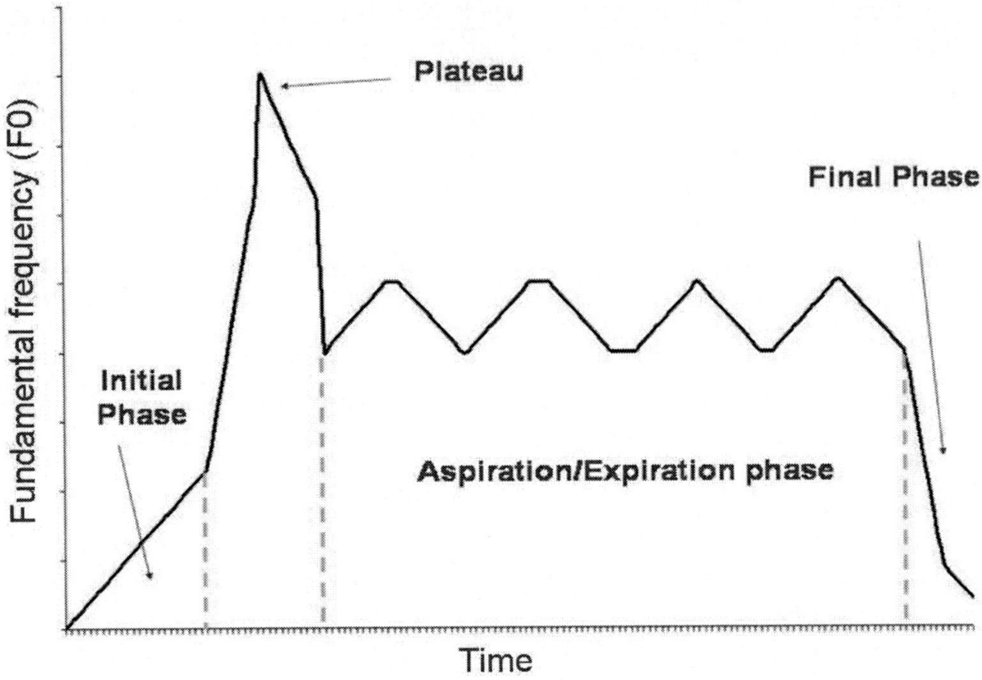

Figure 1. The general shape or *narrative* of a crying cycle in typically developing children.

2. Evolutionary Trajectory Of Crying

A cry is a signal available to infants from the very early stages of life. In a recent study, Gingras, Mitchell and Grattan (2007) reported that a fetal homologue of crying, lasting about 15 seconds, was observed. One of the most replicated findings about crying in early infancy concerns what is called "the cry curve". Crying increases during the first two months of life, with a peak usually found around the sixth week and a decline during the following months (Bell & Ainsworth, 1972; St.James-Robertson, 1989; Barr et al., 1991). In general, soon after birth, the cry becomes an automatic reaction to signal biological needs (hunger, pain, visceral colic); typically it also elicits soothing behavior from caregivers (e.g., cuddling or moving the child rhythmically) that are universally utilized across different cultures. These responses are the result of cultural norms (Barr et al., 1991) and caregiver characteristics (Frodi, 1985); infant cry characteristics influence responses to crying as well (Gustafson & Green, 1989; Zeifman, 2003). The caregiver's adequate behavioral response, which ideally satisfies the newborn's needs, is a mandatory step for good future relations. Deviations in the signal and/or misunderstanding the message can compromise infant care, parental effectiveness, and undermine the budding relationship (LaGasse et al., 2005). Not surprisingly, the needs of an infant do not remain stagnant; on the contrary, the baby's needs generally follow a course of development, as does the expression of crying. Initial cries requesting basic wants soon evolve into solicitations rooted outside of biology. Day by day, the reasons for crying episodes become more social. Whatever the reasons, these bouts typically serve to bring or keep the caregiver in the infant's proximity.

Around the 3rd month, episodes of crying can result from a sudden change in environmental stimulation; for example, when the caregiver goes out of the visual field of the child or when the caregiver stops singing or talking. In these scenarios, restoring the environmental stimulation or distracting the baby with new stimuli often succeeds in stopping the crying. Generally speaking, behaviors that cause distress or offer consolation to the child often match the subtle aspects of crying being expressed at the moment. These different aspects of crying and caregiver responses help define the nature of their relationship (Dunn, 2002), and also reflect: (i) the new competence of the child to face the world; (ii) the child's ability to modulate internal stimuli; (iii) and other factors such as parental age and personality (Ziefman, 2003) and infant age (Schuetze, Zeskind, & Eiden, 2003).

At 8 months, babies can have a specific relationship with their caregivers and a better understanding of the world around them; on the whole, infants are more aware of their needs and they are also more aware of the implications of their cries than earlier. During this stage, to be aware of the power of their cries means that babies are responsive to the effects that their crying can produce, specifically changes in the behavior of others and especially that of their caregiver. Infants also develop, at about 7 or 8 months, both a stronger attachment to the mother and an increased sense of ''stranger fear'' (Bell & Ainsworth, 1972; Trevarthen, Aitken, Papoudi, & Robarts, 1998). Usually stranger fear is expressed through the ''stranger fear cry,'' a specific modality of crying activated when the caregiver is not in sight and another person is closely approaching the child. At 12 months, the cry is an effective and efficient communicative routine, with a narrative and a turn-tacking structure. In short, crying is a base and a guide for the development of language and will be, for the rest of life, a primary communicative approach to express deep and strong feelings (Rothganger, 2003).

3. Parental Reaction to Human Cries

Crying is the very first beahvior with a communictaive valence, and it represents an early signal that the neonate can use to express its needs and wants. For this reason it is important to understand how parents react to this signal. Research during the last several decades has focused on three main aspects: (i) responses of adults to infant crying, (ii) effects of those parental responses on infant crying, (iii) differences between parents and non-parents in their responses to infant crying.

(I) Responses of Adults to Infant Crying

In the last several decades many studies have focused on how the frequency and duration of cyring episodes modulate adult responses. For example researchers have reported that parental responses are the results of cultural norms (Barr et al., 1991), caregiver characteristics (Frodi, 1985), and morphological characteristics of the infant cry (Gustafson & Green, 1989; Zeifman, 2003). Cry pitch also can influence caregivers' perception: higher frequency cries are often perceived as more aversive and distressful than lower frequency cries. A particular type of cry, characterized by low frequency and typical of children with Down syndrome, is often perceived as less urgent than the moderate frequency cries usually encountered in typically developing children. On the other hand, cries of pre-term infants (considered a high-risk population) are typically of higher frequency and for that reason are considered more urgent than moderate frequency cries. Another example: the cries of children with visceral colic are characterized by higher frequency and are also perceived as more distressful (Huffman et al., 1998).

These patterns have been confirmed using an experimental procedure in which acoustic parameters (frequency and duration) of crying episodes were modified and then participants where asked to listen and judge the different stimuli. The results confirmed that frequency plays a crucial role in determining the urgency of a person's response. Another important acoustic variable is the duration of the pauses during a crying episode. Zeskind and colleagues (1992) modified the length of the expiratory phase and pauses in some crying episodes. Participants who were asked to judge those stimuli regarded shorter pauses as more activating, informative, and also distressful.

Irwin (2003) has investigated modality effects on cry perception. In her study, she examined whether perceivers can detect more distress in the acoustic or visual signals within the cry. Perceiver ratings differed for high- and low-distress cries at each infant age on the basis of facial and vocal action, but not bodily movement. Perceivers rated the cry sound as more distressed and the cry face as less distressed with increasing infant age. The author speculated that information about distress is available to perceivers in both the crying infant's face and voice.

(II) Effects of Parental Responses to Infant Crying

In a naturalistic study, Bell and Ainsworth (1972) showed that the promptness of maternal response to crying was related to children's individual differences in their amount of crying and with more favourable outcomes for children. These same results were also described by Moss (1974). Other experimental studies (Korner & Grobstein, 1966; Korner & Thoman, 1970) have analyzed the effectiveness of different interventions. In general, it seems that maternal warmth and promptness of maternal response to cries are important predictors of outcome. Many studies report that a caregiver's responsiveness to infant cries play an important role in the development of the child's personality, temperament, and cognitive and linguistic skills. Some authors suggest that crying should be interpreted as a biosocial phenomenon that directly reflects the status of the nervous system and indirectly mediates development through parental intervention (Lester, 1984; LaGasse et al., 2005). Some support for this interpretation is provide by data gathered in a study of preterm infants in which parents were asked to rate the aversiveness of an infant's cry (Lester, Boukydis, & Garcia Coll, 1995). Infants of mothers who better identified their infant's cry as more aversive or less had higher Bayley mental scores and language scores at 18 months than infants whose mothers misperceived their infant's cry (Lester, 1984; LaGasse et al., 2005). It has been speculated that agreement between the cry signal and parent perception optimizes child development (La Gasse, 2005).

(III) Differences between Parents and Non-Parents in Their Responses to Infant Crying

Adult brain activation varies enormously in response to infant vocalization; specifically, it is affected by the sex and parental status of the adult. In a study by Seifritz and colleagues (2003), functional magnetic resonance imaging (fMRI) was used to analyze brain response to infant crying and laughing in mothers and fathers of young children and in female and male non-parents. Interestingly, they found that women but not men, independent of their parental status, showed neural deactivation in the anterior cingulate cortex, as indexed by decreased blood oxygenation level– dependent signal, in response to both types of infant vocalization. Different patterns emerged in other brain regions, controlling for the role of parental experience. In the amygdala and in the limbic regions connected, parents showed stronger activation from crying, whereas non-parents showed stronger activation from laughing. These results suggest that sex and experience change the brain response pattern. The authors of this study speculated that a "successful recognition and evaluation of infant vocalizations can be critical for bonding mechanisms and for offspring well-being and survival. Thus, the modulation of responses by experience seems to represent an adaptive mechanism that can be related to reproductive fitness" (Seifritz et al., 2003).

A number of studies have investigated the differences between parents and non-parents. Fleming and colleagues (2003), analyzing endocrine responses in response to infant cries, made an interesting point. In order to determine the responsiveness of experienced fathers, new fathers and non-fathers toward infant cues, they proposed an experimental procedure for which participants were asked to listen to infant cries and other control stimuli, and affective and endocrine responses were measured prior to and after the cry presentations. In particular, they measured salivary testosterone, cortisol and plasma prolactin concentrations. Their results showed that fathers hearing the cry stimuli felt more alert and sympathetic compared to non-fathers. The baseline level of hormones was predictive of the general affectivity of the men toward the infants and was not influenced by prior experience. More specifically (i) adult males (both fathers and non-fathers) with lower testosterone levels had higher sympathy to infant cries than adult males with higher testosterone levels and (ii) fathers with higher prolactin levels were more alert and more positive in response to the cries then fathers with lower levels of it. Another interesting result of this study was related to the level of increase in hormones. In particular, (i) a greater percentage increase in testosterone was reported for fathers hearing the cry stimuli compared to fathers not hearing the cry stimuli and (ii) a greater percentage increase in prolactin levels was reported for experienced fathers hearing the cries compared to first-time fathers or to non-fathers hearing control stimuli. Finally, after accounting for the variance related to parity and experience, both experience and testosterone continued to contribute to the variance in fathers' affective responses to infant cries. This pattern of results led the authors to conclude that human fathers are more responsive to infant distress signal then non-fathers and that both hormones and caregiving experience play an important role in this pattern.

The two studies just described suggest that both direct experience and biological alterations can affect how adults react to infant cries. Others studies have also noted how parents appear more skilled then non-parents. For example, parents are more able to identify episodes of cry with a higher level of fundamental frequency (hyperphonation), often related to expression of pain (Green, Jones & Gustafson, 1987), than non-parents. This result was also replicated with a Japanese sample, which is interesting because in Japan the expression of crying is often culturally inhibited (Adachi, Murai, Okada, & Nihei, 1985).

Others differences between parents and non-parents are related to the amount of information they need to recognise the cause of the cry: parents need less information, (Green et al, 1987). Furthermore parents know more soothing strategies than non-parents (Zeskind & Lester, 2001). A similar finding was described by Gustafson and colleagues (2000) after using a simulation experiment in which mothers and non-mothers were asked to sooth a manikin resembling an infant. They found that mothers and non-mothers alike began their response with some combination of five different behaviours: (1) pick up the infant; (2) put the infant to their shoulder; (3) verbal stimulation; (4) tactile stimulation (e.g., patting or stroking), and (5) vestibular stimulation (e.g., rocking or swaying). Moreover mothers were somewhat better at guessing the exact cause of the cries, and they spent a greater proportion of their time engaged in activities that might soothe the infant's distress (Gustafson et al., 2000).

4. Cries in Children with Atypical Development

A number of studies that examined cries of infants with a specific medical conditions related to neurological damage were conducted in the twenty-year period from the 1960 to the 1980. Since the instrumentation of that time was limited by today's standards, those early studies gave a description of crying that included only a limited number of acoustic characteristics. In general, those studies demonstrated an association between crying and neurological status. In particular, they highlighted how the fundamental frequency (f0) was particularly sensitive to neurological insult with both higher levels overall and greater variability resulting. The fundamental frequency seems particularly influenced by neurological damage. Among these studies, some identified brain anomalies associated with a higher level of f0, whereas other anomalies were associated with a lower level of f0. In particular, higher levels of f0, more biphonation (f0 instability), and less duration were associated with brain damage (Fisichelli & Karelitz, 1966; Sirvio & Michelsson, 1976), Krabbe's Disease (Thoden and Michelsson, 1979), Meningitis (Michelsson, Sirvio, & Wasz-Hockert, 1977), and Asphyxia (Michelsson, 1971). On the other hand, lower levels of f0, were described in children with Down syndrome (Wasz-Hockert, Lind, Vuorenski, Partanen, & Valanne, 1968), children with hypothyroidism (Michelsson & Sirvio, 1976), and children with Trisomy 13, 18, 21 (Michelsson, Tupperainen, & Aula, 1980).

Many of the early researchers also examined cry characteristics in infants at risk for poor outcomes based on potential neurological insult (e.g., prematurity). Overall, groups of infants at-risk showed higher and more heterogeneity of fundamental frequency and fewer utterances but increased short utterances, suggesting increased tension and instability of neural control of the vocal tract and poorer capacity of the respiratory system. More recently cry studies have examined the effects of potential prenatal insult during pregnancy (e.g., drug exposure). These studies suggest that drug-exposed infants also show increased fundamental frequency, shorter utterances, a higher level of dysphonation, hyperphonation, and more dysregulation—all signs that indicating poor neural control of the vocal track and respiration (see LaGasse et al., 2005). Among groups of at-risk children, premature infants are often studied. For example, Corwin and colleagues, (1992) showed short cry utterances and lower developmental outcome (measured at 30 months) in preterm infants. Higher f0 and shorter duration in preterms infants has been described as well (Michelsson, Jarvenpaa, & Rinne, 1983, Lester, 1987).

A number of studies have emphasized that anomalies in cry characteristics can be related to neurological compromise. These findings suggest that undetected neurological damage may be found by analyzing cries, even when no other symptoms seem to be present. In this view, atypical cries may be considered an early indicator of developmental risk. The kind of cry and its perception could thus aid the identification of neonatal risk. Starting from this point of view, some researchers have begun to analyze episodes of crying in children with Autism Spectrum Disorder (ASD). Considering the tight connection between crying and the functioning of the brainstem and limbic system (both areas highly compromised in ASD children), it seems reasonable to expect some anomalies in the expression of cry in ASD infants. Moreover ASD afflicts individuals by compromising their communicative and social skills and their activity repertoire, and crying can be viewed as both the first communicative system and the first social structure in human development. The analysis of acoustic features of crying episodes has found a number of differences among children with ASD and matched controls. In particular, in ASD children episodes of cry were characterized with shorter duration, less waveform modulation, and more dysphonation (Esposito, Venuti, & Giusti, 2004). In a more recent study (Esposito & Venuti, 2007), the shape of the "narrative structure" of cry cycles in infants with ASD has been described (see fig. 2). This specific *narrative* of a cycle of cry in ASD children has showed some anomalies in the 4 phases, specifically: (i) the initial phase was often shorter than usual; (ii) the *plateau* phase presented a series of repetitive peaks with high frequency; (iii) the *aspiration/expiration* phase was usually not present and when present was shorter than expected; and the last phase (iv) was also shorter then for the matching control cases. The authors speculated that these differences can lead to caregivers misinterpreting the child's needs and create problems in the child-caregiver relationship.

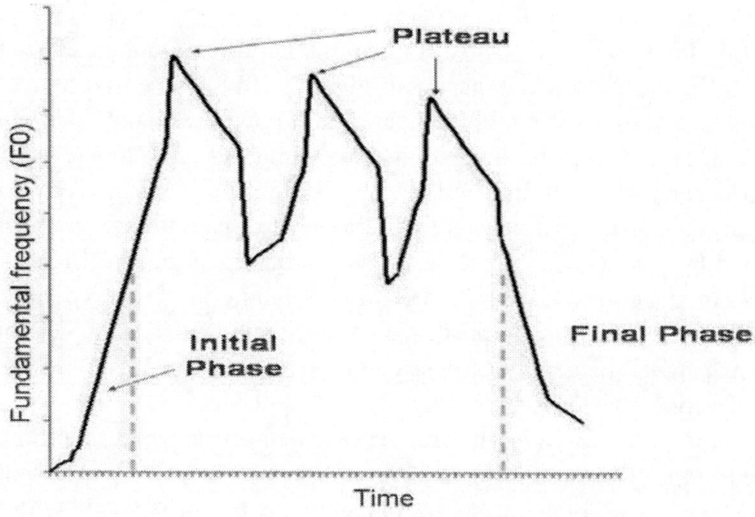

Figure 2. The general shape or *narrative* of a crying cycle in children with Autism Spectrum Disorder.

5. How Cries are Perceived in Children with Atypical Development: the Case of Autism Spectrum Disorder

In typical situations, parents understand the level of distress of a crying episode. They pay attention to the sound (in particular evaluating the intensity and the height of the pitch), evaluate the facial expression of the child, and take the environmental situation into account (such as the hour of the day, the time since the previous meal, etc.). Furthermore, when a child has a specific, previously diagnosed neurological condition, and if the parent has received appropriate training from a specialist, those parents can correctly interpret the distress signals of their child even though their child's cries are quite atypical. An excellent example of this process of accommodation, where the parent can understand a signal after training, is provided by the Cri-du-Chat syndrome. The Cri-du-Chat syndrome (also called deletion 5p syndrome) is a rare genetic disorder due to a missing portion of chromosome 5. The condition affects an estimated 1 in 20,000 to 50,000 live births. The disorder is found in people of all ethnic backgrounds and is slightly more common in females by a 3-1 ratio. The peculiarity of this syndrome (form which it gets its name) is the characteristic cry sound, which sounds just like a meowing kitten and is characterized by cries of very high pitch and short duration. Although the meaning of an episode of cry-du-chat is difficult to impossible to understand at first, parents of children with this disorder can, after adequate training, come to understand their child's needs and wants. But what happens when parents cannot adequately understand their children's cries? An instructive example occurs when a parent interacts with a child with neurological deficits, but before those deficits are diagnosed. This situation often happens in the case of children with ASD (Esposito & Venuti, 2008), for whom diagnoses are usually provided only after 24 months of age.

In later interviews with parents whose children have been diagnosed with ASD, the parents often report that they had great difficulty decoding the emotional signals of their children, especially during the first year. They report, in particular, problems with understanding the causes of crying episodes. Such misunderstandings regarding why their infant is crying can initiate a vicious cycle. The caregiver fails to recognize the child's needs, and this results in inadequate feedback to the child.

A number of studies (Venuti, Giusti, LaFemina, Esposito, Domini, 2002, Esposito et al., 2004; Venuti & Esposito, 2007; Esposito & Venuti, 2008) have investigated how parents perceive crying in children with ASD compared to typical developing children and children with intellectual disabilities. In a first study (Venuti et al., 2002), an interview was administrated to parents of children with ASD and those of typically developing children. Qualitative analysis showed that negative patterns with respect to crying episodes were more often mentioned by parents of ASD children, who often mentioned difficulty understanding those episodes. In a successive study (Esposito & Venuti, 2008), an experimental procedure was designed to test whether the atypical structure of crying episodes typical of children with ASD could bias parents' perception. In particular, a ''Listen-and-Response'' experiment was carried out. Twelve episodes of crying at different ages (13 and 20 months) from retrospective home video of children with ASD and from matching control group children were presented to participants. Participants were asked to listen to the 12 stimuli, randomly presented, and then answer three questions: (1) guess the age of the child who was crying; (2)

guess the reasons why the child was crying, (3) and describe what they felt while hearing the cries.

The results of this study showed some specificity of ASD crying episodes. In particular, participants assigned younger ages to ASD cries. Nevertheless, when listening to ASD crying episodes, participants felt more negative states. In contrast, more positive mental states were felt when listening to crying episodes of children in the other two groups. These different patterns may be interpreted as resulting from an incorrect decoding of the acoustic stimulus. In particular, because of the acoustic characteristics (few peaks, small modulation, small rhythm, and absence of turn-taking), the crying episodes of the children with ASD are difficult to interpret and for this reason may evoke mental states of uneasiness (Esposito & Venuti, 2008). This suggestion agrees with Zeskind and Marshall (1988) who found that shorter pauses were perceived to be more arousing and aversive.

Some important implications follow from these results. In particular, the authors speculated that the relationship between caregivers and their children with ASD may be prey to a vicious cycle (Venuti, 2003; Venuti & Esposito, 2007). This vicious cycle, pictured in Fig.3, could start from a series of brain anomalies present in ASD children since birth (and possibly even before). Given these hypothesized brain anomalies, the various acoustic qualities of a crying episode may not be easily understood by the caregiver. Problems in understanding their infant's cries creates distress and can make the caregivers uneasy. The distress leads caregivers to provide their children with inadequate feedback, which is not effective in addressing the cause of specific crying episodes. As a result, caregivers do not receive an adequate response from their children and so start to feel inadequate, not able to provide their children with a sense of well being. Sensing something amiss, caregivers may attempt to modify their parenting skills. For their part, children who cannot adequately communicate with their caregivers may engage in such compensatory behaviors as isolation, stereotyped behavior, hyper or hypocinesia, etc.). Thus something related to a neurological disorder (in this example, crying) becomes a starting point for a problem in interaction and sets the tone for the overall relationship between the caregiver and child with ASD, undermining the development of intersubjectivity processes for the child with ASD.

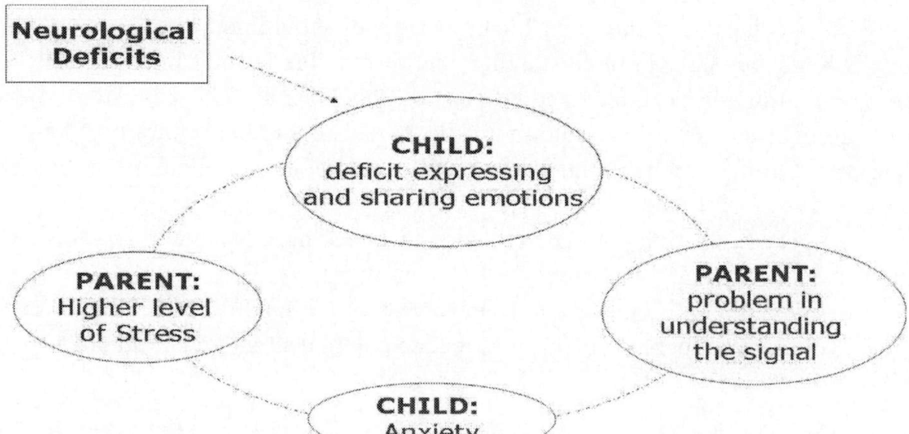

Figure 3. The vicious cycle described in children with Autism Spectrum Disorder

Conclusion

The aim of this chapter was to describe expressions of distress, specifically crying, during early stages of development in infancy. In particular, we wanted to briefly describe the physiology of human crying and its evolutionary trajectory. Then, keeping in mind the communicative valence of crying episodes, our intention was to discuss parental reactions to human cries, focusing on how adults respond to infants crying and how their responses affect infant crying, and also whether or not parents and non-parents differ in their response to crying. Finally, we described some results of studies concerning the cries of children with atypical development and whether or not acoustic anomalies in the cries of children with atypical development can lead to parental misperception of the signal itself.

The core idea of this chapter was that cries serve as an important signal of distress, but moreover, they play a crucial role in human development, representing both the first communicative and the first social structure in infant development. Before neonates smile or visually fixate on objects, they can communicate with the environment by crying. They can use cries to signal their caregiver and make their primary (Murray, 1979) and affective, social, and cognitive needs known.

This behavior, activating the central nervous system (CNS) of both infant and caregiver, creates a state of reciprocal attention and regulates the infant-caregiver relationship. Moreover, it guarantees the building of a specific tie that assures the survival of the infant. Crying starts early communication between caregiver and infant and, based on the maternal (or paternal) skill to give a meaning to the child's cries, their parents' behavior assures the infant about caregiver proximity, thus the infant acquires a sense of reliance in the external environment. Furthermore the strict connection that exists between the cry expression and the central nervous system, gives to the cry the status of an important early indicator of mental health. The cry behavioral system can be altered in two ways: (i) the child's cries can be atypical or (ii) the caretaker's reactions to cries can be atypical. Both these two possibilities need to be considered in order to assure an infant's ideal development. Moreover, although many studies have focused on the acoustic or social features of children's cries, less emphasis has been given to the ways parents face episodes of cry. Especially during the first months after the birth, pediatricians and other health personnel should dedicate more attention to the difficulty parents may have in understanding and responding to their infant's cries. In general we believe that training programs should start during pregnancy to educate new-parents on the language of cries. With this additional skill, parents could better monitor their children's cries and report to their pediatrician any anomalies that could be related to potential medical problems.

Moreover, cry evaluation could be included in screening tools that assess the neurological activity of the new-born and in order to activate early intervention programs with families. In this view, intervention with families, to help parents understand their children's crying, could help them avoid interactional problems and reduce parental stress and child anxiety.

References

Adachi, T., Murai, N., Okada, H., & Nihei, Y. (1985). Maternal perception of infant cries. *Japanese Journal of Educational Psychology*. 33,146-151.

Barr, R.G., Konner, M., Bakeman, R., & Adamson L. (1991). Crying in !kung San Infants: a test of cultural specificity hypothesis. *Developmental Medicine and Child Neurology*. 33, 601-610.

Bell, S.M., & Ainsworth, M.D.S. (1972). Infant crying and maternal responsiveness. *Child Development*. 43, 1171-1190.

Corwin, M. J., Lester, B. M., Sepkoski, C., McLaughlin, S., Kayne, H.., & Golub, H. L. (1992). Effects of in utero cocaine exposure on newborn acoustical cry characteristics. *Pediatrics*. 89, 1199-1203.

Doussard-Roosevelt, JA., & Porges SW., (1999). The role of neurobehavioral organization in stress responses: a polyvagal model. In M. Lewis, & D. Ramsey, (Eds). *Soothing and stress* (pp. 57–76). New Jersey, Lawrence Erlbaum Associates.

Dunn, J. (2002). Emotional development in early childhood: A social relationship perspective. In R. Davidson, H. H. Goldsmith, & K. Scherer (Eds.). *The handbook of affective science* (pp. 332–346). Oxford, UK: Oxford University Press.

Esposito G., & Venuti, P. (2007). Is this a cry? A study on early communication signals in children with Autistic Spectrum disorder (ASD). *Proceedings of X International Workshop on Cry Research*. Dragor, Denmark.

Esposito G., & Venuti P. (2008). How is crying perceived in children with Autistic Spectrum Disorder? *Research in Autism Spectrum Disorders*. 2(2), 371-384.

Fisichelli, V.R., & Karelitz, S., (1966). Frequency spectra of the cries of normal infants and those with Down's Syndrome. *Psyconomic Science*. 6, 195-196.

Fleming, A.S., Corter, C., Stallings, J., & Steiner, M. (2002). Testosterone and prolactin are associated with emotional responses to infant cries in new fathers. *Hormones & Behaviour*. 42, 399-413.

Frodi, A. (1995). When emphathy fails. Avversative infant crying and child abuse. In Lester B.M., Boukydis C.F.Z. (Eds). *Infant crying: theoretical and research perspectives* (pp. 263-277). New York: Plenum Press.

Gingras, J.L., Mitchell, E.A., & Grattan, K.E. (2005). Fetal homologue of infant crying. *Archives of Disease in Childhood: Fetal Neonatal*. 90, 415-418.

Golub, H.L. (1989). A physioacoustic model of the infant cry. In Lester Mb, Boukydis CFZ (Eds). *Infant crying: Theoretical and research perspectives* (pp. 59-82). New York: Plenum Press.

Green, J.A., Jones, L.E., & Gustafson, G.E. (1987). Perception of cries by parents and non-parents: Relation to cry acoustics. *Developmental Psychology*. 23, 370-382.

Gustafson, G.E., & Green, J.A. (1989). On the Importance of Fundamental Frequency and Other Acoustic Features in Cry Perception and Infant Development. *Child Development*. 60(4), 772-780.

Gustafson, G., Wood, R., & Green, J., (2000). Can we hear the causes of infants' crying? In R., Barr, B., Hopkins, & J. Green (Eds). *Crying as a sign, a signal, and a symptom* (pp 8-22). London: Mac Keith Press.

Huffman, L.C., Bryan, Y.E., del Carmen, R., Pedersen, F.A., Doussard-Roosevelt, J.A., & Porges, S.W. (1998). Infant Temperament and Cardiac Vagal Tone: Assessments at Twelve Weeks of Age. *Child Development*. 69(3), 624-635

Irwin, J.R., (2003). Parent and Non-parent Perception of the Multimodal Infant Cry. *Infancy*. 4, 503-516.

Korner, A.E, & Grobstein, R.. (1966). Visual alertness as related to soothing in neonates: Implications for maternal stimulation and early deprivation. *Child Development*. 37, 867-876.

Korner, A.E, & Thoman, E.B. (1970). Visual alertness in neonates as evoked by maternal care. *Journal of Experimental Child Psychology*. 10, 67-79.

LaGasse, L., Neal, A.R., & Lester, B.M., (2005). Assessment of Infant Cry: acoustic Cry analysis and parental perception. *Mental Retardation and Development disabilities: Research Review*. 11, 83-93.

Lester, B.M. (1987). Prediction of developmental outcome from acoustic cry analysis in term and preterm infant. *Paediatrics*. 80, 529-534.

Lester, B.M., Boukydis, C.F., & Garcia Coll C.T. (1995). Developmental outcome as a function of the goodness of fit between the infant's cry characteristics and the mother's perception of her infant's cry. *Pediatrics*. 95, 516 –521.

Lester, B.M. (1984). A biosocial model of infant crying. In: Lipsitt L., Rovee-Collier C., (Eds). *Advances in infant research*.

Michelsson, K., Jarvenpaa, A.L., & Rinne, A. (1983). Sound spectrographic analysis of pain cry in preterm infants. *Early Human Development*. 8,141–149.

Michelsson, K, & Sirvio, P. (1976). Cry analysis in congenital hypothyroidism. *Folia Phoniatrica*. 28, 40–47.

Michelsson, K. (1971). Cry analyses of symptomless low birth weight neonates and of asphyxiated newborn infants. *Acta Paediatrica Scandinava Supplement*. 216, 9–45.

Michelsson, K., Sirvio, P., & Wasz-Hockert, O. (1977). Pain cry in full-term asphyxiated newborn infants correlated with late findings. *Acta Paediatrica Scandinava*. 66, 611-616.

Michelsson, K., Tupperainen, N., & Aula, P. (1980). Cry analysis of infant with karyotype abnormality. *Neuropediatrics*.11, 365-376.

Moss, H.A. (1974). Communication in mother-infant interaction. In L. Krames, P. Plin, & T. Alloway (Eds). *Advances in the study of communication and affect* (vol. 1, pp. 171-191). New York: Plenum Press.

Murray, A.D. (1979). Infant crying as elicitor of parental behaviour: An examination of two models. *Psychological Bulletin*. 86, 191-215.

Rothganger, H., (2003). Analysis of the sounds of the child in the first year of age and a comparison to the language. *Early Human Development*. 75, 55-69.

Schuetze, P., Zeskind, P.S., & Eiden, R.D. (2003). The perceptions of infant distress signals varying in pitch by cocaine-using mothers. *Infancy*. 4, 65– 83.

Seifritz, E., Esposito, F., Neuhoff, J.G., Luthi, A., Mustovic, H., Dammann, G., von Bardeleben, U., Radue, E.W., Cirillo, S., Tedeschi, G., & Di Salle, F. (2003). Differential sex-independent amygdala response to infant crying and laughing in parents versus nonparents. *Biological Psychiatry*. 12(54), 1367-1375.

Sirvio, P., & Michelsson, K. (1976). Sound-spectrographic cry analysis of normal and abnormal newborn infants: A review and a recommendation for standardization of the cry characteristics. *Folia Phoniatrica*. 28, 161–173.

St James-Roberts, I., (1989). Persistent crying in infancy. *Journal of Child Psychology and Psychiatry*. 30, 189–95.

Thoden, C.J., & Michelsson, K. (1979). Sound spectrographic cry analysis in Krabbe's Disease. *Developmental Medicine and Child Neurology*. 21, 400–401.

Trevarthen, C., Aitken, K., Papoudi, D., & Robarts, J. (1998). *Children with autism: Diagnosis and interventions to meet their needs*. London: Jessica Kingsley .

Venuti, P., Esposito, G., Giusti, Z. (2004). A qualitative analysis of crying and vocal distress in children with autism. *Journal of Intellectual Disability Research*. 48(4&5) 338.

Venuti, P., & Esposito, G. (2007). Come piangono i bambini con disturbo dello spettro autistico? [How do children with Autism Spectrum Disorder cry?] *Psicologia Clinica dello Sviluppo*. 12(2). 325-344.

Venuti, P., (2003), *L'Autismo: Percorsi d'intervento*. [Autism: Therapeutical Practice] Roma, Carrocci.

Venuti, P., Giusti, Z., La Femina, F., Esposito, G., & Domini, F. (2002). Cry qualitative analysis in autistic children through home video. *Proceedings of VIII International Workshop on Cry Research*. Padova, Italy.

Wasz-Hockert, O., Lind, J., Vuorenski, V., Partanen, T., & Valanne, E. (1968). The infant cry: A spectrographic and auditory analysis. *Clinical Development and Medicine*. 29, 1–42.

Wolff, P., (1969). The natural history of crying and other vocalizations in early infancy. In B. Foss (Ed). *Determinants of infant behaviour* (vol. 4). London: Mathuen.

Zeskind, P.S., & Marshall, T.R. (1988). The Relation between Variations in Pitch and Maternal Perceptions of Infant Crying. *Child Development*. 59(1), 193-196.

Zeskind, P.S., Klein, L., & Marshall, T.R. (1992). Adult's perceptions of experimental modifications of durations of pauses and expiratory sounds in infant crying. *Child Development*. 59, 193-196.

Zeskind, P.S., & Lester, B. M. (2001). Analysis of infant crying. In L. T. Singer, & P. S. Zeskind (Eds). *Biobehavioral assessment of the infant* (pp. 149–166). New York: Guilford Publications Inc.

Ziefman, D.M. (2003). Predicting adult responses to infant distress: Adult characteristics associated with perceptions, emotional reactions, and timing of intervention. *Infant Mental Health Journal*. 24, 597-612.

Reviewed by Prof. Roger Bakeman
Georgia State University

In: Children and Language: Development, Impairment … ISBN 978-1-60692-395-5
Editor: Michael A. Reed

Chapter 9

DOES LANGUAGE EXPERIENCE INFLUENCE THE ACQUISITION OF LEXICON? INSIGHTS FROM THE INTELLECTUAL DISABILITY FIELD

***Bruno Facon*[1*] *and Thérèse Bollengier*[2]**
[1]Université Lille Nord de France F-59653 Villeneuve d'Ascq cedex
Unité de Recherche sur l'Evolution des Comportements et des Apprentissages (EA 1059)
[2]Service de psychologie Circonscription Education Nationale de Roubaix France

ABSTRACT

Correlational, quasi-experimental and experimental research conducted with typical children has shown that language input strongly influences the development of vocabulary and syntax. Another approach to this issue, based on the pathological method, is reviewed in the present chapter. This approach consists in studying participants with intellectual disability because they present a "natural" (i.e., unprovoked) dissociation between their general developmental level and their educational experience. Indeed, compared to intellectually average children of the same mental age, children and adolescents with intellectual disability have had more learning opportunities simply because, given their chronological age, they have lived longer. In particular, and all things being equal, they have participated more often in educational or leisure activities and have a far greater language experience, including more verbal interactions with their parents, grandparents, educators, teachers and all their other caregivers. This language experience related to age may well give them, among other things, an advantage with regard to the acquisition of additional vocabulary. Indeed, if interindividual differences in lexical development are caused, at least in part, by differences in language input, then CA-related language experience should give adolescents or children with intellectual disability a vocabulary *advantage* over typical children of comparable cognitive level. In the present literature review, the classical approaches (i.e., correlational, quasi-

* Correspondence concerning this chapter may be sent to Bruno Facon, Université Lille Nord de France, 35 rue Sainte Barbe, B. P. 70460, 59208 Tourcoing CEDEX, France. E-Mail : bruno.facon@univ-lille3.fr or bruno.facon@laposte.net.

experimental and experimental) used to study the relationship between the language learning environment and the acquisition of lexicon are successively presented. The pathological method is then considered and illustrated with the aim of showing that the study of children and adolescents with intellectual disability might be an innovative way to examine the relationship between language experience and language development.

1. Language and Experience: The Three Traditional Ways

The Correlational Approach

A large body of evidence points to the influence of the language learning environment on the child's acquisition of vocabulary and syntax. Intercultural studies show, for example, that cultural context influences the style and the content of adult-child verbal interactions which, in turn, determine the nature and the rate of the child's first language acquisitions (Bates, Devescovi, & Wulfeck, 2001; Bornstein & Cote, 2005; Choi, 2000; Choi & Gopnik, 1995; Devescovi *et al.*, 2005; Lieven, 1994; Tardif, 1996; Tardif, Shatz, & Naigles, 1997). Studies comparing the verbal development of children coming from families of different socioeconomic status also reveal large differences in the learning rate and the scope of verbal skills, whether it be in comprehension or in production (Arriaga, Fenson, Cronan, & Pethick, 1998; Bornstein, Haynes, & Painter, 1998; Dollaghan *et al.*, 1999; Farkas & Beron, 2004; Hart & Risley, 1995; Huttenlocher, Vasilyeva, Cymerman, & Levine, 2002; Snow, 1999). Moreover, it appears that the observed differences fade when the characteristics of maternal speech are held constant (Hoff, 2003), thus suggesting that the relationship between SES and child's language development is mediated by the nature of verbal input provided by the parents.

Of course, the relationship between parental SES and child language or, more generally, between language development and features of verbal input or educational practices of parents (e.g., Hoff & Naigles, 2002; Huttenlocher, Haight, Bryk, Seltzer, & Lyons 1991; Pan, Rowe, Singer, & Snow, 2005; Tamis-LeMonda, Bornstein, & Baumwell, 2001; Weizman & Snow, 2001) cannot be interpreted in a causal manner. It could be attributed as well to effects of genotype and of correlations (passive, evocative and active) between genotype and the verbal environment (see, Scarr, 1992; Scarr & McCartney, 1983). However, there are some natural situations for which a biological (i.e., genetic) or a reciprocal explanation of the relationship between child's language level and the characteristics of his linguistic environment cannot be put forward. For example, first-born children, who initially benefit from an individualized linguistic environment, show at least a temporary advantage over later-born children with respect to vocabulary and syntax (Berglund, Eriksson, & Westerlund, 2005; Hoff-Ginsberg, 1998; Pine, 1995). Also, progress by bilingual children in one and the other of their two languages is a function of the degree of exposition in each of them on an everyday basis (Patterson, 2002; Patterson & Pearson, 2004; Pearson, Fernandez, Lewedeg, & Oller, 1997). Furthermore, the relationship between infants' lexical development and current maternal utterances is significantly weaker when the mothers are not at home as full-time caregivers (i.e., work outside the home), a phenomenon indicating that early maternal input indeed contributes to the child's language development (Dunham & Dunham, 1992).

The Quasi-Experimental Approach

Quasi-experimental studies conducted in the school environment or in day care centers also provide valuable information. Time-period comparisons show, for example, that the development of vocabulary and/or syntax is more important during the school year than during summer vacation, a coherent result given the richer character of verbal input provided by school in comparison with that available in most families (Hayes & Grether, 1983; Heyns, 1978; Huttenlocher, Levine, & Vevea, 1998). Another approach, based on the between-grades regression discontinuity design, also indicates a strong effect of schooling on vocabulary (Cahan & Cohen, 1989). Indeed, the regression line of vocabulary scores on chronological age of pupils *within* each school grade shows a sharp discontinuity with those of the adjacent grades. Yet, since the oldest pupils in the lower grade are nearly as old as the youngest in the higher grade, their vocabulary should be of comparable size, and the regression lines shouldn't present any between-grade discontinuity. In fact, this latter is the consequence of the difference of schooling experience (i.e., one year) between the youngest pupils of any grade and that of the oldest pupils of the immediately preceding grade, experience which favorably influences the vocabulary level. In the same way, and although the methodological approach is different, a recent study by Huttenlocher *et al.* (2002) shows that the syntactic progress of four years old children over the school year is positively correlated with the complexity of teacher speech, even though the children's and teacher's syntactic skills are uncorrelated at the start of the year. Studies related to the influence of early day care center quality on language development give congruent results. They reveal significant relationships between indexes of quality (e.g., child-staff ratio, group size, caregiver training and education, amount of verbal interaction between children and caregivers) and language skills of the children, even when controlling for family background (McCartney, 1984; NICHD Early Child Care Research Network, 1999). Consequently, selection or reciprocal effects cannot be invoked to explain the results.

The Experimental Approach

Another line of evidence arises in experimental studies in which verbal input is systematically manipulated and participants randomly assigned to either the treatment or the control group. The manipulation can be "global", consisting of an increase in *non specific* verbal models provided to the child during activities favorable to adult-child verbal interactions, such as *dialogic or shared reading*. In this case, substantial syntax and vocabulary differences between experimental and comparison or control groups are classically observed (Arnold, Lonigan, Whitehurst, & Epstein, 1994; Lonigan & Whitehurst, 1998; Sénéchal, 1997; Sénéchal, Thomas, & Monker, 1995; Valdez-Menchaca & Whitehurst, 1992; Whitehurst *et al.*, 1994, 1988). The manipulation can also be more differentiated, aiming at learning of specific linguistic forms (e.g., two-word semantic relations, adjective-noun combinations, compound sentences, wh-questions, irregular past tense or passive voice). In this context, experimental subjects generally show impressive improvement with regard to mastery of target structures (Camatara & Nelson, 2006; Fey, Cleave, Long & Hughes, 1993; Hart & Risley, 1968, 1974, 1975; Nelson, 1977, 2000; Saxton, Kulcsar, Marshall, & Rupra,

1998; Scherer & Olswang, 1984; Valian & Casey, 2003; Vasilyeva, Huttenlocher, & Waterfall, 2006).

Correlational, quasi-experimental and experimental studies provide coherent evidence in support of a strong influence of verbal learning experience on the development of children's language skills. This does not mean, however, that research on this question should cease. Indeed, there are contradictory results which, for the moment, preclude definitive conclusion. For example, some linguistic differences in child's language growth attributed to cultural context are not always confirmed (Caselli *et al.*, 1995), and the same goes for the birth-order effect (Bornstein, Leach, & Haynes, 2004). Also, the variance explained by SES varies greatly from study to study (Hoff, 2006) and experimental studies sometimes give ambiguous results (see, for a review, Valian & Casey, 2003). These contradictions are probably related to differences in instruments and procedures, sample characteristics (e.g., age of participants) or size, reliability of measures or variance of independent variables and, consequently, must lead us to conduct methodologically improved studies. A diversification of angles of approach would also be interesting. Indeed, the more differentiated the array of evidence, the more plausible the inferences drawn from the data, particularly if methodological weaknesses inherent to each approach are uncorrelated (see, Ceci, 1991).

2. Toward a Fourth Way: The Pathological Approach A Fruitful Methodological Approach in Many Respects

One way to diversify the study of the relationship between language and experience might be to adopt the pathological method, that is, to study disorders caused by disease or accident, not in order to contrast the *pathological* with the *normal* but, on the contrary, to throw light on the normal. The works of Jean Baptiste Bouillaud and Pierre Paul Broca have, for example, shown the decisive role that this method had at the beginning of modern neurosciences (Young, 1990). It is also via this approach that French psychology, stimulated by Théodule Ribot, made its transition from the philosophical analysis to the scientific study of psychological phenomena (Nicolas, 2002). The contribution of the pathological method was well illustrated by Oléron (1957, 1977), Furth (1964, 1971), Hatwell (1966/1985, 2003) or Gouin Decarie (1969) in the field of sensory or motor deficiencies. But the study of children with intellectual disability also proved to be useful in many respects. For example, recent research on Williams syndrome opened a new angle on the thorny problem of the relationship between language and cognition and, more generally, the links between genes, brain and behavior (Bellugi, Adolphs, Cassady, & Chiles, 1999; Bellugi, Lichtenberger, Jones, Lai, & George, 2000; Karmiloff-Smith, Brown, Grice, & Paterson, 2003; Mervis, 2003; Mervis & Morris, 2007; Thomas & Karmiloff-Smith, 2003). However, beyond these interesting and controversial questions, the study of children and adolescents with intellectual disability might also be an innovative means to examine the relationship between language experience and language development. Indeed, children and adolescents with intellectual disability present a "natural" (i.e., unprovoked) dissociation between their cognitive level and their educational experience. More precisely, compared to intellectually average children of the same mental age (MA), they have had more learning opportunities simply because, given their chronological age, they have lived longer. In particular, and all things being equal, they have a far greater language experience because they have had more verbal interactions with their parents, grandparents, educators, teachers and all their other caregivers. This language experience related to age may well give them, among other things, an advantage with regard to the acquisition of vocabulary. Indeed, if inter-individual differences in lexical development are caused, at least in part, by differences in language input, then CA-related language experience should give, to adolescents with intellectual disability, a vocabulary *advantage* over typical (or even retarded) children of comparable cognitive level.

Beyond Conjectures: Some Preliminary Results

This prediction has, in practice, already been tested and confirmed in several preliminary studies demonstrating that when the cognitive level of children and adolescents is held constant, chronological age exerts a significant effect on receptive vocabulary, vocabulary richness or the ability to define words with accuracy and precision (Facon, Bollengier, & Grubar, 1993; Facon & Facon-Bollengier, 1997, 1999a, 1999b; Facon, Facon-Bollengier, & Grubar, 2002; Facon, Grubar, & Gardez, 1998).

In the study by Facon et al. (1993), the *Test de Vocabulaire en Images*, the French version of the Peabody Picture Vocabulary Test (Légé & Dague, 1974) and Raven's Colored Progressive Matrices (Raven1981) were administered to three groups of participants *matched on MA* (30 intellectually average participants age 5 years and two groups of 30 participants with intellectual disability, one composed of 10-year-olds, the other, 16-year olds). In accordance with results of nearly all comparative studies of the last five decades conducted on performance in various cognitive tasks (e.g., reasoning, attention, short term or working memory, etc.) of participants with and without intellectual disability matched on MA (e.g., Hooper *et al.*, 2008; Hulme & Mackenzie, 1992; Iarocci & Burack, 1998; Numminen, Lehto, & Ruoppila, 2001; Numminen, Service, & Ruoppila, 2002; Weiss, Weisz, & Bromfield, 1986; Weisz & Yeates, 1981; Weisz & Zigler, 1979; Vicari, Bellucci, & Carlesimo, 2001; Vicari & Carlesimo, 2002, 2006), participants with intellectual disability in the Facon *et al.* study would have had to obtain scores comparable, if not inferior, to those of typical children on *both* tests. In fact, statistical analyses did reveal no significant differences among the three groups on Raven's Matrices, but there was a strong linear relationship between CA and performance on the *Test de Vocabulaire en Images* (Figure 1). Thus, despite the MA matching, the greater the mean CA of the group, the greater the mean receptive vocabulary. This finding was interpreted as an effect of the language experience correlated with CA insofar as receptive vocabulary, contrary to processes tapped by Raven's Matrices, can be learned in numerous everyday situations.

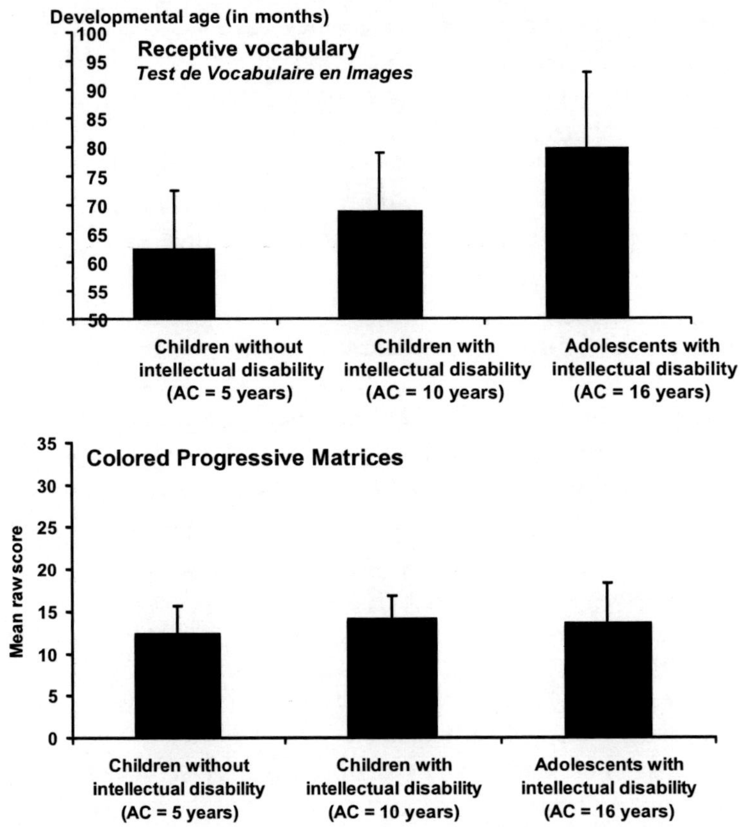

Figure 1. Means and standard deviations of the three groups for the vocabulary test (top panel) and Ravens Matrices (bottom panel). Bars indicate standard deviations. Adapted with permission from Facon, Bollengier, and Grubar (1993).

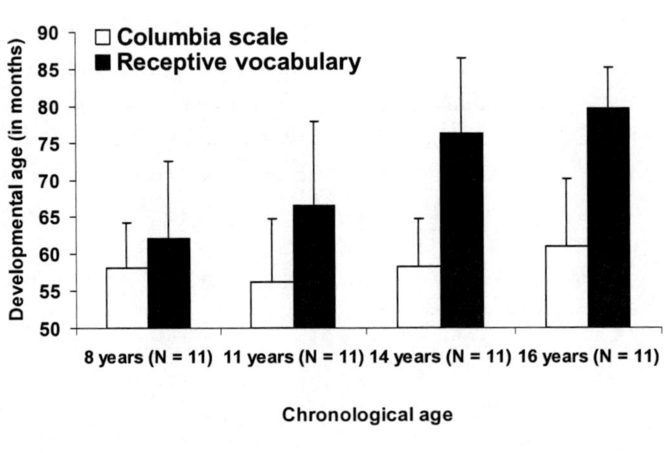

Figure 2. Means and standard deviations of four groups of participants with intellectual disability on the receptive vocabulary test (Test de Vocabulaire en Images) and the Columbia Mental Maturity Scale. Bars indicate standard deviations. Adapted with permission from Facon and Facon-Bollengier (1997).

These results were confirmed in a further study by Facon and Facon-Bollengier (1997) in which a similar relationship between chronological age and receptive vocabulary was observed among children and adolescents with intellectual disability who were matched for MA on the Columbia Mental Maturity Scale, a test of categorization coming within the fluid component of human intelligence (Figure 2). Moreover, it was also shown, in another study conducted by these same authors, that the influence of CA-related experience was, beyond receptive vocabulary, also observed using numerous other verbal measures (Facon & Facon-Bollengier, 1999a). In that study, a sample of about a hundred participants with intellectual disability ages 6 to 20 years were given a battery of verbal tasks including four verbal subtests extracted from the Wechsler Preschool and Primary Scale of Intelligence [WPPSI] and the Wechsler Intelligence Scale for Children Revised [WISC-R], two tests of receptive vocabulary, and The Test of Vocabulary Richness.[1] The cognitive level of participants was estimated using several tests of fluid intelligence such as Raven's Matrices and the Columbia Mental Maturity Scale. While the relationship between chronological age and fluid intelligence was not significant, results showed, once again, a strong relationship between age and performance on verbal tasks (Figure 3). Thus, chronological age does not relate only to receptive vocabulary of adolescents and young adults with intellectual disability. Their ability to define words or to conceptualize verbally is also age-related.

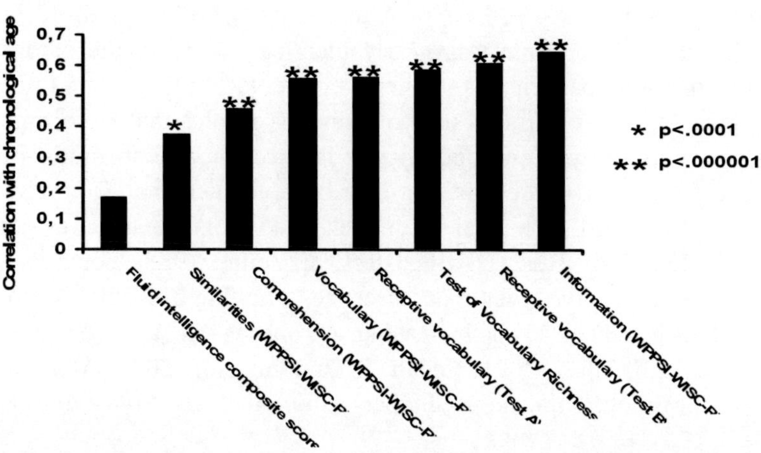

Figure 3. Strength of correlation between chronological age and performance on various verbal tasks of participants with intellectual disability aged 6 to 20 years. The nonsignificant correlation between chronological age and the fluid intelligence composite score is due, of course, to the sampling procedure.[2] Adapted with permission from Facon and Facon-Bollengier (1999a).

[1] Information items from the WPPSI and the WISC-R were combined to avoid ceiling or floor effects, a procedure also applied with the other WPPSI and WISC-R verbal subtests included in the study (Comprehension, Vocabulary and Similarities). For each of the 30 items of the Test of Vocabulary Richness, the participant was asked to give two instances of the same conceptual category; for example, "give me the name of two vegetables" (item 3), "give me the name of two insects" (item 10), "give me the name of two geometric forms" (item 17) or "give me the name of two trades" (item 30).

In order to avoid a too strong correlation between chronological age and the fluid intelligence score, young participants recruited for the study were mostly mildly disabled whereas adolescents and young adults were mostly moderately or severely disabled.

Taken together, these results clearly suggest the existence of a strong relationship between chronological age and vocabulary of persons with intellectual disability, even when their cognitive level is held constant. Nevertheless, additional data are needed before generalizing. For example, the possible influence of etiology must be considered in the interpretation of results because participants in the three studies were selected without regard to etiology. Thus, it is not certain that the relationship between chronological age and vocabulary performance holds for more homogeneous groups of persons with the same or similar etiologies. Indeed, a growing number of studies with specific etiological groups (e.g., Down syndrome, Fragile X, Williams syndrome), shows that persons of a common etiology often display a similar profile of behavioral or cognitive strengths and weaknesses and a specific developmental trajectory (Dykens & Hodapp, 2001, 2007; Dykens, Hodapp, & Finucane, 2000; Hodapp & Burack, 2006; Hodapp & Dykens, 2001, 2007; Rondal, Hodapp, Soreci, Dykens, & Nota, 2004). It is therefore necessary to determine whether or not the effect of chronological age-related experience on vocabulary is dependent on etiology. This question was investigated in a study that included only Down syndrome participants and thus kept the variables *age* and *etiology* orthogonal (Facon, Grubar, & Gardez, 1998). The sample included 29 participants with Down syndrome drawn from community-based schools. Age range was approximately 6 to 14, with a mean of 10 years. All participants were tested individually during one session with the Columbia Mental Maturity Scale followed by a receptive vocabulary test. As can be seen in Figure 4, although the developmental level achieved on the Columbia Scale was nearly identical whatever the chronological age, the performance of the older participants on the receptive vocabulary test was greater than that of the younger ones, which confirms results of previous studies that were conducted regardless of the etiology of disability. Consequently, the latter cannot be attributed to etiology-related effects. In addition, even if there is considerable evidence that Down syndrome subjects perform at the same level as mental age-matched controls, retarded or not, on vocabulary tasks (e. g., Fowler, 1990; Rosin, Swift, Bless, & Vetter, 1988), some studies indicate that vocabulary exceeds cognitive level in adolescence, a finding probably due to greater diversity of educational experiences with increasing chronological age (Chapman, 1999, 2006; Chapman & Hesketh, 2000, 2001; Glenn & Cunningham, 2005; McDuffie, Chapman, & Abbeduto, 2008; Miolo, Chapman, & Sindberg; 2005; Roberts, Price, & Malkin, 2007).

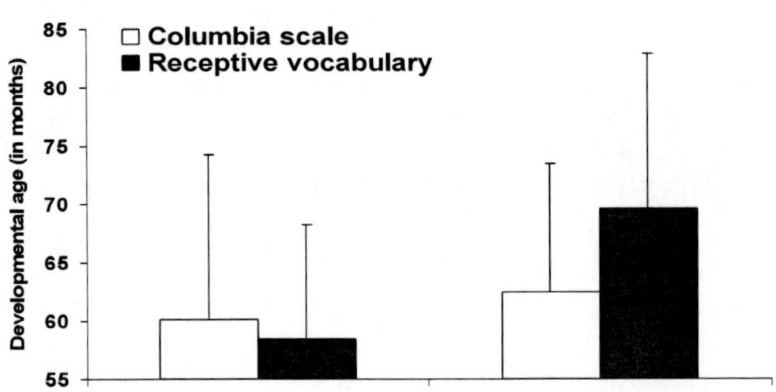

Figure 4. Means and standard deviations of participants with Down syndrome on the receptive vocabulary test (*Test de Vocabulaire en Images*) and the Columbia Mental Maturity Scale. Bars indicate standard deviations. Adapted with permission from Facon, Grubar, and Gardez (1998).

Finally, the question of the moderating influence of the degree of intellectual deficiency on the relationship between age and vocabulary was considered in a study based on the WISC-R data of 1101 participants with moderate or mild intellectual disability aged 8 to 17 years. In this study, a multiple regression analysis was conducted using as dependent variables raw scores on four verbal subtests (Information, Vocabulary, Similarities and Comprehension). Raw scores on the six other subtests (Picture Completion, Picture Arrangement, Block Design, Object Assembly, Arithmetic and Coding) were used as non-verbal measures of cognitive level and, for this reason, were entered *before* chronological age in the regression equation. Results showed that even with non-verbal cognitive level statistically controlled, chronological age was strongly related to verbal performance for participants with moderate intellectual disability as well as for those with mild intellectual disability. However, the standardized regression coefficients were significantly greater for those with mild disability (Figure 5), meaning perhaps that given their lower cognitive level, participants with moderate intellectual disability are less able to take advantage of their life experience.

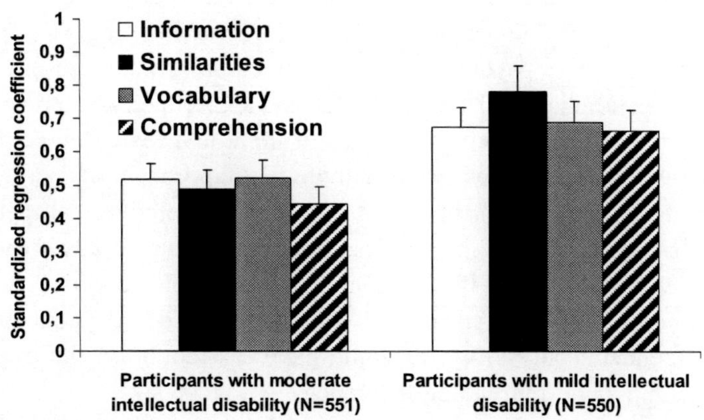

Figure 5. Standardized regression coefficients of four verbal subtest scores of the WISC-R vs. chronological age, with scores on the non-verbal subtests entered first in the equation. Bars indicate standard errors. Adapted with permission from Facon and Facon-Bollengier (1999b).

3. Some Comments and Further Research Perspectives

The studies here reviewed indicate the existence of a strong relationship between chronological age and several lexical skills of children and adolescents with intellectual disability (receptive vocabulary, ability to define words or to conceptualize verbally). This relationship appears to be independent of etiology and can be observed among participants with either mild or moderate intellectual disability. But, more importantly, this relationship obtains even when the cognitive level of participants is held constant. The information supplied in the articles consulted for the present review show that all things being equal, and particularly the cognitive level of participants, chronological age still "explains" on the order of 15 to 20 percent of the variance of vocabulary measures. According to statistical standards (e.g., Cohen, 1988), this value corresponds to a moderate, and thus non-negligible, effect size which is to be understood in light of results of most comparative studies involving mental age-matched groups. Indeed, when participants with intellectual disability are compared with

MA-matched participants, for example typical children, they show similar or lower performance, rarely better, on almost any dependent measures (e.g., Hooper et al., 2008; Hulme & Mackenzie, 1992; Iarocci & Burack, 1998; Numminen et al., 2001, 2002; Perkins & Small, 2006; Weiss, Weisz, & Bromfield, 1986; Weisz & Yeates, 1981; Weisz & Zigler, 1979; Vicari et al., 2001; Vicari & Carlesimo, 2002, 2006). Consequently, the adolescents with intellectual disability included in the above-mentioned studies should have, at best, lexical performance comparable to that of the children because they are at the same cognitive level. In this respect, our interpretation is that given their chronological age, the adolescents have greater language experience and, for this reason, obtain higher scores on lexical tasks than children of same mental age.

This type of results increases the array of evidence on the relationship between verbal input and lexical development. Indeed, if such a relationship really exists, the lexical performance of subjects with intellectual disability of similar cognitive level must be correlated to chronological age, simply because language experience is, all thing being equal, necessarily correlated with age. The research studies summarized in the present chapter suggest, in our view, the usefulness of combining several methodological approaches in order to understand and explain a psychological phenomenon. In the present case, it can be considered that correlational, quasi-experimental and experimental studies conducted with typical children on the relationship between verbal input and lexical development permitted the prediction of results obtained with the pathological approach, and are likely to explain them. In addition, data collected on this question using the pathological method allow us, in turn, to validate lessons drawn from studies of typical subjects based on more classical approaches. From this standpoint, if it had not been possible to prove the existence of a chronological age effect on the vocabulary development of MA-matched children and adolescents with intellectual disability, it would have cast doubt on the true meaning of the link between verbal input and individual differences in lexicon size.

The studies here presented are more a starting point than a culmination. First, replications with more etiological groups would permit generalization of the results. For example, the fact that persons with other etiologies differ from Down syndrome subjects in their trajectories of development or in their cognitive and linguistic profiles (e.g., Abbeduto, Warren, & Conners, 2007; Gerenser, Forman, & Child, 2007; Price, Roberts, Vandergrift, & Martin, 2007) might throw into question the present conclusions. Likewise, some syndrome-specific behaviors, e.g., maladaptive behaviors in Fragile X syndrome (Hall, Debernardis, & Reiss, 2006; Hall, Lightbody, & Reiss, 2008; Reiss & Dant, 2003), might diminish the child's capacity to elicit engaging and positive reactions from others and, thus, reduce the range of learning experiences. Because of this, the influence of chronological age-related experience would surely be less important than for individuals demonstrating low rates of such behaviors. Conversely, this age effect could be of a far more important size among subjects exhibiting a high degree of sociability –such as individuals with William's syndrome, who are reputed to be unusually sociable, friendly, and empathic. For that matter, it has been showed that children with Williams syndrome capitalize on their developing language abilities for social purposes (Jones et al., 2000). Thus, the CA-related experience effect on their linguistic abilities could be stronger than for other etiologic subgroups with intellectual disability.

Second, it would be useful to further diversify the dependent variables. For example, if it now seems likely that CA-related experience increases the performance of adolescents with intellectual disability on frequency-based tests of object- or event-related vocabulary, such as the Peabody Picture Vocabulary Test, CA's influence appears negligible on tests evaluating the mastery of abstract relational words such as the Boehm Test or the Vocabulary subtest of the Test for Auditory Comprehension of Language (see, Fazio, Johnston, & Brandl, 1993; Miolo et al., 2005). The use of measures of syntactic development would also be interesting. The few studies on this issue indicate that CA-related experience does not appear to affect the syntactic performance of adolescents with intellectual disability (Facon et al., 2002). In our opinion, this phenomenon is not due to the fact that syntax is an autonomous and innate component of language and, thus, is less influenced than vocabulary by the experience accumulated with chronological age. Rather, the acquisition of syntax, like that of abstract relational words, is perhaps more constrained by cognitive level than the acquisition of vocabulary. It is possible that the chronological age effect is cancelled or at least greatly diminished by the less efficient working memory of persons with intellectual disability. Indeed, since a great number of studies emphasize the link between working memory and syntactic development (Adams & Gathercole, 2000; Fowler, 1998; Miolo & Chapman, 1999; Montgomery, 2003; Rondal & Edwards, 1997; Van Daal, Verhoeven, & Van Leeuwe, 2008), it is quite conceivable that one or more working memory deficits counteract the effect of CA-related experience on syntax development in intellectual disability.

A third line of research could productively focus on responses to items of vocabulary tests. If CA-related experience influences the lexical performance of adolescents with intellectual disability, it would be interesting to know whether this experience increases the likelihood of success on *all* items or only on *some* of them. In this second case, an interaction would be observed between chronological age and the item response profiles of the participants.

CONCLUSION

All scientific approaches have methodological weaknesses. The correlational approach does not permit conclusions in terms of causation because of the “third variable” problem and that of the “direction of effect”. Quasi-experimental research designs do not enable one to draw firm causal inferences because participants are not randomly assigned to the different conditions planned by the investigator. Thus, selection biases are real possibilities and thus preclude definitive conclusions. In the same way, even if the systematic manipulation of independent variables and the randomization of participants allow us to eliminate most alternative explanations and confer a high degree of internal validity on the study (Shadish, Cook, & Campbell, 2002), the results often lack generalizability and external validity. The pathological approach is not itself without flaws. The localization, the extend and the outcome of damage caused by a disease or an accident are often difficult to specify. From this standpoint, the “natural experiments” are never quite so simple. Moreover, the damage may creates substitute mechanisms and specific idiosyncratic psychological functions such that the functions examined among disabled individuals are not necessarily comparable to those which can be observed among typical individuals (Reuchlin, 1979). What appears unaltered or intact in spite of the disorders noted elsewhere is possibly something different resulting from a reorganization of the whole system. Stated otherwise,

> "the notion that an ability is necessarily intact in a [...] disorder when behavior falls within the normal range fails to consider the psychological processes underlying overt behavior. This kind of reasoning negates the role of development in producing phenotypic outcomes and treats the end-state cognitive system as if it were a normal system with some components missing and others intact. In other words, it is based on the neuropsychology model of brain damage to previously normal adults and can, in our view, be very misleading when applied to developmental disorders" (Karmiloff-Smith et al., 2003, p. 228).

If these different methodological approaches still coexist today in scientific psychology in spite of their respective biases, it is surely because they are useful in some respects. In our view, they must be used conjointly in order to target the fullest range of psychological phenomena. In scientific research, the combination of several angles of study is always preferable to adopting the narrow attitude of the blind man facing the elephant. As stated by Ceci (1991, p. 718),

> "[...] if studies using different methodologies, different mental measures, and different samples all converge on the same conclusion and if these studies possess uncorrelated weaknesses, then one can infer that their collective power is greater than that of their individual conclusions."

Acknowledgements

We thank John M. Belmont for his helpful comments on this chapter.

References

Abbeduto, L., Warren, S. F., & Conners, F. A. (2007). Language development in Down syndrome: From the prelinguistic period to the acquisition of literacy. *Mental Retardation and Developmental Disabilities Research Reviews*, *13*, 247-261.

Adams, A.-M., & Gathercole, S. E. (2000). Limitations in working memory: Implications for language development. *International Journal of Language and Communication Disorders*, *35*, 95-116.

Arnold, D. H., Lonigan, C. J., Whitehurst, G. J., & Epstein, J. N. (1994). Accelerating language development through picture book reading: Replication and extension to a videotape training format. *Journal of Educational Psychology*, *86*, 235-243.

Arriaga, R. K., Fenson, L., Cronan, T., & Pethick, S. J. (1998). Scores on the MacArthur Communicative Development Inventory of children from low- and middle-income families. *Applied Psycholinguistics*, *19*, 209-225.

Bates, E., Devescovi, A., & Wulfeck, B. (2001). Psycholinguistics: A cross-language perspective. *Annual Review of Psychology*, *52*, 369-396.

Bellugi, U., Adolphs, R., Cassady, C., & Chiles, M. (1999). Towards the neural basis for hypersociability in a genetic syndrome. *NeuroReport*, *10*, 1653-1657.

Bellugi, U., Lichtenberger, L., Jones, W., Lai, Z., & George, M. (2000). The neurocognitive profile of Williams syndrome: A complex pattern of strengths and weaknesses. *Journal of Cognitive Neuroscience*, *72*, 7-29.

Berglund, E., Eriksson, M., & Westerlund, M. (2005). Communicative skills in relation to gender, birth order, childcare and socioeconomic status in 18-month-old children. *Scandinavian Journal of Psychology*, *46*, 485-491.

Bornstein, M. H., & Cote, L. R. (2005). Expressive vocabulary in language learners from two ecological settings in three language communities. *Infancy*, *7*, 299-316.

Bornstein, M. H., Haynes, O. M., & Painter, K. M. (1998). Sources of child vocabulary competence: A multivariate model. *Journal of Child Language*, *25*, 367-394.

Bornstein, M. H., Leach, D. B., & Haynes, O. M. (2004). Vocabulary competence in first- and secondborn siblings of the same chronological age. *Journal of Child Language*, *31*, 855-873.

Cahan, S., & Cohen, N. (1989). Age versus schooling effects on intelligence development. *Child Development*, *60*, 1239-1249.

Camarata, S. M., & Nelson, K. E. (2006). Conversational recast intervention with preschool and older Children. In R. J. McCauley & M. E. Fey (Eds.), *Treatment of language disorders in children* (pp. 237-264). Baltimore, MD: Paul H. Brookes Publishing Company.

Caselli, M. C., Bates, E., Casadio, P., Fenson, J., Fenson, L., Sanders, L., & Weir, J. (1995). A cross-linguistic study of early lexical development. *Cognitive Development*, *10*, 159-199.

Ceci, S. J. (1991). How much does schooling influence general intelligence and its cognitive components? A reassessment of the evidence. *Developmental Psychology*, *27*, 703-722.

Chapman, R. S. (1999). Language and cognitive development in children and adolescents with Down syndrome. In J. F. Miller, L. A. Leavitt & M. Leddy (Eds.), *Improving the Communication of People with Down Syndrome* (pp. 41-60). Baltimore, MD: Paul H. Brookes Publishing Company.

Chapman, R. S. (2006). Language learning in Down syndrome: The speech and language profile compared to adolescents with cognitive impairment of unknown origin. *Down Syndrome Research and Practice*, *10*, 61-66.

Chapman, R. S., & Hesketh, L. J. (2000). Behavioural phenotype of individuals with Down syndrome. *Mental Retardation and Developmental Disability Research Reviews*, *6*, 84-95.

Chapman, R. S., & Hesketh, L. J. (2001). Language, cognition, and short-term memory in individuals with Down syndrome. *Down Syndrome Research and Practice*, *7*, 1-7.

Choi, S. (2000). Caregiver input in English and Korean: Use of nouns and verbs in book-reading and toy-play contexts. *Journal of Child Language*, *27*, 69-96.

Choi, S., & Gopnik, A. (1995). Early acquisition of verbs in Korean: A cross-linguistic study. *Journal of Child Language*, *22*, 497-529.

Cohen, J. (1988). *Statistical power analysis for the behavioral sciences* (2nd ed.). Hillsdale, NJ: Laurence Erlbaum Associates.

Devescovi, A., Caselli, M. C., Marchione, D., Pasqualetti, P., Reilly, J., & Bates, E. (2005). A crosslinguistic study of the relationship between grammar and lexical development. *Journal of Child Language*, *32*, 759-786.

Dollaghan, C. A., Campbell, T. F., Paradise, J. L., Feldman, H. M., Janosky, J. E., Pitcairn, D. N., & Kurs-Lasky, M. (1999). Maternal education and measures of early speech and language. *Journal of Speech, Language and Hearing Research*, *42*, 1432-1443.

Dunham, P., & Dunham, F. (1992). Lexical development during middle infancy: A mutually driven infant-caregiver process. *Developmental Psychology*, *28*, 414-420.

Dykens, E. M., & Hodapp, R. M. (2001). Research in mental retardation: Toward an etiologic approach. *Journal of Child Psychology and Psychiatry*, *42*, 49-71.

Dykens, E. M., & Hodapp, R. M. (2007). Three steps toward improving the measurement of behavior in behavioral phenotype research. *Child and Adolescent Psychiatric Clinics of North-America*, *16*, 617-630.

Dykens, E. M., Hodapp, R. M., & Finucane, B. (2000). *Genetics and mental retardation syndromes: A new look at behavior and interventions*. Baltimore, MD: Paul H. Brookes Publishing Company.

Facon, B., Bollengier, T., & Grubar, J.-C. (1993). Overestimation of mentally retarded persons' IQs using the PPVT: A re-analysis and some implications for future research. *Journal of Intellectual Disability Research*, *37*, 373-379.

Facon, B., & Facon-Bollengier, T. (1997). Chronological age and Peabody Picture Vocabulary Test performance of persons with mental retardation: New data. *Psychological Reports*, *81*, 1232-1234.

Facon, B., & Facon-Bollengier, T. (1999a). Chronological age and crystallized intelligence of people with intellectual disability. *Journal of Intellectual Disability Research*, *43*, 489-496.

Facon, B., & Facon-Bollengier, T. (1999b). Chronological age and performance of persons with mental retardation on verbal subtests of the Wechsler Intelligence Scale for Children-revised, French version. *Psychological Reports*, *85*, 857-862.

Facon, B., Facon-Bollengier, T., & Grubar, J.-C. (2002). Chronological age, receptive vocabulary and syntax comprehension in children and adolescents with mental retardation. *American Journal on Mental Retardation*, *107*, 91-98.

Facon, B., Grubar, J.-C., & Gardez, C. (1998). Chronological age and receptive vocabulary of persons with Down syndrome. *Psychological Reports*, *82*, 723-726.

Farkas, G., & Beron, K. (2004). The detailed age trajectory of oral vocabulary knowledge: Differences by class and race. *Social Science Research*, *33*, 464-497.

Fazio, B. B., Johnston, J. R., & Brandl, L. (1993). Relation between mental age and vocabulary development among children with mild mental retardation. *American Journal on Mental Retardation*, *97*, 541-546.

Fey, M. E., Cleave, P. L., Long, S. H., & Hughes, D. L. (1993). Two approaches to the facilitation of grammar in children with language impairment: An experimental evaluation. *Journal of Speech & Hearing Research*, *36*, 141-157.

Fowler, A. E. (1990). Language abilities in children with Down syndrome: evidence for a specific syntactic delay. In D. Cicchetti & M. Beeghly (Eds.), *Children with Down syndrome* (pp. 302-328). New York: Cambridge University Press.

Fowler, A. E. (1998). Language in mental retardation: Associations with and dissociations from general cognition. In J. A. Burack, R. M. Hodapp & E. Zigler (Eds.), *Handbook of mental retardation and development* (pp. 290-333). Cambridge, UK: Cambridge University Press.

Furth, H. G. (1964). Research with the deaf: Implications for language and cognition. *Psychological Bulletin, 62*, 145-164.

Furth, H. G. (1971). Linguistic deficiency and thinking: Research with deaf subjects 1964-1969. *Psychological Bulletin, 76*, 58-72.

Gerenser, J., Forman, B., & Child, T. (2007). Speech and language deficits in children with developmental disabilities. In J. W. Jacobson, J. A. Mulick & J. Rojahn (Eds.), *Handbook of Intellectual and Developmental Disabilities* (pp. 563-579). New York: Springer.

Glenn, S., & Cunningham, C. (2005). Performance of young people with Down syndrome on the Leiter-R and British Picture Vocabulary Scales. *Journal of Intellectual Disability Research, 49*, 239–244.

Gouin Decarie, T. (1969). A study of the mental and emotional development of the thalidomide child. In B. M. Foss (Ed.), *Determinants of infants behavior* (vol. 4, pp. 167-187). London, UK: Methuen.

Hall, S. S., Debernardis, G. M., & Reiss, A. L. (2006). Social escape behaviors in children with fragile X syndrome. *Journal of Autism and Developmental Disorders, 36*, 935-947.

Hall, S. S., Lightbody, A. A. & Reiss, A. L. (2008). Compulsive, self-injurious and autistic behavior in Fragile X syndrome. *American Journal on Mental Retardation, 113*, 44-53.

Hart, B. M., & Risley, T. R. (1968). Establishing use of descriptive adjectives in the spontaneous speech of disadvantaged preschool children. *Journal of Applied Behavior Analysis, 1*, 109-120.

Hart, B. M., & Risley, T. R. (1974). Using preschool materials to modify the language of disadvantaged children. *Journal of Applied Behavior Analysis, 7*, 243-256.

Hart, B. M., & Risley, T. R. (1975). Incidental teaching of language in the preschool. *Journal of Applied Behavior Analysis, 8*, 411-420.

Hart, B. M., & Risley, T. R. (1995). *Meaningful differences in the everyday experiences of young American children*. Baltimore, MD: Paul H. Brookes Publishing Company.

Hatwell, Y. (1985). *Piagetian reasoning and the blind.* New York : American Foundation for the Blind [translated from : Y. Hatwell (1966). *Privation sensorielle et intelligence. Effets de la cécité précoce sur la genèse des structures logiques de l'intelligence.* Paris : Presses Universitaires de France].

Hatwell, Y. (2003). *Psychologie cognitive de la cécité précoce / Cognitive psychology of early blindness.* Paris: Dunod.

Hayes, D. P., & Grether, J. (1983). The school year and vacations: when do students learn? *Cornell Journal of Social Relations, 17*, 56-71.

Heyns, B. (1978). *Summer learning and the effects of schooling*. New York: Academic Press.

Hodapp, R. M., & Burack, J. A. (2006). Developmental approaches to children with mental retardation: A second generation? In D. J. Cohen & D. Cicchetti (Eds.), *Developmental psychopathology: Risk, disorder, and adaptation* (Vol. 3, 2nd ed., pp. 235-267). Hoboken, NJ: John Wiley & Sons.

Hodapp, R. M., & Dykens, E. M. (2001). Strengthening behavioral research on genetic mental retardation syndromes. *American Journal on Mental Retardation, 106*, 4-15.

Hodapp, R. M., & Dykens, E. M. (2007). Behavioral effects of genetic mental retardation disorders. In J. Rojahn, J. W. Jacobson & J. A. Mulick (Eds.), *Handbook of intellectual and developmental disabilities* (pp. 115-131). New York: Springer Publishing Company.

Hoff, E. (2003). The specificity of environmental influence: Socioeconomic status affects early vocabulary development via maternal speech. *Child Development, 74*, 1368-1378.

Hoff, E. (2006). How social contexts support and shape language development. *Developmental Review*, *26*, 55-88.

Hoff, E., & Naigles, L. (2002). How children use input to acquire a lexicon. *Child Development*, *73*, 418-433.

Hoff-Ginsberg, E. (1998). The relation of birth order and socioeconomic status to children's language experience and language development. *Applied Psycholinguistics*, *19*, 603-629.

Hooper, S. R., Hatton, D., Sideris, J., Sullivan, K., Hammer, J., Schaaf, J., Mirrett, P., Ornstein, P. A., & Bailey, D. P. Jr. (2008). Executive functions in young males with fragile X syndrome in comparison to mental age-matched controls: baseline findings from a longitudinal study. *Neuropsychology*, *22*, 36-47.

Hulme, C., & Mackenzie, S. (1992). *Working memory and severe learning difficulties*. Hove, UK: Lawrence Erlbaum Associates.

Huttenlocher, J., Haight, W., Bryk, A., Seltzer, M., & Lyons, T. (1991). Early vocabulary growth: Relation to language input and gender. *Developmental Psychology*, *27*, 236-248.

Huttenlocher, J., Levine, S. C., & Vevea, J. (1998). Environmental input and cognitive growth: A study using time period comparisons. *Child Development*, *69*, 1012-1029.

Huttenlocher, J., Vasilyeva, M., Cymerman, E., & Levine, S. (2002). Language input at home and at school: Relation to child syntax. *Cognitive Psychology*, *45*, 337-374.

Iarocci, G., & Burack, J. A. (1998). Understanding the development of attention in persons with mental retardation: Challenging the myths. In J. A. Burack, R. M. Hodapp & E. Zigler (Eds), *Handbook of mental retardation and development* (pp. 349-381). New York: Cambridge University Press.

Jones, W., Bellugi, U., Lai, Z., Chiles, M., Reilly, J., Lincoln, A., & Adolphs, R. (2000). Hypersociability in Williams syndrome. *Journal of Cognitive Neuroscience, 12*, 30-46.

Karmiloff-Smith, A., Brown, J. H., Grice, S., & Paterson, S. (2003). Dethroning the myth: Cognitive dissociations and innate modularity in Williams syndrome. *Developmental Neuropsychology*, *23*, 229-244.

Légé, Y., & Dague, P. (1974). *Test de Vocabulaire en Images / Picture Vocabulary Test*. Paris: Editions du Centre de Psychologie Appliquée.

Lieven, E. V. M. (1994). Crosslinguistic and cross cultural aspects of language addressed to children. In C. Gallaway & B. J. Richards (Eds.), *Input and interaction in language acquisition* (pp. 74-106). Cambridge, UK: Cambridge University Press.

Lonigan, C. J., & Whitehurst, G. J. (1998). Relative efficacy of parent and teacher involvement in a shared-reading intervention for preschool children from low-income backgrounds. *Early Childhood Research Quarterly*, *13*, 263-290.

McCartney, K. (1984). Effect of quality of day care environment on children's language development. *Developmental Psychology*, *20*, 244-260.

McDuffie, A., Chapman, R. S., & Abbeduto, L. (2008). Language profiles of adolescents and young adults with Down syndrome and Fragile X syndrome. In J. E. Roberts, R. S. Chapman & S. F. Warren (Eds.), *Speech and language development and intervention in Down syndrome and Fragile X syndrome* (pp. 117-172). Baltimore, MD: Paul H. Brookes Publishing Company.

Mervis, C. B. (2003). Williams syndrome: 15 Years of psychological research. *Developmental Neuropsychology*, *23*, 1-12.

Mervis, C. B., & Morris, C. A. (2007). Williams syndrome. In J. L. Ross & M. M. M. Mazzocco (Eds.), *Neurogenetic developmental disorders: Variation of manifestation in childhood* (pp. 199-262). Cambridge, MA: The Massachusetts Institute of Technology Press.

Miolo, G., & Chapman, R. S. (1999). *Predicting sentence comprehension in children: A comparison of three measures of working memory capacity.* Symposium for Research on Children's Language Disorders. Madison, WI, June.

Miolo, G., Chapman, R. S., & Sindberg, H. (2005). Sentence comprehension in adolescents with Down syndrome and typically developing children: Role of sentence voice, visual context, and auditory-verbal short-term memory. *Journal of Speech, Language, and Hearing Research, 48*, 172-188.

Montgomery, J. W. (2003). Working memory and comprehension in children with specific language impairment: What we know so far. *Journal of Communication Disorders, 36*, 221-231.

Nelson, K. E. (1977). Facilitating children's syntax acquisition. *Developmental Psychology, 13*, 101-107.

Nelson, K. E. (2000). Methods for stimulating and measuring lexical and syntactic advances: Why fiffins and lobsters can tag along with other recast friends. In L. Menn & N. B. Ratner (Eds.), *Methods for studying language production* (pp. 115-148). Mahwah, NJ: Lawrence Erlbaum Associates.

NICHD Early Child Care Research Network (1999). Child outcomes when child care center classes meet recommended standards for quality. *American Journal of Public Health, 89*, 1072-1077.

Nicolas, S. (2002). *Histoire de la psychologie française. Naissance d'une nouvelle science / History of French psychology. Birth of a new science.* Paris: In Press Editions.

Numminen, H., Lehto, J. E., & Ruoppila, I. (2001). Tower of Hanoi and working memory in adult persons with intellectual disability. *Research in Developmental Disabilities, 22*, 373-387.

Numminen, H., Service, E., & Ruoppila, I. (2002). Working memory, intelligence, and knowledge base in adult persons with intellectual disability. *Research in Developmental Disabilities, 23*, 105-118.

Oléron, P. (1957). *Recherches sur le développement mental des sourds-muets / Studies of the mental development of deaf-mutes.* Paris: Centre National de la Recherche Scientifique.

Oléron, P. (1977). *Language and mental development.* Oxford, UK: Lawrence Erlbaum Associates [Translated form P. Oléron (1972). *Langage et développement mental.* Bruxelles: Pierre Mardaga Editeur].

Pan, B. A., Rowe, L. M., Singer, J. D., & Snow, C. E. (2005). Maternal correlates of growth in toddler vocabulary production in low-income families. *Child Development, 76*, 763-782.

Patterson, J. L. (2002). Relationships of expressive vocabulary to frequency of reading and television experience among bilingual toddlers. *Applied Psycholinguistics, 23*, 493-508.

Patterson, J. L., & Pearson, B. Z. (2004). Bilingual lexical development: Influences, contexts, and processes. In B. A. Goldstein (Ed.), *Bilingual language development and disorders in Spanish-English speakers* (pp. 77-104). Baltimore, MD: Paul H. Brookes Publishing Company.

Pearson, B. Z., Fernandez, S. C., Lewedeg, V., & Oller, D. K. (1997). The relation of input factors to lexical learning by bilingual infants. *Applied Psycholinguistics*, *18*, 41-58.

Pine, J. M. (1995). Variation in vocabulary development as a function of birth order. *Child Development*, *66*, 272-281.

Perkins, E. A., & Small, B. J. (2006). Aspects of cognitive functioning in adults with intellectual disabilities. *Journal of Policy and Practice in Intellectual Disabilities*, *3*, 181–194.

Price, J., Roberts, J., Vandergrift, N., & Martin, G. (2007). Language comprehension in boys with fragile X syndrome and boys with Down syndrome. *Journal of Intellectual Disability Research*, *51*, 318–326.

Raven, J. (1981). *Progressive Matrices*. Issy-les-Moulineaux: Editions Scientifiques et Psychologiques.

Reiss, A. L., & Dant, C. C. (2003). The behavioral neurogenetics of fragile X syndrome: Analyzing gene-brain–behavior relationships in child developmental psychopathologies. *Development and Psychopathology*, *15*, 927-968.

Reuchlin, M. (1979). *Les méthodes en psychologie / The methods in psychology*. Paris: Presses Universitaires de France.

Roberts, J. E., Price, J., & Malkin, C. (2007). Language and communication development in Down syndrome. *Mental Retardation and Developmental Disabilities Research Reviews*, *13*, 26–35.

Rondal, J.-A., & Edwards, S. (1997). *Language in mental retardation*. London, UK: Whurr Publishers Ltd.

Rondal, J.-A., Hodapp, R. M., Soreci, S., Dykens, E. M., & Nota, A. (2004). *Intellectual disabilities: Genetic, behaviour and inclusion*. London, UK: Whurr Publishers Ltd.

Rosin, M. M., Swift, E., Bless, D., & Vetter, D. K. (1988). Communication Profiles of adolescents with Down syndrome. *Journal of Childhood Communication Disorders*, *12*, 49-64.

Saxton, M., Kulcsar, B., Marshall, G., & Rupra, M. (1998). The longer-term effects of corrective input: An experimental approach. *Journal of Child Language*, *25*, 701-721.

Scarr, S. (1992). Developmental theories for the 1990s: Development and individual differences. *Child Development*, *63*, 1-19.

Scarr, S., & McCartney, K. (1983). How people make their own environments: A theory of genotype → environment effects. *Child Development*, *54*, 424-435.

Scherer, N. J., & Olswang, L. B. (1984). Role of mothers' expansions in stimulating children's language production. *Journal of Speech & Hearing Research*, *27*, 387-396.

Sénéchal, M. (1997). The differential effect of storybook reading on preschoolers' acquisition of expressive and receptive vocabulary. *Journal of Child Language*, *24*, 123-138.

Sénéchal, M., Thomas, E., & Monker, J. A. (1995). Individual differences in 4-year-old children's acquisition of vocabulary during storybook reading. *Journal of Educational Psychology*, *87*, 218-229.

Shadish, W. R., Cook, T. D., & Campbell, D. T. (2002). *Experimental and quasi-experimental designs for generalized causal inference*. Boston, MA: Houghton Mifflin Company.

Snow, C. E. (1999). Social perspectives on the emergence of language. In B. MacWhinney (Ed.), *The emergence of language* (pp. 257-276). Mahwah, NJ: Lawrence Erlbaum Associates.

Tamis-LeMonda, C. S., Bornstein, M. H., & Baumwell, L. (2001). Maternal responsiveness and children's achievement of language milestones. *Child Development*, *72*, 748-767.

Tardif, T. (1996). Nouns are not always learned before verbs: evidence from Mandarin speakers' early vocabularies. *Developmental Psychology*, *32*, 492-504.

Tardif, T., Shatz, M., & Naigles, L. (1997). Caregiver speech and children's use of nouns versus verbs: A comparison of English, Italian, and Mandarin. *Journal of Child Language*, *24*, 535-565.

Thomas, M. S. C., & Karmiloff-Smith, A. (2003). Modeling language acquisition in atypical phenotypes. *Psychological Review*, *110*, 647-682.

Valdez-Menchaca, M. C., & Whitehurst, G. J. (1992). Accelerating language development through picture book reading: A systematic extension to Mexican day care. *Developmental Psychology*, *28*, 1106-1114.

Valian, V., & Casey, L. (2003). Young children's acquisition of wh-questions: The role of structured input. *Journal of Child Language*, *30*, 117-143.

Van Daal, J., Verhoeven, L., & Van Leeuwe, J. (2008). Working memory limitations in children with severe language impairment. *Journal of Communication Disorders, 41,* 85-107.

Vasilyeva, M., Huttenlocher, J., & Waterfall, H. (2006). Effects of language intervention on syntactic skill levels in preschoolers. *Developmental Psychology*, *42*, 164-174.

Vicari, S., Bellucci, S., Carlesimo, G. A. (2001). Procedural learning deficit in children with William syndrome. *Neuropsychologia*, *39*, 665-677.

Vicari, S., & Carlesimo, G. A. (2002). Children with Intellectual Disabilities. In A. D. Baddeley, M. D. Kopelman & B. Wilson (Eds.), *The handbook of memory disorders* (pp. 501-520). New York: John Wiley & Sons.

Vicari, S., & Carlesimo, G. A. (2006). Short-term memory deficits are not uniform in Down and Williams syndromes. *Neuropsychology Review*, *16*, 87-94.

Weiss, B., Weisz, J. R., & Bromfield, R. (1986). Performance of retarded and nonretarded persons on information-processing tasks: Further tests of the similar structure hypothesis. *Psychological Bulletin*, *100*, 157-175.

Weisz, J. R., & Yeates, K. O. (1981). Cognitive development in retarded and nonretarded persons: Piagetian tests of the similar structure hypothesis. *Psychological Bulletin*, *90*, 153-178.

Weisz, J. R., & Zigler, E. (1979). Cognitive development in retarded and nonretarded persons: Piagetian tests of the similar sequence hypothesis. *Psychological Bulletin*, *86*, 831-851.

Weizman, Z. O., & Snow, C. E. (2001). Lexical input as related to children's vocabulary acquisition: Effects of sophisticated exposure and support for meaning. *Developmental Psychology*, *37*, 265-279.

Whitehurst, G. J., Arnold, D. S., Epstein, J. N., Angell, A. L., Smith, M., & Fischel, J. E. (1994). A picture book reading intervention in day care and home for children from low-income families. *Developmental Psychology*, *30*, 679-689.

Whitehurst, G. J., Falco, F. L., Lonigan, C. J., Fischel, J. E., DeBaryshe, B. D., Valdez-Menchaca, M. C., & Caulfield, M. (1988). Accelerating language development through picture book reading. *Developmental Psychology*, *24*, 555-559.

Young, R. M. (1990). *Mind, brain, and adaptation in the nineteenth century: Cerebral localization and its biological context from Gall to Ferrier.* New York: Oxford University Press.

In: Children and Language: Development, Impairment … ISBN 978-1-60692-395-5
Editor: Michael A. Reed

Chapter 10

LATE TALKERS: CHILDREN WITH DEVELOPMENTAL DYSPHASIA (LONGITUDINAL FOLLOW-UP)

Olga Dlouha[1]
Charles University in Prague, First Faculty of Medicine and
General Teaching Hospital, Phoniatric Department, Prague, Czech Republic

ABSTRACT

This study reports longitudinal follow-up of 300 children with developmental dysphasia. Their expressive disturbances are a manifestation of their auditory decoding impairment. These children were investigated on battery of tests of spoken language, of phonological processing and of different audiometric procedures, in order to register all the information necessary to be able judge the speech-language development. The tests focused on diagnosis of central auditory disorder, confirmed the difficulties in association area in children with developmental dysphasia. In speech perception, the temporal processing is one of the functions necessary for the discrimination of phonemes, and of similar words. Our results confirmed long-term problems of children with developmental dysphasia with central auditory perception disorder.

INTRODUCTION

The literature on auditory-phonological processing presents the heterogenity of SLI (specific language impairment). A child with a receptive or expressive language disorder, or both, and no other developmental disability has specific language impairment, a condition also called language-learning impairment, developmental language disorder, developmental dysphasia, or developmental aphasia. Children with SLI are usually late talkers and most - 67% to 84% are boys. At 3 or 4 years old, most children with SLI have a limited vocabulary and speak in short phrases rather than sentences.

[1] Mailing Address: Associated Professor Olga Dlouha, MD, PhD, Phoniatric Dept., First Faculty of Medicine and General Teaching Hospital, Zitna 24, 120 00 Prague 2, Czech Republic; olga.dlouha@lf1.cuni.cz

In Czech language we usually use the term developmental dysphasia. Some studies have focused on children with severe comprehension problems, asking to what extent their difficulties are auditory or linguistic. Others have concentrated on searching for a link between defective speech production and abnormal speech perception. Identification of speech sounds appears to be a problem in all groups. Several reviewers have documented a number and variety of cognitive tasks that are difficult in children with SLI [1]. Developmental dysphasia denotes inability to acquire normal expression and comprehension of language in the absence of peripheral hearing impairment, neurological disorder and mental retardation. The use of the term of developmental dysphasia implies that the child´s perceptual ability for auditory speech events underlies his impairment for the acquisition of auditory symbols. At the heart of developmental dysphasia, there is disorder of auditory perception. Central auditory deficit may result in or coexist with difficulties in other CNS-based skills, such as speech-language impairment, attention deficit, learning and developmental disabilities.

Concerning developmental dysphasia, the typical clinical picture is delayed speech-language development, with specific disorders within all structures; disorder of the distinctive features of phonemes, disorders in the sequential arrangement of syllables (transpositions and reductions), problems with grammar (with word categories and with syntax), and problems with semantic and association language functions. These children experience typical speech comprehension problem, varying in intensity; they also have typical auditory decoding deficits, integration deficit, associative deficit and out-put organisation deficit of speech. Many of these children are unable to recognize acoustic contours and to identify keywords from a spoken message. These children often behave as if peripheral hearing loss was present, despite normal hearing. In some children, problems with perception are so conspicuous that the children appear as having a hearing disorder as they do not understand common conversation and elicit impression of the desorientation.

The neurological examination confirm diffuse lesion of CNS: more often slight hypotonic syndrome with a delay in maturation of cerebellar function, in some cases slight dyskinetic syndrome or signs of spasticity-pyramidal irritation (lower extremities). Generally, the children have problems mostly with muscle coordination, especially with graphomotor functions. The CNS imaging techniques (CT and NMR of the brain) neither unable further subdivision of the dysphasia or bring any other explanation concerning the etiopathogenesis (as opposed to CT and NMR results in patients with aphasia, enabling further differentiation according to localization of the organic lesion).

During the impaired EEG records, the children are also affected either by impairment or by a stagnation of the speech-language development. EEG abnormalities within developmental dysphasia are less severe, but fully correspond to changes within Landau-Kleffner syndrome: the acquired epileptic aphasia of children [2, 3].

Disorders of speech comprehension are typical of all patients with central auditory processing disorders (CAPD). In speech perception, temporal processing is one of the functions necessary for the discrimination of phonemes, and of similar words. The existence of cognitive functions disorders is much more important than difficulties directly involved in speech production. Impairments have been reported both within receptive and expressive language and, more specifically, in morphosyntax and naming [4].

Central auditory processing disorder is an auditory processing deficit caused by deficiency in those skills that are subserved by the central auditory mechanism in the brainstem and brain. Many children will suffer from only one subtype of CAPD, others may suffer from combined subtype profiles. Concerning primary subtypes; based upon presumed anatomical site of dysfunction, include auditory decoding deficit, integration deficit and prosodic deficit. Secondary subtypes include auditory association deficit and out-put organization deficit [5].

Central auditory tests go beyond standard tests of hearing to examine how well the auditory system uses or interprets the information that the ear sends it. The term "auditory processing" refers to "what we do with what we hear" [6]. Concerning dichotic speech tests, dichotic listening involves the presentation of stimuli to both ears simultaneously, with information presented to one ear being different from that presented to the other. Depending on the test itself, the listener may be required to repeat everything that is heard (binaural integration). The information presented to each ear is composed of a portion of the entire message, necessitating integration of the information order for the listener to be able to perceive the whole message [7].

Like all auditory evoked potentials, the long latency auditory evoked potentials (LAEP), and wave P3 are nonspecific for disease, but provide information about auditory system function. LAEPs were studied in children with speech-language disorders. The author [8] explain the P3 (300) positive peak as a first phase of the language processing and they also consider the manifestation of the hemisphere dominance. The electrophysiological changes recorded correspond with the character of the respective speech disorders: it is apparent that the long latency auditory evoked potentials can be used to study the disorders of speech comprehension and their pathology is related to the role of the temporal processing of the auditory stimuli.

Material

It is not correct to make a diagnosis of developmental dysphasia according to our opinion using one type of examination. We must combine the electrophysiological examination with behavioural auditory tests. The group of 300 children (212 boys and 88 girls – figure 1), of age 4-8 years was being monitored. The relationship of handedness: 247 right-handed and 53 left-handed (figure 2). The mean age of children suffering from dysphasia was 6 years 2 months, follow-up period 1-5 years.

Family history: positive family history was confirmed in 185 children. Sex of risk relatives – overbalancing representation of male relatives, as it is with majority of speech-language disorders. Perinatal history: a positive perinatal risks were found in 145 children (risk pregnancy in 59, immaturity in 26 children, patological delivery - in 19, respiratory di-stress syndrome in 41 cases (figure 3). Disorders of phonemic discrimination and of verbal comprehension were found in majority of cases. Auditory decoding deficits, phonological, lexical and syntactic deficits and associative deficit were diagnosed. Pure tone audiometry was normal in all cases. Developmental dysphasia (DD) is occasionally complicated by other diagnoses. In a group of 300 children were mentioned these complications: stuttering (balbuties) and dysarthria (figure 4).

Children within this age (6 to 7 years) were being best diagnosed in view of the fact of possibility to accomplish the widest possible spectrum of examinational methods. Majority of our children with developmental dysphasia underwent detailed special examination –

evaluation of phonological awareness, of central auditory dichotic tests and of cortical auditory evoked potentials.

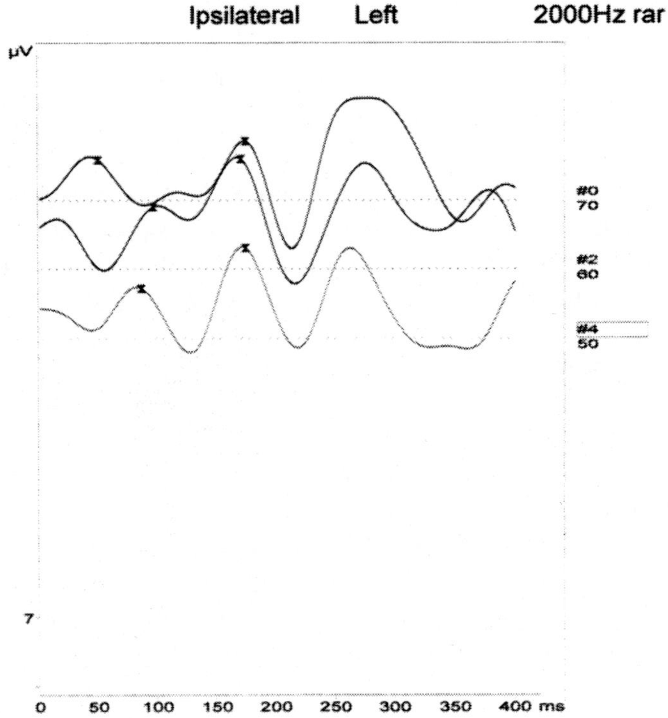

Figure 1. Children with developmental dysphasia (DD)

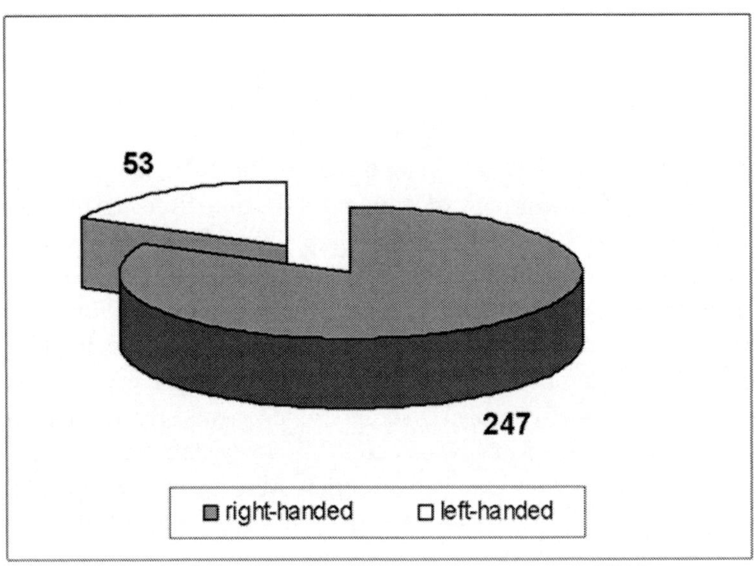

Figure 2. The relationship of handedness

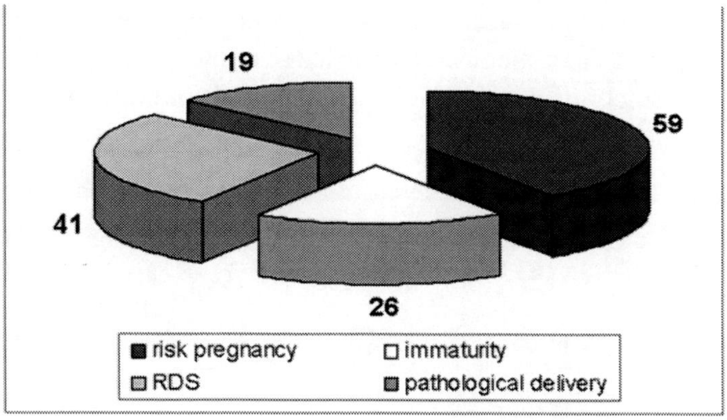

Figure 3. Perinatal history – positive risks in group of DD children

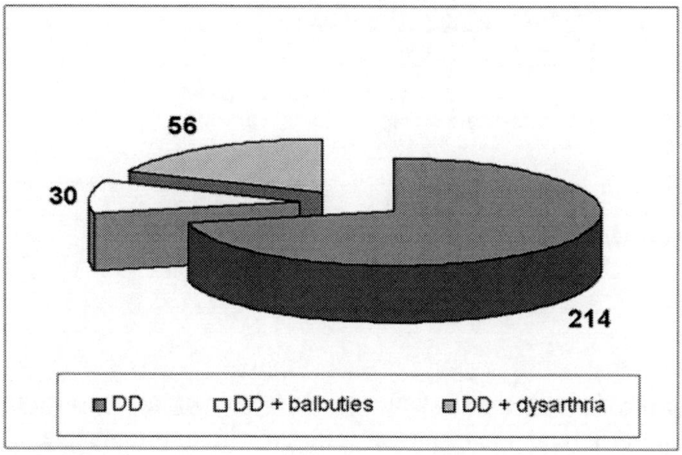

Figure 4: Combination of diagnoses

1. The Special Test of Phonological Awareness for Pre-School Children

Introduction

It means presenting phoneme pairs different in one distinctive feature; the words were chosen according to distinctive features of sounds of Czech language. The test was used for multiple examinations of 300 children aged 4-8 years with developmental dysphasia. These children exerted problems in the tests requiring understanding of phonological constants (figure 5). The total number of words included in the test is 120 (mono- and disyllabic ones) with 15 pairs of phonological oppositions presented for each distinctive feature assessed. All the words are lined up into acoustically similar pairs with different meaning. There are 4 distinctive features assessed in the test: voiced-voiceless, continuity-discontinuity, nasality-non-nasality, compactness-diffusivity of vowel sounds. In comparison with results of children of appropriate age, dysphasic children have disturbed ability to differentiate phonemes. While being tested, the child makes a selection from the presented pair of pictures in time limit given. The precondition of the testing is the knowledge of the meaning of the words used. The test also enables assessment of the current level of short-term memory – the children repeat the words by the sample recorded.

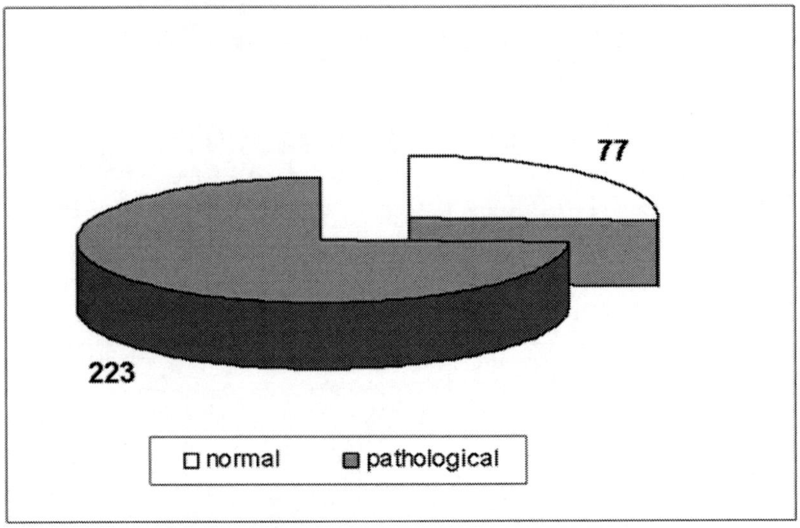

Figure 5. Phonological awareness in children with DD

Results

Children with physiologic speech-language development accomplish this test as early as at the age of 5 years. Although the results in children with developmental dysphasia approach the norm for 6-7 years, mainly in voiced-voiceless consonant distinctive feature, the approaching of 100% is slower at a later age (8-9 years), in terms of the total result (with other distinctive features), compared with a control group. The results remain close to the lower limit of the norm for a long time. The examination of older dysphasic children suggests that the deficiency in voice x voiceless consonant distinctive characteristics results in the risk of the development of congenital learning disorders dyslexia and dysorthography (regarding central auditory processing disorder).

2. Central Auditory Dichotic Language Tests in Children with Developmental Dysphasia

Introduction

We have made an effort to construct speech tests in our mother language that would capturing and analyzing central auditory perception functions in children as well as in adults. As we have observed on a long-term basis children with developmental dysphasia (at the our Phoniatric Department), that show typical problems with speech comprehension, we have focused on comparison of the tests results in these children with developmental dysphasia and in children with normal speech-language development (mean especially chronological age). The tests aim at taking into account the dichotic listening possibilities using simple words (two-syllable words), in which case the central integration, temporal processing and linked short-term memory quality can be evaluated, as well as association ability of the children, as the case may be. Two-syllable words were chosen from a children's vocabulary; the nouns and verbs (type: CVCV – consonant, vowel, consonant, vowel), average word duration is 886 ms. Three types of tests (tests 1-3) were used, the total of 60 two-syllable words devided to pairs in decades (test No 1: 20 words=10 pairs…). The assigned words were presented in the dichotic binaural manner, simultaneously to both ears above the threshold value at 60 dB HL using the two-channel audiometer. The interstimulation pauses were 5 seconds long. The child had to repeat the order of these mentioned words - the task was to repeat both words. Requirements for testing are represented by normal hearing sensitivity, average intellect, knowledge of these mentioned words and age limitation.

The set observed by us was formed by 90 children with developmental dysphasia in the age of 6 - 7 years: 67 boys and 23 girls, 78 right-handed and 12 left-handed. Control group of 20 children with normal speech-language development was matched for age and gender.

Receptive ability is the understanding of the spoken word – retrieving and processing sounds in the language storage centers of the brain and discriminating the differences between sounds in words (like cat versus pat). Expressive ability is how we learn to formulate grammatically and syntactically correct sentences.

Reproduction of the content heard must be recorded with the greatest accuracy possible during the examination in order to evaluate language abilities of the children - all the observations presented were performed by the same person in order to increase objectivity of the evaluation. The results evaluate the percentage rate of success of the words recognized (e.g. 7 out of 10 = 70%).

Results

Results of the dichotic speech test in 90 children with developmental dysphasia in the age of 6 - 7 years are provided in the table: average rate of success of these children was 56% in test 1, 64% in test 2, and 63% in test 3. Rate of success of the control group was 92%, 93%, and 92% (figure 6, table 1). Highly significant differences ($p<0.001$) were confirmed by statistical evaluation using the pair t-test. The average number of correct responses was significantly lower in DD children than in children from control group (of chronological age and normally developed). The language – impaired children obtained lower scores at all targets (than controls). Results in our group of pre-school DD children confirmed disability to synthesize 2 two-syllabic words during dichotic listening. These children are unable to create simple sentences from different two words presented simultaneously to both ears. Some of children suffering from specific language impairment perceived only 1 word from two-word sentence during dichotic tests.

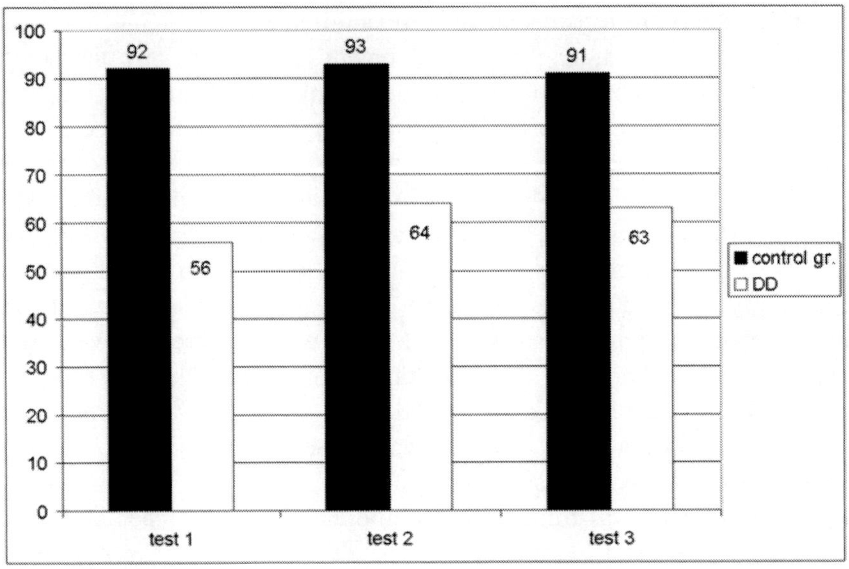

Figure 6. Results (in %) of central dichotic tests – comparison of children with DD versus control group

Table 1. Results (in %) of the dichotic speech test 1-3 in 90 children with SLI in the age of 6 - 7 years. Statistical analysis (pair t-test) - p<0.001

	Test 1		Test 2		Test 3	
	mean	std dev	mean	std dev	mean	std dev
control N = 20	92.00	9.51	93.25	8.62	91.75	11.50
SLI N = 90	56.39	17.62	63.83	17.10	63.00	17.90

Results of the tests in children with developmental dysphasia confirmed integration problems in the central perception area and the short-term memory disorder. The expressions perceived were often reproduced with reduction of the number of syllables or with syllable shifts (e.g. the stone falls - palls, the woman washes - wowashes, the horse jumps - humps, the wasp bites - biwasp, the lamp blinks - dings, the fish swims - swimmfi, the aunt calls - calla, the wind blows - windows, the car hoots - caroots etc. – mentioned translation from Czech language). In identical tasks, children of the same age from the control group showed only minimum problems in composing two-syllable expressions from dichotic listening (rate of success more than 90%). The results in 8-9 year children with developmental dysphasia suggest improved integration of the auditory ability: in Tests 1-3, these children already coped with their handicap in dichotic listening, observed at the age 6-7 years. However, in a harder test with more syllables. Test 4: dichotic presentation of parts of the sentence; children with residual symptoms of developmental dysphasia do not manage more demanding tasks (table 2).

Table 2. Statistical analysis - SLI children 7-8 y. old - pair t-test, results in % p=0.001

	Test 1		Test 2		Test 3		Test 4	
	mean	SD	mean	SD	mean	SD	mean	SD
control group N = 12	99.58	1.44	99.58	1.44	100.0	0.0	87.50	9.41
SLI group N = 30	80.71	19.11	81.50	18.76	83.83	17.25	56.50	14.21

Conclusion

The first results of this type of dichotic testing in children with developmental dysphasia confirm the expected assumption within the framework of the speech comprehension (perception) disorder, in the sense of the central auditory processing disorder (CAPD): deficit in speech sounds decoding, integration deficit for the demands of the stimuli temporal sequence, the short-term (working) memory disorder, all lead to general reduction of the communication perceived and to association problems [6,7]. Already in the course of common examination, the speech comprehension disorder is striking in such children, sometimes even connected with attention outages. Small children with developmental dysphasia in the age of 6 - 7 years exhibit weak auditory consciousness, and thus in words with limited entropy they cannot use the contingent possibility of redundance. Older children with residual forms of specific language disorder do not show such a typical symptomatology in their spontaneous speech expression, however, difficulties still remain in them especially on the phonological level and on the auditory differentiation level of distinctive phonemes features: they suffer from developmental learning disorders, dyslexia and dysortographia. The test type presented can contribute also to diagnostics of hidden language difficulties of such children. Older children clearly use their auditory experiences better, as well as their auditory consciousness, and the ability to associate up to confabulations. The differential - diagnostic contribution of the tests (confirmation of the speech comprehension disorder and the central auditory function disorder relationship) does not lie only in the area of developmental speech-language disorders but the tests can serve to evaluate the speech development stage, as well as to evaluate the rate of success of speech rehabilitation. Tests focused on the central auditory processing disorder diagnostics, on the integration deficit, also confirm difficulties in the linked association area in children with specific language disorder. In speech perception, temporal processing represents one of the functions necessary to recognize the phonemes. Temporal characteristics of auditory stimuli are critical for children with developmental dysphasia. In respect of these findings, the developmental speech-language disorders are classified by some authors among the central auditory processing disorders [4,5,10]. Damages caused by the temporal sequence perception disorders probably occur in the left, speech-dominant hemisphere. Recently, classification according to the perception deficit also occurred within the framework of non-uniform terminology in the area of developmental speech-language disorders. The relationship between damaged speech comprehension and the deficit in speech expression has been sought, in which case the speech expressive disorders represent manifestation of worsened decoding of input acoustic information. As no unchanging criteria are available here, generalization is very difficult and shows marked dependence on the age in which the children are diagnosed and observed. Usage of further test types will contribute to evaluation of the central auditory function and of the relationship with central speech-language disorders.

A final point to note is that there may be quite wide individual variation in the severity of discourse comprehension problems seen in children with developmental dysphasia. Our results are useful in intervention, by specifying which parameters make it easier or more difficult for children to process language.

3. Cortical Auditory Evoked Potentials in Children with Developmental Dysphasia Introduction

Like all auditory evoked potentials, the long latency auditory evoked potentials (LAEPs), are nonspecific for disease, but provide information about auditory system function. It is apparent that the cortical auditory potentials can be used to study the disorders of speech comprehension and their patology is related to the role of the temporal processing of the auditory stimuli. All studies presuppose that the children suffering from developmental speech disorders have also a speech perception disorder related to the defective temporal processing of the speech stimuli (figures 7, 8 – normal characteristics of LAEPs).

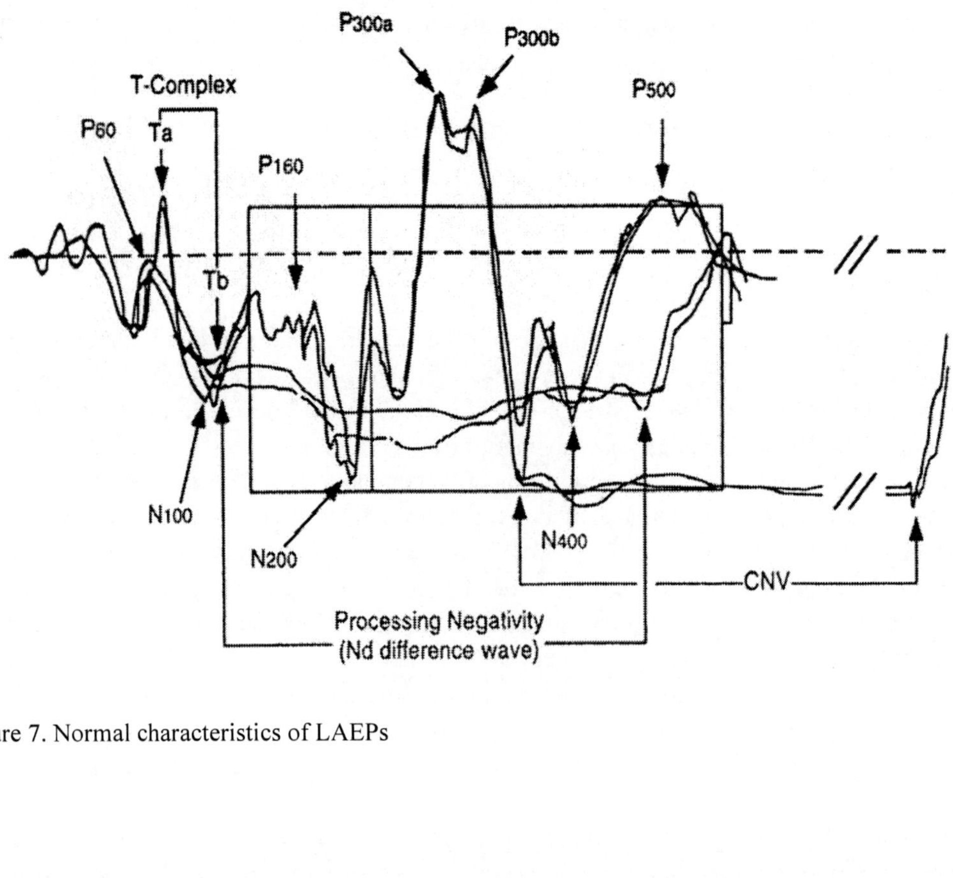

Figure 7. Normal characteristics of LAEPs

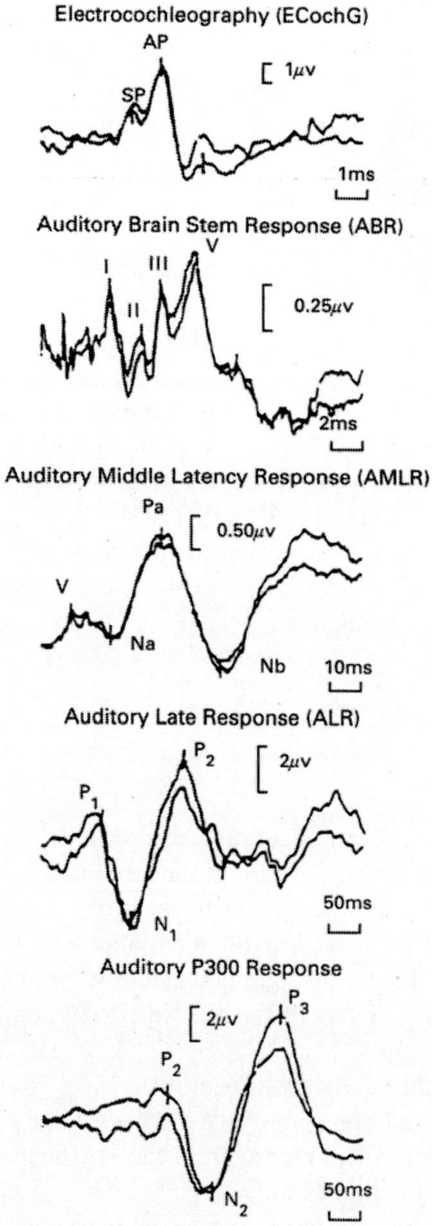

FIGURE 4.12. Waveforms for major auditory evoked potentials.
Latency and amplitude scales for each AER noted in right portion of figure. (AP = action potential; SP = summating pontential; uv = microvolts; I, II, III, and V = waves, numbered sequentially; N and P are negative and positive voltage indicators, respectively.)

SOURCE: With permission from Hall, J.W., *Handbook of Auditory Evoked Pontentials*, Needham Heights, MA: Allyn & Bacon, 1992, page 105.

Figure 8. Normal characteristics of LAEPs

Material and Method

LAEPs were studied in children with speech-language disorders to compare the maturation of speech and tonal-evoked components. Long latency auditory evoked potentials were observed in a considerable part of children with developmental dysphasia.

All individuals were audiologically normal according to pure-tone audiometry and tympanometry.

Study 1

In this study 30 subjects with developmental dysphasia from 6 to 7 years of age were examinated. We used verbal stimuli (two-syllabic Czech word, duration 400 ms) and we recorded especially P3 cognitive potential; ERA Madsen 2250.

Study 2

In this study 33 subjects with developmental dysphasia from 6 to 10 years of age were examinated. These subjects were devided to 2 groups - group A: 6-7 y. old children with developmental dysphasia, group B: 9-10 y. old children with developmental dysphasia. We used tone burst 2 kHz stimuli; Evoselect ABR diagnostic system.

Both tone and speech stimuli were presented monoaurally at a level 70 dB SPL. The LAEPs were recorded from 4 electrodes. All results were compared with results of children with normal speech-language development.

Results

Study 1

The responses to verbal stimuli were not recorded or were found with decreased amplitudes and with prolonged latency, almost in the left dominant hemisphere. When testing the hypotheses on differences between the values of the P3 latencies in children with dysphasia (the P3 was chosen for testing as the most important response with respect to the stimulation by verbal stimuli), the following relationships were found:

a) tonal stimulation – no significant difference was found between the P3 latencies on the right versus left side,

b) verbal stimulation – statistically significant differences were confirm in the records of the P3 latencies from the left and right sides between the studied group and the match-control group (at 1% significance level). The record from the left hemisphere was statistically the most significant (p - 0.001) – graph 1, 2; table 3,

c) when comparing the results after tonal and verbal stimulation – no significant difference was found in the P3 latency values on the right side. However, at the left side the statistically significant difference (1%) was confirmed; after the verbal stimulation the P3 latencies are longer on the left side compared to tonal stimuli (figure 9).

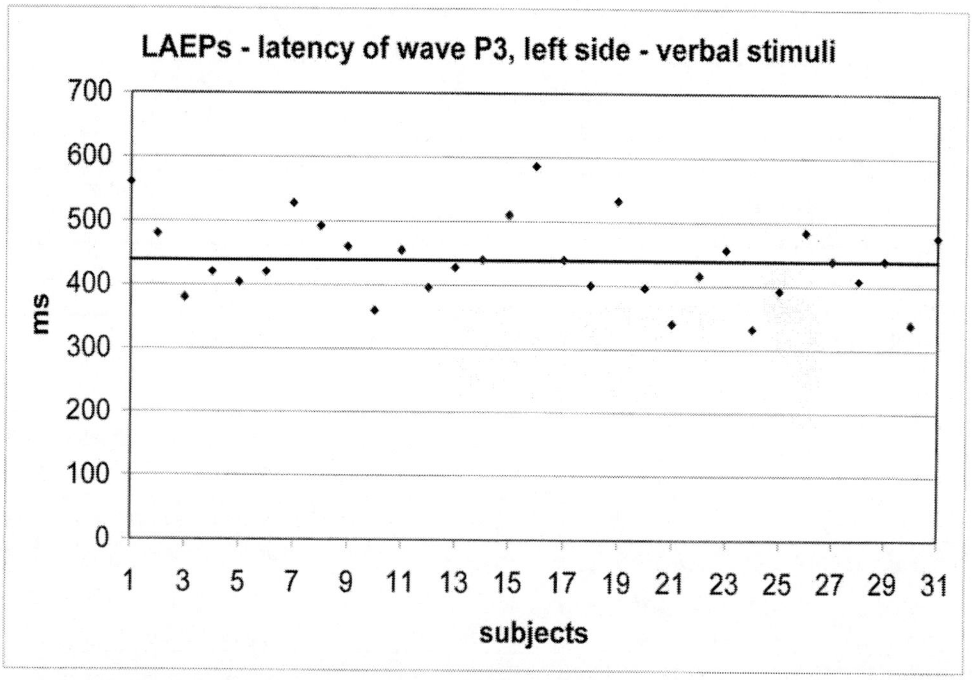

Graph 1. LAEPs, P3 latencies – verbal stimuli

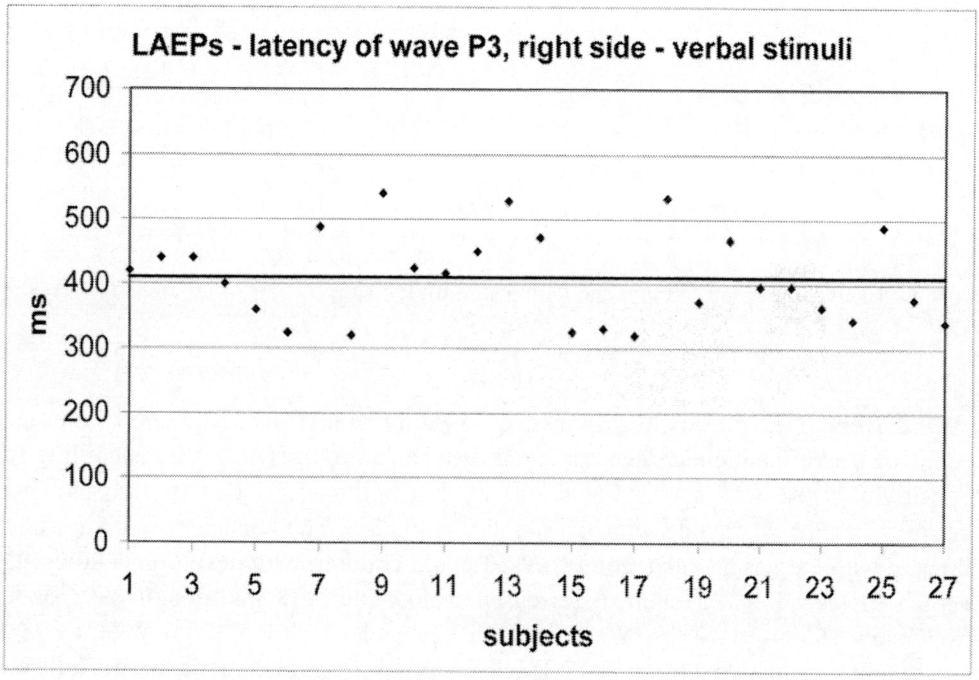

Graph 2. LAEPs, P3 latencies – verbal stimuli

Table 3. LAEPs – latency of wave P3 (ms) - verbal stimuli

Group	Latency – dx	n	Latency – sin	n
Control	**321 +- 22**	**10**	**311 +- 28**	**10**
Dysphasia	**410 +- 68**	**27**	**440 +- 62**	**31**

tonal stimuli

Group	Latency – dx	n	Latency – sin	n
Control	**327 +- 30**	**16**	**335 +- 25**	**16**
Dysphasia	**380 +- 60**	**17**	**382 +- 78**	**17**

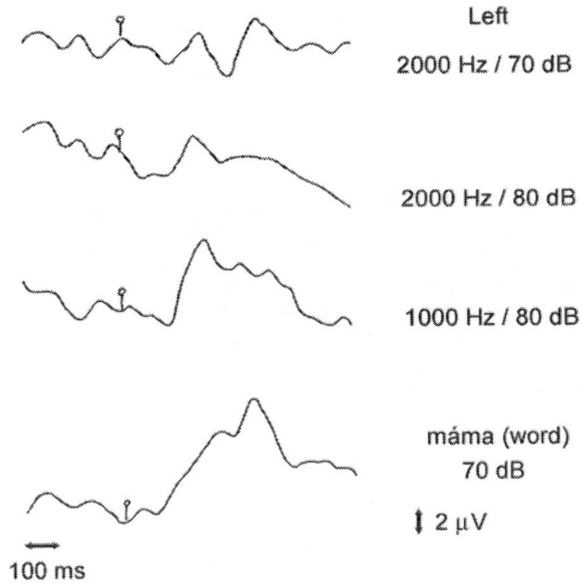

Figure 9. LAEPs - comparison of tonal nad verbal stimuli; left side

Study 2

Grand average waveforms in response to 2 kHz tone burst; recorded latencies are shown in graphs of above mentioned developmental dysphasia groups (A and B) according to age. The positivity of P2 waves was significant for both groups; P2 was the most distinctive. These waves are already stable without side differentiation. The latencies are being shortened within age: with increasing age (group B: 9-10 y. old children with developmental dysphasia) converged to the adult. P2 latency decreased from about 235 ms at 6-7 years of age to approximately 160 ms at 10 yrs. We recorded P2 latencies – group A: graph 3, 4 – average: left side 237 ms, right side 235 ms; P2 latencies – group B: graph 5, 6 – average: left side 162 ms, right side 164 ms. Fig. 10, 11: results of 6 y. old boys with developmental dysphasia

Figures 12, 13: results of 10 y. old boys with developmental dysphasia – all waves (P1, P2, P3) are stabilized.

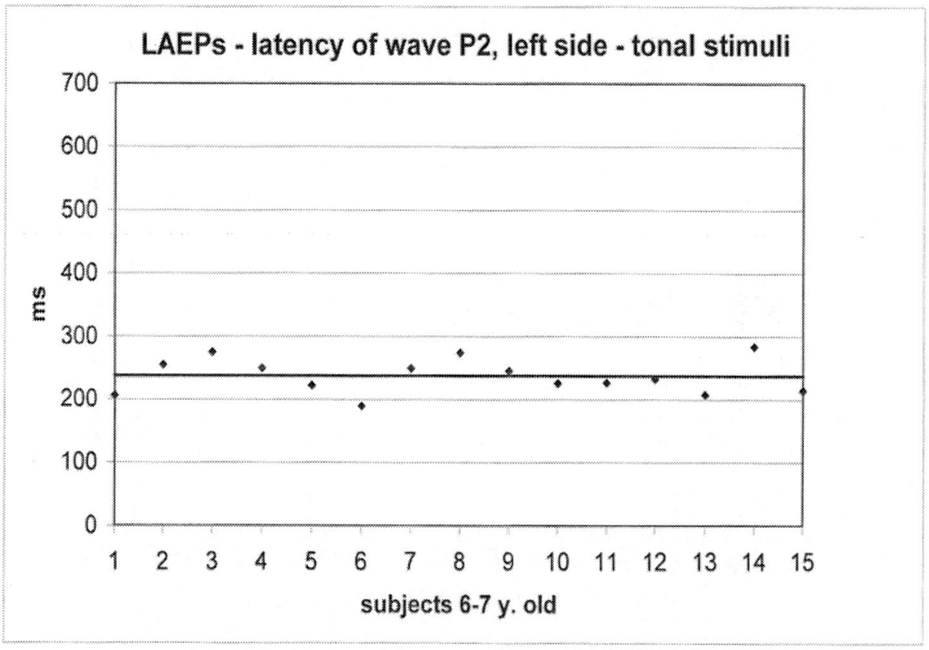

Graph 3. LAEPs, P2 latencies – group A: average: left side 237 ms, right side 235 ms

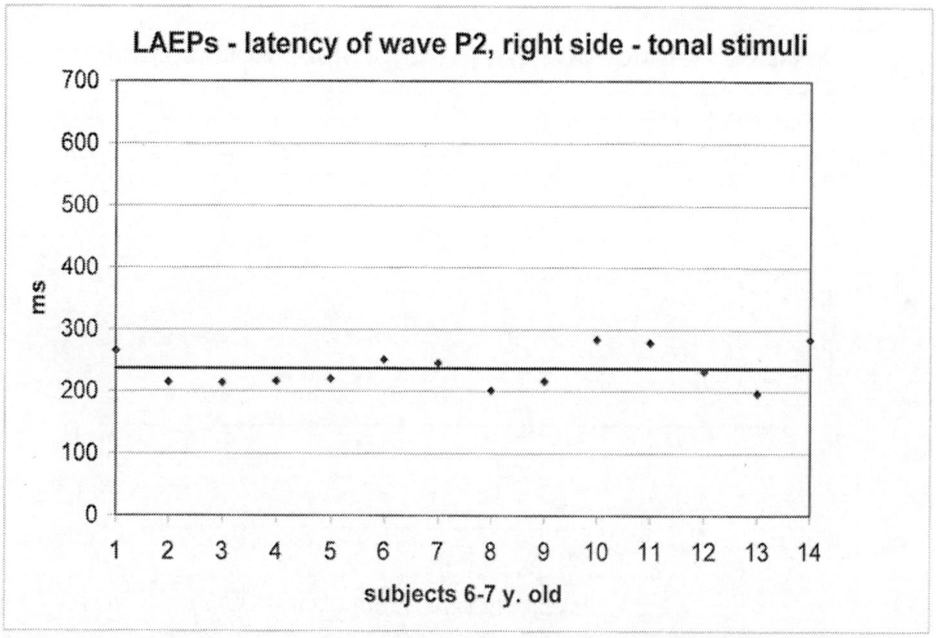

Graph 4. LAEPs, P2 latencies – group A: average: left side 237 ms, right side 235 ms

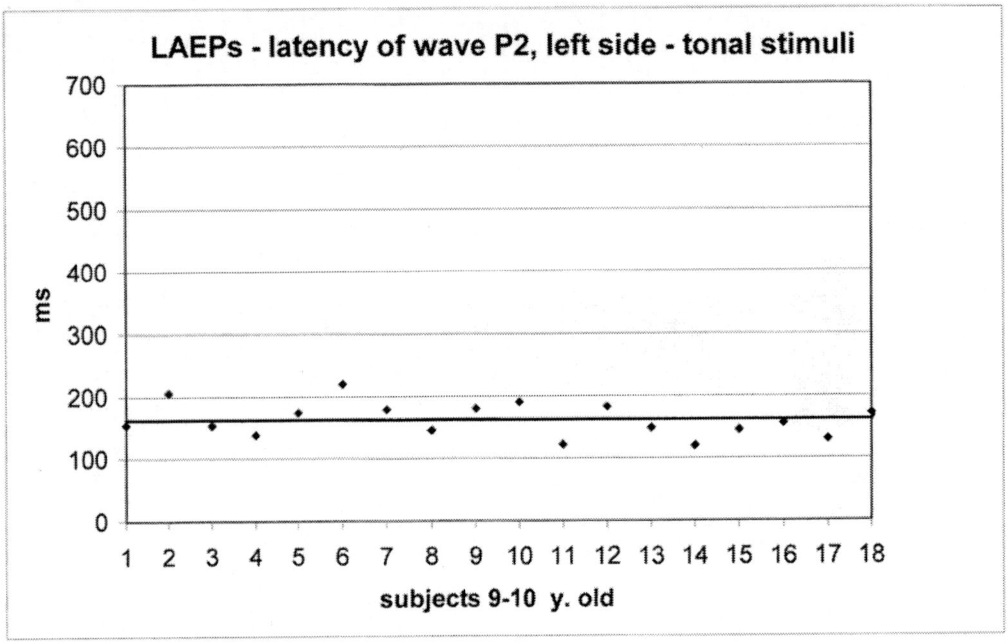

Graph 5. LAEPs, P2 latencies – group B: average: left side 162 ms, right side 164 ms

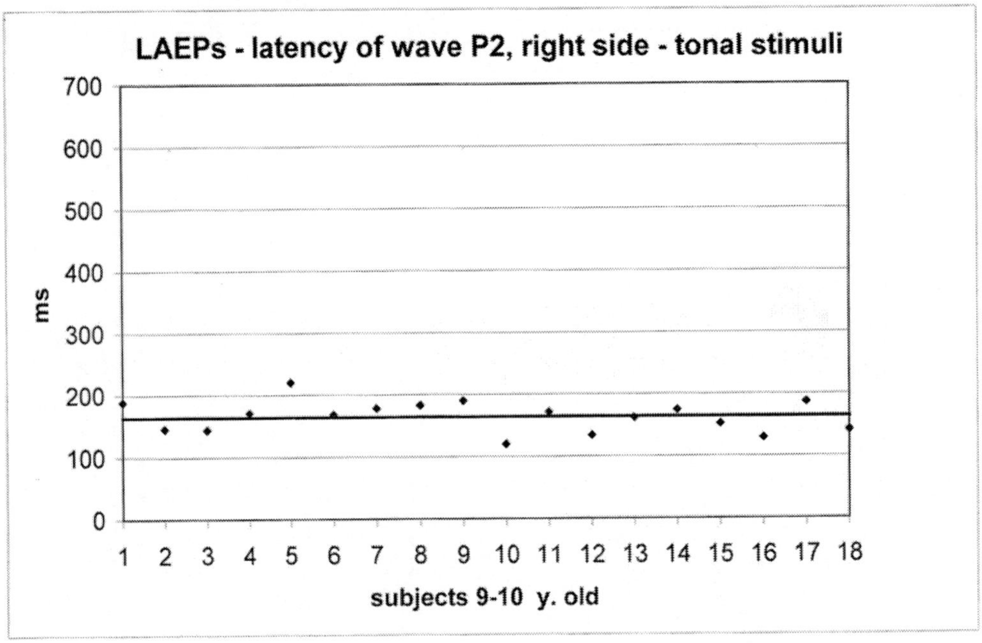

Graph 6. LAEPs, P2 latencies – group B: average: left side 162 ms, right side 164 ms

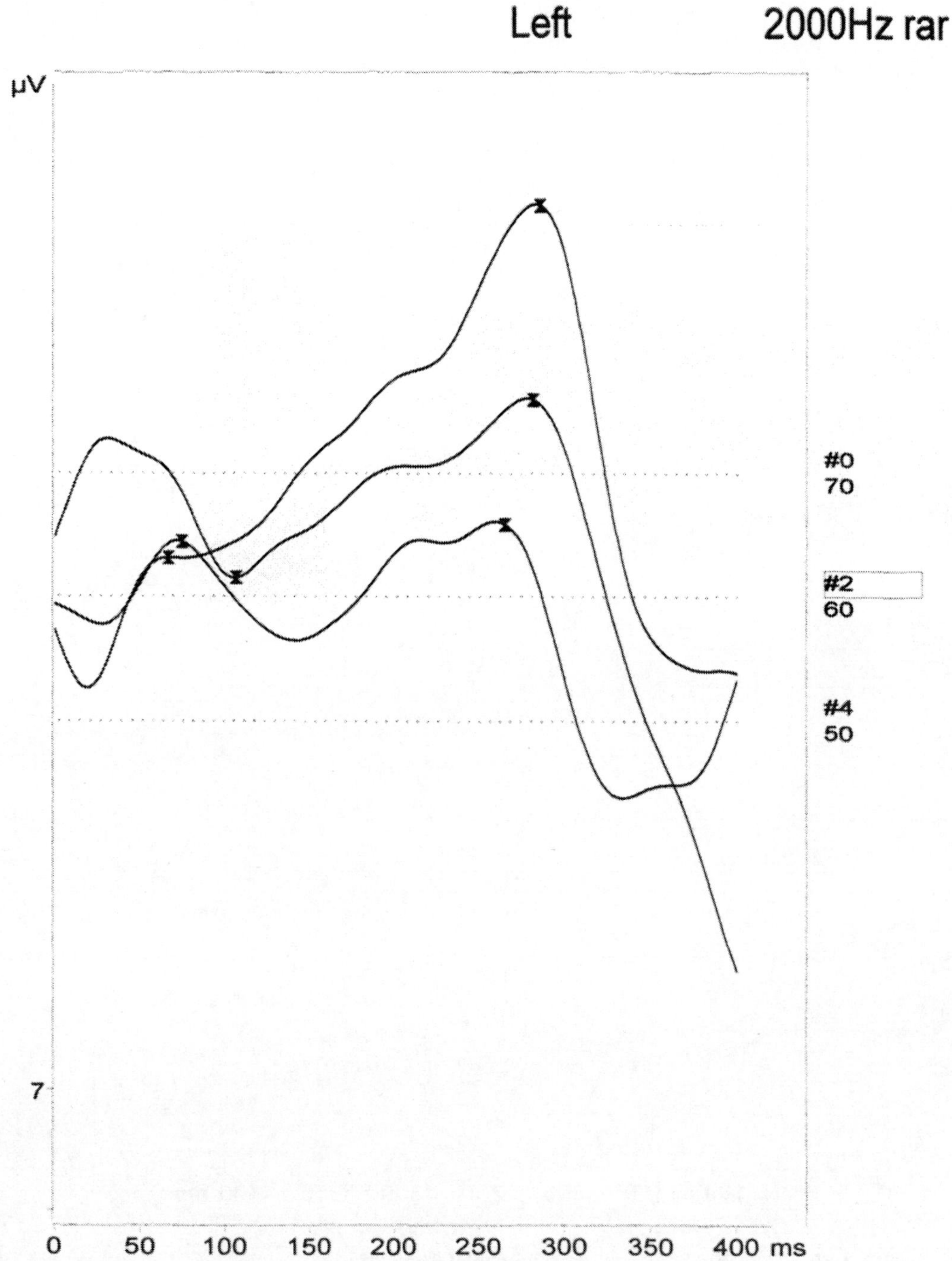

Figure 10. LAEPs of 6 y. old boys with developmental dysphasia

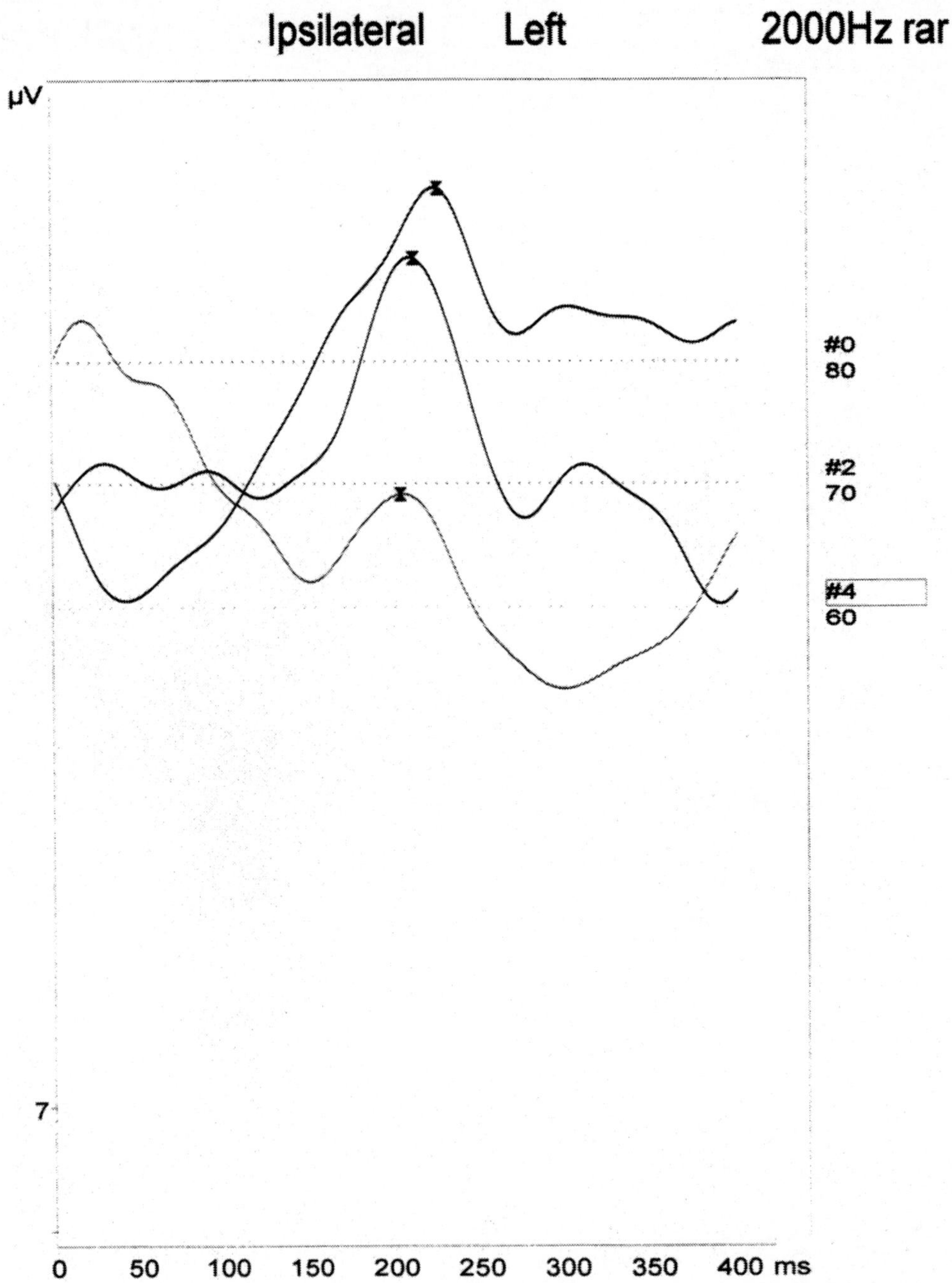

Figure 11. LAEPs of 6 y. old boys with developmental dysphasia

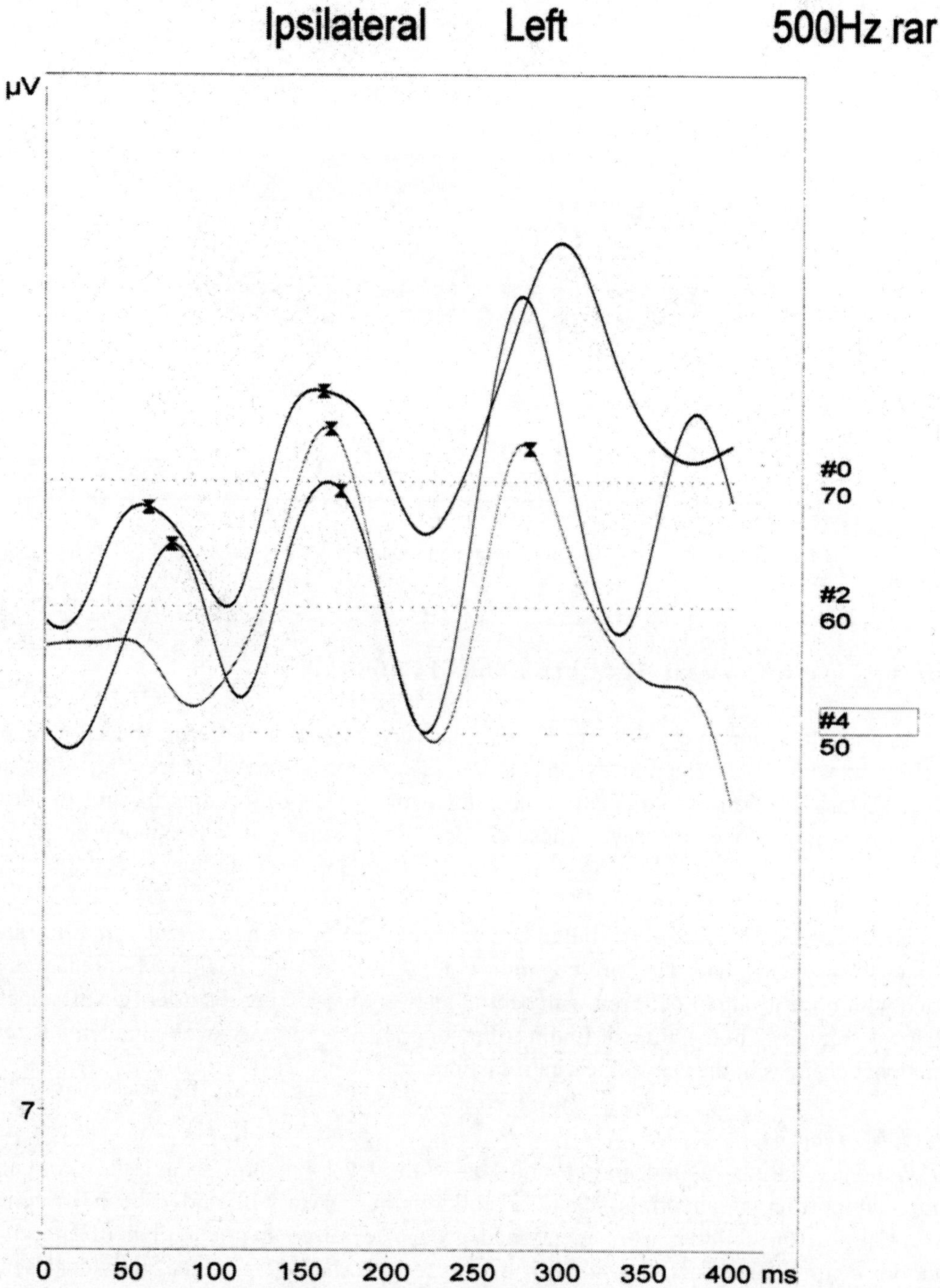

Figure 12. LAEPs of 10 y. old boys with developmental dysphasia – all waves (P1, P2, P3) are stabilized

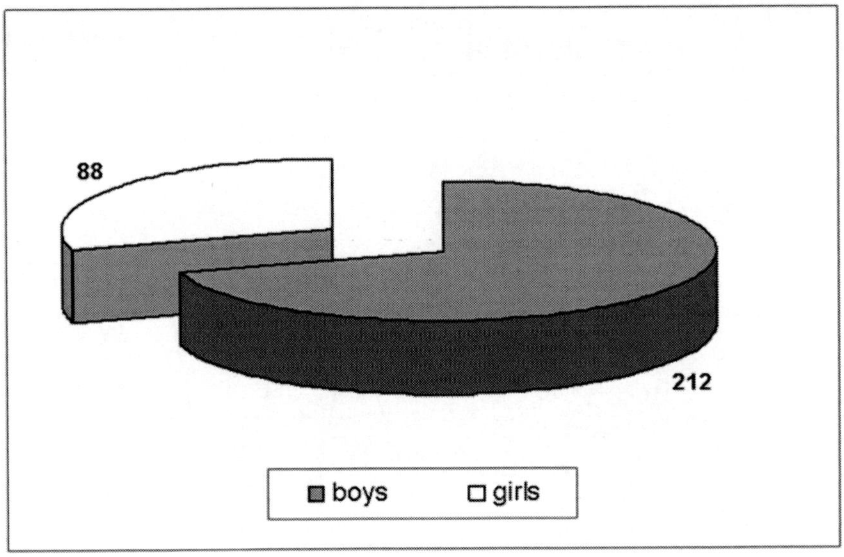

Figure 13. LAEPs of 10 y. old boys with developmental dysphasia – all waves (P1, P2, P3) are stabilized

Conclusions to Cortical Auditory Evoked Potentials

As a result of our study, we suppose that the very important matter in speech perception in children with developmental dysphasia is a disorder in temporal processing of acoustic signals. Many of these children are unable to recognize acoustic contours and to identify keywords from a spoken message. These children often behave as if peripheral hearing loss was present, despite normal hearing. With auditory training, common language skills of these children can be improved.

The occurrence of waves is limited and is influenced by the age. Great variability in P1, P2 and P3 latencies, and their prolongation compared to normal healthy children, was also found within the group of children with central auditory processing disorder (CAPD). Despite the great variability in the clinical findings the long latency auditory evoked potentials reflect functional changes in the central hearing function.

The EEG records

Obtained during monitoring of children with developmental dysphasia contain an important portion of abnormalities (223 children in our group) and especially epileptic abnormalities (66 children from mentioned group) localized in the region of speech and auditory centres which correspond with the respective characters of the individual speech-language disorders. These are children who also manifest clinical signs of epilepsy; in our group 6 children were affected; there occurred absence in 5 children, in 1 child tonic- clonic seizures were present - [3, 9].

General Conclusion

A longitudinal study was conducted to document and compare evolution of children with developmental speech-language impairment. Our results indicate the relationship between developmental dysphasia and central auditory processing disorder (CAPD): our dysphasic children have auditory processing deficit: not only integration, but also associative deficit. Deficiency within the ability to perform tasks that require inter-hemispheric communication and inefficient intra-hemispheric cooperation.

Speech-language comprehension disorders are typical in all patients with central auditory processing disorder. It is important to realize the matter of perception of the acoustic signal in connection with time. The temporal processing is a decisive factor for the myriad of auditory perceptions, including speech and music perception.

Temporal processing in speech perception is one of functions, which are necessary to distinguish between the fine stimuli, such as voicing, and other. In other words, to distinguish between the distinctive features of the phonemes or to distinguish between similar words.

The results of phonological awareness remain close to the lower limit of the norm for a long time. The hypothesis of the worst results in voiced-voiceless consonants and compactness-diffusivity distinctive features, seen generally in children with developmental dysphasia, was confirmed. However, the results are always proportional to the intensity and the duration of rehabilitation care and to the individual characteristics of a child (e.g. concentration ability during the test). The examination of older dysphasic children suggests that the deficiency in voice versus voiceless consonant distinctive characteristic results in the risk of development of congenital learning disorders dyslexia and dysortografia (regarding central auditory processing disorder). The difficulties within final realisation of sounds in dysphasic children persist despite improvement of their auditory differentiation – later on, the children have difficulties predominantly in the semantic domain (not being able to follow the story line and reproduce even a short story).

The judgement of temporal order does not occur at ear, it rather represents a central auditory function. Using a variety of acoustic stimuli, an inter-stimulus interval of only 2 ms is required for the normal listener to perceive two sounds instead of only one. However, this interval must be 17 ms long to identify correctly which sound appeared as the first one. If the listener needs more than 15 to 20 ms to realize the sequence of two consecutive stimuli, the examiner should check the central auditory system for pathologic changes. The first 100 to 250 ms of an auditory stimulus presentation is the most critical consequence for stimulus recognition. As a result of our study, we suppose that the very important matter in speech perception in children with developmental dysphasia is a disorder in temporal processing of acoustic signals. This presumption has also been confirmed by the results of examinations of the long latency auditory evoked potentials presented in this paper.

The potentials records display prolongation of the P3 latencies (as cognitive potentials) especially after stimulation with verbal stimuli. Great variability in the responses, probably related to a variation in the bioelectrical activity, which can be seen also in abnormal native EEG records; this can be found in the results. Children with developmental dysphasia have most difficulties in processing of the speech signal. The abnormalities or epileptic seizures in the region of speech and hearing centres probably explain the cause of the central speech and auditory disorders. The mechanisms of the speech comprehension disorder in developmental dysphasia and in Landau-Kleffner syndrome are quite similar and it is evident that these EEG changes cause disorders in comprehension and verbal expression abilities. Etiopathogenesis is unclear, however a disorder of integration auditory and speech connections due to the defect in myelinization, delayed maturation of the unknown origin, or due to the relationships of pre- and postsynaptic elements is expected [9].

We suppose that this initiate evaluation corresponds with approach to developmental dysphasia at our workplace. With an auditory training producing improved speech-language abilities in everyday context, this would be the strongest support yet for the view that linguistic difficulties in these children are secondary to more fundamental auditory limitations. Special hearing and speech-language treatment can be improved auditory and auditory-related skills to create long-term benefit for children with developmental dysphasia. In comparison and evaluation of results of special tests during our therapy were confirmed good successes in word recognition, in phonological analysis and in central auditory function. With auditory training, common language skills of these children can be improved [10]. The level of pragmatic language, i.e. the comprehension of spoken language in real communication, is being developed, too.

ACKNOWLEDGEMENT

The research has been supported by the Project IGA MZ CR 9105-3/2006

REFERENCES

[1] Bishop, DVM. *Uncommon understanding.* East Sussex: Psychology Press, 1999.

[2] Echenne, B. Epileptic electroencephalographic abnormalities and developmental dysphasia. *Brain Dev (Tokyo).* 1992, 14: 216-225.

[3] Dlouha, O.; Nevsimalova, S. EEG changes and epilepsy in developmental dysphasia. *Clinical Neurophysiology at the Beginning of the 21st Century; Supplements to Clin Neurophysiol.* 2000, 53: 271-274.

[4] Bellis, TJ. *Assessment and management of central auditory processing disorders in the educational setting.* Singular Publishing Group, Inc. 1996.

[5] Chermak, GD; Musiek F. *Central auditory processing disorders. (New perspectives)* Singular Publishing Group, Inc. San Diego. London. 1997.

[6] Ferre, JM. Understanding childrenś central auditory disorders. *Abstracts, 25th World Cogress of the International Association of Logopedics and Phoniatrics. Montreal, 2001.*

[7] Dlouha O.; Novak A; Vokral J. Central auditory processing disorder (CAPD) in children with specific language impairment (SLI). Central auditory tests. *Int J Pediatr Otorhinolaryngol.* 71(6), 2007, 903-907.

[8] Mc Pherson, DL. *Late potentials of the auditory system.* Singular Publishing Group, Inc. San Diego, London 1996.

[9] Dlouha O. *Vyvojove poruchy reci. (Developmental Language Disorders).* Prague. 2003.

[10] Kuhn-Inacker H; Weinmann S. Training the temporal order perception – A concept of supporting the language perception of children with central auditory processing disorders (CAPD), Sprache-Stimme-Gehor 24 (2000), 119-125.

Reviewed by: Prof. Sona Nevsimalova2, MD, DrSc. Charles University in Prague, First Faculty of Medicine and General Teaching Hospital, Department of Neurology, Prague,

[2] Czech Republic. 120 00 Prague 2, Katerinska 30, Czech Republic. sona.nevsimalova@lf1.cuni.cz

Short Communications

In: Children and Language: Development, Impairment … ISBN 978-1-60692-395-5
Editor: Michael A. Reed

Short Communication A

EARLY MIDDLE EAR EFFUSION AND CENTRAL AUDITORY PROCESSING AT AGE SEVEN

Dale L. Johnson[1], Constance D. Baldwin[2] and David P. McCormick[3]
[1]University of Houston
[2]University of Rochester School of Medicine and Dentistry
[3]University of Texas Medical Branch, Galveston

ABSTRACT

This study examined the relation of middle ear effusion MEE) in the first three years of life to central auditory processing at age seven. Ears were examined on a regular basis frequently in the home over the first three years and a count of days with bilateral MEE was used to quantify ear status. Central auditory processing was assessed with SCAN, Screening Test for Auditory Processing Disorders. With a sample of 76 children studied prospectively from birth there were significant correlations between MEE and all four SCAN measures. A possible link between SCAN and attention problems was also examined using the Test of Variables of Attention (TOVA). Three of 16 possible correlations were significant, suggesting a weak relation between attention and SCAN.

EARLY MIDDLE EAR EFFUSION AND CENTRAL AUDITORY PROCESSING AT AGE SEVEN

Middle ear effusion (MEE) is a common illness of infancy and early childhood when it frequently causes temporary hearing loss. In the great majority of cases, the hearing loss is quite brief, but in some cases it can last most of a child's early life, and, as the child does not hear clearly, may have an effect on language development. It is to be expected that if the child cannot hear well, aspects of language development would be impaired. Several kinds of language development need to be examined. Our research on MEE resulted in two reports on MEE and language. The first at child age 5, found significant correlations between early MEE and scores on the Carrow Elicited Language Inventory (Carrow, 1974) and Goldman-Fristoe Articulation Test (Goldman & Fristoe, 1986) (McCormick, Baldwin, Klecan-Aker, Swank,& Johnson, 2001). Correlations of MEE with the Carrow Auditory Visual Abilities in Quiet Test (Carrow-Wolfolk, 1981) were also significant when modified by stimulation provided in the home environment. Children were less affected by MEE if the home environment was more stimulating. The same research group published a study of MEE and language at age seven (Johnson, McCormick & Baldwin, 2008). Using the Test of Auditory Analysis Skill (Rosner, 1975), Goldman-Fristoe Test of Articulation (Goldman & Fristoe, 1986), and Clinical Evaluation of Language Fundamentals-Revised (Semel, Wiig, & Secord, 1987) no significant correlations were found. Comparing the results from child ages 5 and 7 the authors suggest that children had outgrown earlier language deficits caused by MEE.

These mixed results did not examine all aspects of language development, and the present report explores another component, central auditory processing.

Central auditory processing disorder (CAPD) has been defined as "the impaired ability to discriminate, recognize, or comprehend information presented auditorily " (Keith, 1986, p. 3) and it is not due to peripheral hearing impairment (McFarland & Cacace, 1995).. It has also been defined as a deficiency in one or more of the following processes: sound localization and lateralization, auditory discrimination, auditory pattern recognition, temporal aspects (resolution, masking, integration, ordering) of audition, and auditory performance decrements with competing and degraded acoustic sounds (ASHA, 1996). When CAP is not functioning optimally, it is referred to as a disorder, CAPD and is thought to be implicated in the development of school and social problems. It has been found to be related to attention deficit disorder and language disorder (Lam & Sanchez, 2007). There is some evidence that from 2% to 7% of children have CAPD (Musiek, Gollegly, Lamb,& Lamb, 1990).

Several studies have reported on the relation between MEE and CAP, with mixed results. Some had sample sizes too small to be considered (Asbjernsen, et al., 2000; Emerson, Crandall, Seikal, & Chermak, 1997; Gravel & Wallace, 1992; Webster, Bamford, Thyer, & Ayles, 1989). One prospective study reported mixed results for children at 5 to 8 years of age. They found significant impairment for a high MEE group on the speech-in-noise test, but not on the other five measures (Schilder, Snik, Straatman, & van den Broek. (1994). No study with an adequate sample size reported consistent CAP relations with MEE.

The CAP measures are somewhat controversial. Some evidence has been reported that there may be a sociocultural bias. Woods, Pena, and Martin (2004) found that Mexican American children scored slightly lower than Anglo American children on the Filtered Words subtest of SCAN. It seems quite likely that if English were not the only language spoken in the home that there might be effects on English-language development.

The SCAN tests are more complex than most language tests. They all require that the child subject give the tasks total attention, and this is difficult for some children. The possibility that SCAN is essentially a measure of attention rather than language will be explored using data from a widely used electronic measure of attention, the Tests of Variables of Attention (TOVA). One study compared TOVA and SCAN (Riccio, Cohen, Garrison, & Smith, 2005) and found no significant correlations.

This is a study measuring both CAP and attention at 7 years of age in a sample of 76 children who were evaluated carefully for MEE over the first three years of life.

Hypotheses

1) It is hypothesized that MEE will be significantly related to SCAN scores at child age seven.
2) It is hypothesized that SCAN measures will be significantly correlated with measures of attention.

Method

Study Population

In the period 1984-1989, 698 children were recruited from three newborn nurseries in Galveston County, Texas. At the time of enrollment, parents gave informed consent for participation in the project using a form approved by the institutional review boards at the University of Texas Medical Branch in Galveston and the University of Houston. The originally recruited sample consisted of 698 infants; 379 were still active in the study at three years of age, 294 at five years, and 198 at seven years. Language data from 76 children were available for the present study. Attrition was greatest between enrollment and 18 months of age, before our measures of SES (Socio-Economic Status) and HOME (Home Observation of the Measured Environment), and mother's intelligence were administered. Compared to other participants, children who dropped out of the study early (0-3 years) were significantly more likely to be of African-American ethnicity (X^2 = 8.2; $p < 0.02$), and had experienced less MEE, $X^2(1) = 27.1$, $p = 0.001$. Drop-out was not related to gender or birth order of the child. Evidence that the sample had not changed much through attrition may be seen in the SES mean scores, which were 37.4 (SD = 12.5) for the age three sample and 35.3 (SD = 12.4) for the sample at age seven. Further evidence of the normal distribution of scores for this sample, and the normality of the sample, may be seen in the results for the Stanford-Binet Fourth Edition (Thorndike, Hagen & Sattler, 1986) administered to children at ages 3, 5 and 7 (Johnson et al., 2000). Their IQ scores were, 100.6 (SD = 12.2), 98.3 (12.6), and 98.0 (14.00), respectively, which are close to the normative sample IQ of 100.0 (SD = 15.0).

Infants were recruited at birth without respect to gender, ethnicity, or SES. Because language performance would be assessed, children were excluded if English was not the primary language spoken in the home. Other exclusion criteria were the presence at birth of neonatal complications or craniofacial anomalies, lack of a home telephone, or plans to move from the area in the next five years. Subjects with evidence of sensorineural deafness at any age were dropped from the study (n=1). Participation was offered to all who met the eligibility criteria.

Monitoring, Definition and Calculation of Duration of MEE

From the time of recruitment, home visits were scheduled every 2 to 4 weeks to determine the status of the middle ear; i.e., whether symptoms of middle ear effusion were present. The first visit was at age two weeks. Monitoring was discontinued at age 3. If MEE was present parents were informed and if treatment was sought it was obtained from the child's pediatrician who followed her or his usual practice for treatment of the MEE situation.

The middle ear status of the child was assessed by trained research assistants who used tympanometry. The tympanometers were automated screening models that used a 226 Hz probe tone. The following models were used: Ear Scan II (Micro-Audiometrics, Port Orange, FL) at 79% of the visits, model 28 (Grason-Stadler, Littleton, MA) at 19% and other tympanometers at 2%. At each visit, if an abnormal reading was obtained, the test was repeated and the more normal result was used. Tympanometry has been found to be a valid measure of MEE status by Karzon (1991) and by Wiley (1991).

Otitis media with effusion was diagnosed if any one of the following two criteria was documented: (1) otorrhea visible without an otoscope, (2) a type B tympanogram defined as compliance of 0.0 or 0.1 ml. These criteria are similar to those previously reported to be predictive of middle-ear effusion (Le, et al., 1992; Schwartz & Schwartz, 1986).

For children with tympanostomy tubes, MEE was diagnosed if one of the following was documented: (1) otorrhea or (2) a type B tympanogram only if the canal volume indicated that the tube was not patent (i.e., canal volume < 1.0 ml for children < 6 months of age or canal volume < 1.4 ml for children ≥ 6 months). If a type B tympanogram was obtained at three consecutive visits after tube insertion, the tube was considered blocked or extruded and the parents were encouraged to see a physician to document the status of the tubes and ensure that tube function was restored. The project was originally designed to compare tube placement with non-tube placement using random group assignment of infants. After a year we discovered that many children in the tube placement group had not had tubes placed and children in the non-tube placement groups had had tubes placed. As the conditions of random assignment were violated we dropped this component of the study.

At each visit, each ear was evaluated separately and a diagnosis of MEE was made, or the ear was identified as normal as described above. A computer program calculated the percentage of time each child spent with unilateral, bilateral, and combination (unilateral plus bilateral) MEE for a given period. If two consecutive visits showed MEE, the intervening days were counted as days with MEE. If one visit showed MEE, and the next normal status, or vice versa, half of the intervening days were counted as days with MEE. A maximum of 28 days of MEE were calculated from any single abnormal visit.

MEE Measurement

One MEE measure was used in this study: bilateral MEE which consisted of the percent of days with MEE affecting both ears in the first three years (Table 2).

Socioeconomic status (SES)

The Hollingshead Four-Factor Index of Social Status (Hollingshead, 1975) was used. When each subject was seven years of age, SES was measured with the Hollingshead Four-Factor method, which takes into account the educational and social stimulation provided by the parents. The measure has a range of potential scores from 8 to 66. SES was measured as a continuous variable.

Central Auditory Processing Disorder

The test used was the SCAN (Screening Test for Auditory Processing Disorders) (Keith, 1986). The SCAN, which was administered at age 7, has three parts: Fltered Words (FW), in which sounds are filtered out or blurred. Forty monosyllabic, low-pass filtered words are presented monauralally with 20 presented to each ear. Auditory Figure Ground (AFG), in which words are presented against a jumble of noises, as in a cafeteria. Again 40 monosyllabic words are presented in a background of multi-talker babble with a +8 dB signal to noise ratio. Competing Words (CW), in which different words are presented at the same time to each ear. 100 monosyllabic words are presented as 50 dichotic word pairs. In each subtest, the child has to repeat the words that are presented. There is also a Composite score which is a sum of the three subscales. Raw scores were converted to standard scores. SCAN was administered at child age 7. SCAN can be administered in 20 minutes using a portable stereo cassette player in a quiet room. At age five children received audiometric testing and none showed language impairment. It was assumed that the same would be true at age seven.

Test-retest reliability has been reported by Amos and Humes (1998). They found that using a 6 to 7 week retest period with 25 children in the first grade with standard scores the following results were obtained: FW: 0.27, AFG: 0.24, CW: 0.73 and Composite: 0.72. The reliabilities for FW and AFG were not adequate, but that CW and Composite reliabilities were adequate. The results were similar for the third-grade sample. Keith (1986) reported internal consistency alphas that ranged from 0.57 to 0.97.

Test of Variables of Attention

The Test of Variables of Attention (TOVA) (Greenberg, 1991), which is a widely accepted measure of attention, was administered at age seven. The 10-minute version was used. TOVA consists of an electronic button that is pushed when a specified signal appears on a screen. Measures are 1) errors of omission, failure to respond to the target designated, 2) errors of commission, when the response is inappropriate, 3) response time, and 4) variability, or the standard deviation of the mean correct response times. It is a widely accepted measure of child attention (e.g., Fuchs et al., 2004; Rugino & Copley, 2001; Forbes, 1998).

RESULTS

Characteristics of the sample of seven-year old children are given in Table 1. These characteristics may be compared with those for the language study discussed above (Johnson, McCormick, & Baldwin, 2008). In that study there were 179 children, compared with 76 in the present study. Background characteristics were available for 72 and 74 children, with a few children for whom background data were not collected. Socioeconomic status was slightly higher for the earlier study, 36.75 versus 35.32, but this difference is minimal.. The earlier study had a smaller percent of African American children, 32 percent versus 44 percent. A power analysis was carried out prior to data collection. Sample sizes were adequate even considering sample size decreases.

Table 1. Characteristics of the Study Sample

Ethnicity	N
Anglo American	30
African American	32
Mexican American	10
Total	72
Gender	
Female	33
Male	39
Total	72
Socioeconomic Status	
Mean	35.32
Standard Deviation	12.43
Range	11-66
N	74

Means, standard deviations and ranges for MEE and SCAN appear in Table 2.

Table 2. Means, Standard Deviation and Range of MEE and SCAN Scores

	Mean	Standard Deviation	Range
Middle Ear Effusion (MEE)			
Bilateral SCAN	253.86	192.77	0-871
Filtered Words	8.00	4.19	3-17
Auditory Figure Ground	8.28	3.73	3-15
Competing Words	8.08	4.00	3-17
Composite	90.61	22.17	65-156

The correlations between MEE and SCAN scores at age seven were all significant. The results appear in Table 3. As may be seen, although the correlations were significant, none was large. The Composite correlation of -0.27 accounts for only 7.3 percent of the variance.

Table 3. Correlations Between SCAN and Bilateral Middle Ear Effusion (N = 76)

	r	p
Filtered Words	-0.32	.0029
Auditory Figure Ground	-0.33	.0039
Competing Words	-0.35	.0017
Composite	-0.27	.0015

TOVA measures of attention were correlated with SCAN measures. The results are in Table 4. Three correlations of 16 were significant: FW and Commission, AFG and Omission and Composite and Omission. It should be noted, however, that this is not strong evidence for a link between attention and SCAN. Indeed, they seem quite independent.

Table 4. Correlations Between SCAN Data and Tests of Variables of Attention (TOVA)

Filtered Words	r	p
Omission	-0.33	.075
Commission	-0.45	.011*
Response Time	-0.29	.118
Variability	0.35	.053
Auditory Figure Ground		
Omission	-0.45	.011*
Commission	-0.10	.600
Response Time	-0.13	.488
Variability	-0.43	.016
Competing Words		
Omission	-0.28	.131
Commission	-0.02	.903
Response Time	-0.18	.330
Variability	-0.15	.425
Composite		
Omission	-0.37	.042
Commission	-0.97	.697
Response Time	-0.23	.215
Variability	-0.28	.126

* = significant at the .05 level

MEE and TOVA correlations were not significant.

DISCUSSION

The significant correlations between MEE and SCAN were as hypothesized: all were significant. Given our earlier negative results for MEE and several language measures at age seven the present results were somewhat unexpected. Nevertheless, we obtained significant results and must consider how SCAN differs from the other language tests. The same bilateral MEE measure was used in both studies. The only language measure that even approached significance in the previous report study was the Test of Auditory Analysis Skill (TAAS), a measure of phonemic segmentation skills. The items on this test are fairly simple (e.g., "Say 'meat.' Now say it again, but don't say 'm.'" SCAN measures are similar, but words are presented and a response is requested. SCAN questions differ because they are presented under especially challenging conditions Thus, it may be possible that vestiges of earlier MEE-related hearing impairment which we found in earlier years became apparent under these difficult conditions. The implication is that these lingering effects of MEE may interfere with learning in school. However, our research on school achievement found no links to early MEE (McCormick, Johnson, & Baldwin, 2006).

SCAN was also compared with a measure of attention. That three of 16 correlations with TOVA were significant suggests that there is some truth to the contention that SCAN is a measure of attention, but that evidence for this is mixed and weak in the literature and not clearly demonstrated in our study.

LIMITATIONS

The mixed results for reliability of the SCAN measures (Amos & Hume, 1998) cast a shadow over our results. It may be that the obtained low correlations because of the fairly great time between test and retest (6 to 7 weeks).

Another limitation is that the sample for the present study was less than half that for the earlier language study. There were few demographic differences, but we know little or nothing about the children who did not receive the SCAN test. It was difficult to schedule this test as the children had to be alert and the test administered in a quiet room, by a trained speech and hearing graduate student. This combination of requirements seems to have diminished the number of children available for testing.

ACKNOWLEDGEMENTS

The project was largely funded by the National Institute of Child Health and Human Development, grant HD20988. Mary J. Owen, MD and Virgil M. Howie, MD, initiated and carried out the planning, data collection, and early data analyses for this project. We thank data collectors Bev Haas, Dawn Hedgpeth, William Norwood, Carolyn Cunningham, Jennie Dagerath, Kay Whitfield, Stephen Lee, Karen Merkel, Jan Cross, and Sharon Mohr-Sperduti. In addition we are grateful to Heidi Spergel for data entry and Rosina Cobbs for managing the data collection process. Contact author: Dale L. Johnson, 831 Witt Road, Taos, NM 87571. E-mail: dljohnson@uh.edu

REFERENCES

American Speech-Language-Hearing Association (1996). Central auditory processing: Current status of research and implications for clinical practice. *American Journal of Audiology, 5*, 51-54.

Amos,N. E. & Humes, L. E. (1998). SCAN test-retest reliability for first- and third-grade children. *Journal of Speech, Language, and Hearing Research, 41*, 834-845.

Asbjernsen, A., Holmefjord, A., Reiseter, S., Moller, P., Klausen, O., Prytz, B., Boliek, C., Oberzut, J. E. (2000). Lasting auditory attention impairment after persistent middle ear infections: a dichotic listening study. *Developmental medicine and child neurology, 42*, 481-486.

Carrow, E. (1974). *Carrow Elicited Language Inventory*. McAllen, TX: DLM Teaching Resources.

Carrow-Woolfolk, E. (1981). *Carrow Auditory-Visual Abilities Test*. McAllen, TX: DLM Teaching Resources.

Cohen, J. (1988). *Statistical power analysis for the behavioral sciences, 2nd ed.* Hillsdale, NJ: Erlbaum.

Emerson, M. F., Crandall, K. K., Seikel, J. A.,, & Chermak, G. D. (1997). Observations on the use of SCAN to identify children at risk for central processing disorder. *Language, Speech, and Hearing Services in Schools, 28*, 43-49.

Forbes, G. B. (1998). Clinical utility of the Test of Variables of Attention (TOVA) in the diagnosis of attention deficit/hyperactivity disorder. *Journal of Clinical Psychology*, 54, 461-476.

Fuchs, T., Birbaumer, N., Lutzenberger, W.,Gruzellier, J. H., & Kaiser, J. (2003). Neurofeedback for attention deficit/hyperactivity disorder in childreh: a comparison withy methyphendate. *Applied Psychophysiology and Biofeedback*, 28.

Goldman, R., & Fristoe, M. 1986). *Goldman-Fristoe Test of Articulation*. Circle Pines, MN: American Guidance Service.

Gravel, J. S., & Wallace, I. F. (1992). Listening and language at 4 years of age: effects of early otitis media. *Journal of Speech and Hearing Research, 35*, 588-595.

Hollingshead, A. B. (1975). *Four-Factor Index of Social Status*. Unpublished manuscript available through the Department of Sociology, New Haven, CT: Yale University.

Johnson, D. L., Swank, P. R., Owen, M. J., Baldwin, C. D., Howie, V. M., & McCormick, D. P. (2000). Effects of middle ear effusion on child intelligence at three, five and seven years of age. *Journal of Pediatric Psychology, 25*, 5-13.

Johnson, D. L., McCormick, D. P., & Baldwin, C. D. (2008). Early middle ear effusion and language at age seven. *Journal of Communication Disorders*, 41, 20-32.

Karzon, R. G. (1991). Validity and reliability of tympanometric measures for pediatric patients. *Journal of Speech, Language and Hearing Research, 34*, 386-390.

Keith, R. W. (1986). *SCAN: A screening test for auditory processing disorders*. San Antonio, TX: Psychological Corp.

Lam. E., & Sanchez, L. (2007). Evaluation of screening instruments for auditory processing disorder (APD) in a sample of referred children. *Australian and New Zealand Journal of Audiology, 29*,26-39.

Lampe, R. M., Weir, M. R., Spier, J., & Rhodes, M. F. (1985). Acoustic reflectivity in the detection of middle ear effusion. *Pediatrics, 76*, 75-78.

Le, C. T., Daly, K. A., Margolis, R. H., et al. (1992). Clinical profile of otitis media. *Archives of Otolaryngology and Head and Neck Surgery, 11*, 1225-1228.

McCormick, D. P., Baldwin, C. D., Klecan-Aker,J. S., Swank, P. R., & Johnson, D. L. (2001). Association of early bilateral middle ear effusion with language at age 5 years. *Ambulatory Pediatrics, 1*, 87-90.

McCormick, D. P., Johnson, D. L., & Baldwin, C. D. (2006). Relation between early middle ear effusion and school achievement at age 7 years. *Ambulatory Pediatrics, 6*, 280-287.

McFarland, D. J., & Cacace, A. T. (1995). Modality specificity as a criterion for diagnosing central auditory disorder. *American Journal of Audiology, 4*, 36-48.

Mody, M., Schwartz, R. G., Gravel, J. S., & Ruben, R. J. (1999). Speech perception and verbal memory in children with and without histories of otitis media. *Journal of Speech, Language, and Hearing Research, 42*, 1069-1079.

Musiek, F. E., Gollegly, K. M., Lamb, L. E., & Lamb, P. (1990). Selected issues in screening for central auditory dysfunction. *Seminars in Hearing, 11*, 372-384.

Riccio, C. A., Cohen, M. J., Garrison, T., & Smith, B. (2005). Auditory processing measures: correlation with neuropsychological measures of attention, memory, and behavior. *Child Neuropsychology, 11*, 363-372.

Rosner, J. (1979). *Test of Auditory Analysis Skill.* College of Optometry, University of Houston, Houston, Texas.

Rugino, T. A., & Copley, T. C. (2001). Effects of modafinil in children with attention deficit/hyperactivity disorder: a open label study. *Child and Adolescent Psychiatry*, 40, 230235.

Schilder, A. G., Snik, A., Straatman, H., & van den Broek, P. (1994). The effect of otitis media with effusion at preschool age on some aspects of auditory perception at school age. *Ear and Hearing, 15*, 224-231.

Schwartz, D. M., & Schwartz, R. H. (1986). Validity of acoustic reflectometry in detecting middle effusion. *Pediatrics, 79*, 739-742.

Semel, R., Wiig, E. H., & Secord, W. (1987). *Clinical Evaluation of Language Fundamentals-Revised (CELF-R).* San Antonio, TX: Psychological Corporation.

Thorndike, R. L., Hagen, E. P., Sattler, J. M. (1986) *Guide for administering and scoring the Stanford-Binet Intelligence Scale: Fourth Edition*. Chicago: Riverside.

Webster, A., Bamford, J. M., Thyer, N. J., & Ayles, R. (1989). The psychological, educational and auditory sequelae of early, persistent secretory otitis media. *Journal of Child Psychology and Psychiatry, 30*, 529-546.

Wiley, T. L., & Barrett, K. A. (1991). Test-retest reliability of tympanometry. *Journal of Speech and Hearing Research, 34*, 1197-12-6.

Woods, A. G., Pena, E. D., & Martin, F. N. (2004). Exploring possible sociocultural bias on the SCAN-C. *American Journal of Audiology, 13*, 173-184.

In: Children and Language: Development, Impairment … ISBN 978-1-60692-395-5
Editor: Michael A. Reed

Short Communication B

MULTILINGUAL SPECIFIC LANGUAGE IMPAIRMENT (SLI): FUTURE DIRECTIONS FOR RESEARCH

Tanja Rinker and Steffi Sachse
Transfercenter for Neuroscience and Learning (ZNL), Ulm, Germany

ABSTRACT

Children with Specific Language Impairment (SLI) show a significant language deficit with no obvious accompanying condition such as mental retardation, neurological damage, or hearing impairment. While about 6-8% of all children are affected by SLI, it is therefore logical to assume that 6-8% of all multilingual children are affected by SLI as well. In order to diagnose SLI with certainty, SLI must be diagnosed in both languages. While for many languages diagnostic tools exist, there are a large number of languages for which appropriate tests have not yet been designed. Particularly in children with successive bilingual language development, inadequate acquisition of the second language may mask a clinically relevant language impairment or vice versa.

While diagnosis is difficult, the issue of adequate language training or therapy respectively is just as complicated. This situation may be further exacerbated by a general uncertainty of professionals about the effects of multilingual intervention or parent advising regarding the choice of one or two languages. In addition, little is known about the neurophysiological bases and manifestations of multilingual SLI – making appropriate intervention all the more difficult.

In this short communication, we will outline problems and questions with regard to diagnosis and intervention and address future areas of research in the field.

DIAGNOSIS

One major concern is the adequate identification of multilingual children with SLI and the assessment of their language skills. Reasons for the problematic assessment are complex and vary in different countries. Different cultural and social backgrounds may influence the type of bilingualism (simultaneous or successive) and the way a society deals with it.

Some of these approaches are universal and others are specific for instance to the situation in Germany. In Germany, like in other countries, many multilingual children start learning their second language when they enter kindergarten or school between the ages of 3 to 6. The assessment of these children is currently discussed intensively by politicians, educators, and therapists because many children do not have language skills that enable them to cope with the demands of going to school. The main focus when dealing with the assessment of multilingual children is to differentiate children with poor language skills in their second language from children who have problems in both languages and therefore suffer from SLI.

To be able to diagnose SLI in multilingual children, skills in both (or all) languages have to be assessed. A reliable assessment is possible when using standardized language tests. Only in case of failing tests of both languages, language impairment can be diagnosed.

Which Tests Should be Used?

To judge German as the second language, German language tests can be used. Productive and receptive skills of the second language can be assessed. On these tests, a very large proportion of the multilingual children score far below average. Studies report numbers of up to 70 % (Grimm et al., 2004). This high percentage only shows that language skills of these children are clearly behind of the skills of their age-matched monolingual German peers. To identify children with SLI, additional tests for all languages a child speaks are necessary. Unfortunately there are no tests available for most languages multilingual children speak in Germany, e.g. Turkish. It has been suggested to translate a test into another language (Stow & Dodd, 2003). This approach is questionable, because items in language tests are not comparable because of their relevance or difficulty in another language. On one hand, we need tests that measure the same linguistic domain in both languages (e.g. passive vocabulary in both languages). Only if we assess the same domains is it possible to actually compare the skills in both languages. On the other hand, a test that aims to detect SLI should include clinical markers for specific language impairment in both languages (Bedore & Peña, 2008), whereas these markers do not have to involve the same linguistic structures in different languages.

When using tests from other countries the problem of a different language context and use occurs. The language of the home country is not necessarily identical to the language people use in the immigration country, especially if they have lived there for a long time and for more than one generation (Dirim & Gülender, 2002), e.g. the Turkish spoken in Turkey is different from the Turkish spoken by the immigrants that have lived in Germany for many years.

The tests available at this point do not often meet the demands of psychometric tests – they do not provide data for reliability, objectivity and validity and therefore do not allow a reasonable assessment (for tests in Germany, see Roth & Dirim, 2007). To be able to accurately assess language impairment, tests with a high specificity and sensitivity of at least 80 % are needed (Dolloghan, 2004).

So, even if there are tests available for all languages a child speaks, there are still various things to consider. It is important to decide who should perform the tests. Ideally, the person should be bilingual herself or two different persons have be involved in the diagnostic process. Only native speakers can really assess skills of the language in question. However, this will not be possible in every case. One solution is to use computer-based tests. But this only works with receptive skills, when children are asked to point to pictures (e.g. for Turkish and German: CITO-language test, CITO Deutschland, Butzbach)

Which Norms Should be Applied?

Another important issue in the assessment of multilingual children is the question which norms should be applied.

Two approaches are possible when assessing the second language – monolingual or bilingual norms can be used: the bilingual child can either be compared with age-matched peers of his or her first and second language or with other bilingual children.

If monolingual norms of the available language tests are used, they show how a bilingual child is able to speak a language compared to his or her age-matched monolingual peers. In some cases this might be the right approach, e. g. for the assessment of the second language before entering school. Bilingual children should not score far below the monolingual children, otherwise they will be disadvantaged from the very beginning of school.

On the other hand it has to be considered that multilingual language development can be different from monolingual development in many ways (Bialystok, 2001). Applying monolingual norms will then lead to incorrect results (Ünsal & Fox, 2002). This problem can be illustrated with the early stages of language development and diagnosis of language retardation: By the age of two years children should be able to speak at least 50 words, otherwise they are considered „late talkers“ (Dale & Fenson, 1996, Grimm 2003). Research has shown that bilingual children often need longer than monolingual children to reach this criterion and sometimes start to speak a little later than monolingual children (for a review see Bialystok, 2001). To decide if a bilingual child is developing „normally“, we need norms for this special group of children. Research has to be done to be able to develop procedures of assessing early bilingual development. Maybe in the early stages of language development words of both languages have to be considered for the 50 word criterion (Bedore & Peña, 2008, suggest such a total score approach for different linguistic categories) or perhaps bilingual children need more time.

Bilingual norms are very difficult to provide. They are not helpful and even problematic if a large proportion of the bilingual children in one country do not speak the language in a way one would expect. The result of a test would be, that a child is „normal“ compared to his or her bilingual peers but is still not able to speak the language in an adequate way.

Even if it appears to be important to find bilingual norms, e. g. for the mentioned productive vocabulary in two-year-olds, it is very complicated to find a suitable comparison group for standardization. This is because of the various scenarios of language acquisition. Different comparison groups would be necessary.

Summing up the mentioned problems and challenges in diagnosing SLI, a lot of research still needs to be done in order to provide tests in different languages which include similar linguistic structures as well as clinical markers for SLI in different languages and consider a different use of language in different countries (e.g. home country and immigration country). Tests have to provide norms that are suitable for the children that are concerned. Monolingual as well as bilingual norms are necessary. To be able to develop such instruments, extensive standardization studies and further research on bilingualism is necessary.

INTERVENTION/PARENT ADVISING

If a bilingual child is appropriately diagnosed with SLI, many professionals are requested to advise parents regarding the use of one or two languages. In the case of immigrant families speaking a minority language, the advice is often to focus on the majority language in order to integrate children into the school system. This may lead to the situation that if the parents are non-native speakers of the majority language, they are advised to speak in their non-native language to their child, thereby actually reducing their chances of receiving adequate and qualitatively good input.

Often the separation of languages within families is promoted for bilingual children. However, as Thodardottir (2006) points out, there is no indication that code-switching (switching between words, sentences or even within words) is a sign of confusion. On the contrary, a child may be confused by an artificially created one-person, one-language situation.

Another question that is frequently discussed is whether bilingualism has a detrimental effect on SLI. Past studies have been able to show that bilingual language impaired children, for instance, profit just as much from bilingual immersion programs (Bruck, 1982) – therefore, it is not recommended to abandon one language. In fact, monolingual and bilingual children with language impairment show the same grammatical impairments (Håkansson, Salameh, & Nesselbladt, 2003; Paradis, Crago, Genesee, & Rice, 2003) which indicate that multilingualism as such is not a risk factor.

Regarding intervention itself, it is often assumed that treatment in one language (in general the majority language) is sufficient. A single-case study by Thodardottir, Ellis Weismer, & Smith (1997) however, showed that a) bilingual intervention does not slow down language growth and that b) in the acquisition of some words it is even more effective. More research is clearly needed in this area – also in order to assess the transfer of therapy effects from one language to the other.

An international study spanning thirteen countries showed that very few speech-language pathologists provide bilingual intervention (13%) while 26% are bilingual themselves (Jordaan, 2008). Perhaps not surprisingly, the language of the school mostly dictated the language of intervention, closely followed by parental insistence. Another important factor for the choice of language is the language of the community – indicating that the status of the language used is of great importance.

Fredman & Centeno (2006) argue that therapy should ideally be given in both languages of the child, if not possible, at least parents should be advised to maintain their home/native language. According to Thorardottir (2006) monolingual intervention for bilingual children is the reduction of resources available to them which is against the general goal of improving the language abilities of language impaired children. She advises the use of specially trained interpreters where possible, however, the efficacy of this procedure has not been adequately researched as well.

The general set-up of therapy is difficult. The content of intervention has hardly been researched. Therapy of bilingual SLI children is challenging for speech-language therapists and progress should be closely monitored in both languages, if possible.

Overall, the lack of controlled studies in this complex area may contribute to the uncertainty of professionals with regard to the appropriate intervention and parent advising.

Future Directions

In an effort to serve bilingual children with and without SLI better, research should be pursued in the following directions:

- Research linguistic structures that can help discriminate effects of second language acquisition and SLI
- Find markers for bilingual SLI in grammatical development, lexical acquisition, etc.
- Develop diagnostic procedures that apply to bilingual children in general (e.g. Who diagnoses these children? Which norm is appropriate in which context?)
- Provide normative data
- Create tests that identify children with SLI in different linguistic contexts (e.g. successive Turkish-German children growing up in Germany)
- Investigate factors such as parent language politics, the quantity of input in the different languages,
- Controlled studies of effects of intervention (with regards to input, language variance)
- Research the neurophysiological correlates in order to understand the basis of multilingual SLI or to investigate the effects of different approaches of intervention. (with the notable exception of Pihko et al., 2007). Currently, the mechanisms and ways that multilingualism and language impairment interact at the neurophysiological level are still poorly understood.

References

Bialystok, E. (2001). *Bilingualism in development: Language, literacy, and cognition.* Cambridge, UK: Cambridge University Press.

Bruck, M. (1982). Language-disabled children: Performance in additive bilingual education programs. *Applied Psycholinguistics,* 3, 45-72.

Dale, P. S. & Fenson, L. (1996) Lexical development norms for young children. *Behavioral Research Methods, Instruments, and Computers*, 28, 125 – 127.

Dirim, I. & Gülender, S. (2002). Belegte Brötcin. *Grundschule Sprachen*, 8, 34 – 36.

Dolloghan, C. A. (2004). Evedence-based practice in communication disorders: What do we know, and when do we know it? *Journal of Communication Disorders*, 37, 391 – 400.

Grimm, H. (2003). *Störungen der Sprachentwicklung*. Göttingen: Hogrefe.

Grimm, H., Aktas, M., Jungmann, T., Peglow, S., Stahn, D. & Wolter, E. (2004). Sprachscreening im Vorschulalter: Wie viele Kinder brauchen tatsächlich eine Sprachförderung? *Frühförderung interdisziplinär,* 23 (3), 108-117

Håkansson, G., Salameh, E.-K. & Nettelbladt, U. (2003): Measuring language proficiency in bilingual children. Swedish-Arabic bilingual children with and without language impairment. *Linguistics,* 41 (2), 255-288.

Fredman, M., & Centeno, J. G. (Septeber, 2006). *Recommendations to work with bilingual children.* Comité Permanent de Liaison des Orthophonistes /Logopèdes de l'Union Européenne, 6th Congress, Berlin.

Jordaan, H. (2008). Clinical intervention for bilingual children: An international survey. *Folia Phoniatrica et Logopaedica,* 60, 97-105.

Paradis, J., Crago, M., Genesee, F., & Rice, M. (2003). Bilingual children with specific language impairment: How do they compare with their monolingual peers? *Journal of Speech, Language and Hearing Research,* 46, 1-15.

Pihko, E., Mickos, A., Kujala, T., Pihlgren, A., Westman, M., Alku, P., Byring, R. & Korkman, M. (2007). Group intervention changes brain activity in bilingual language impaired children. *Cerebral Cortex,* 17, 849-858.

Roth, H.-J. & Dirim, I. (2007). Erfassung der sprachlichen Performanzen zweisprachig aufwachsender Kinder in Deutschland – Verfahren zur Sprachstandsfeststellung vor und bei Schulbeginn. In: H. Schöler & A. Welling (Eds.), *Handbuch der Sonderpädagogik: Sonderpädagogik der Sprache,* (p. 648 – 665), Göttingen: Hogrefe.

Stow, C. & Dodd, B. (2003). Providing an equitable service to bilingual children in the UK: A review. *International Journal of Language and Comunication Disorders,* 38 (4), 351 – 377.

Thorardottir, E. T., Ellis Weismer, S., & Smith, M.E. (1997). Vocabulary learning in bilingual and monolingual clinical intervention. *Child Language Teaching and Therapy,* 13, (3), 215-227.

Thorardottir, E. T. (2006). Language intervention from a bilingual mindset. *The ASHA Leader, 11*(10), 6-7, 20-21.

In: Children and Language: Development, Impairment … ISBN 978-1-60692-395-5
Editor: Michael A. Reed

Short Communication C

LONGITUDINAL STUDY BETWEEN THE APPARENT PAIN INSENSIBILITY AND THE NON VERBAL COMMUNICATION AND SYMBOLISATION DISORDERS IN AUTISM

Guillaume Bronsard[1], Olivier Bonnot[2], Geneviève Haag and Sylvie Tordjman[4]

[1]Maison départementale de l'adolescent, 169 rue Paradis 13006 Marseille, France
[2]Hôpital Pitié-Salpétrière, 75013 Paris , France
[3]15 rue Emile Duclos, 75015 Paris, France
[4]Hôpital de Rennes, 154 rue de Chatillon, 35000 Rennes, France

ABSTRACT

Numerous clinical reports sustain the hypothesis of the pain insensitivity in autistic children. This insensitivity may be explained by the increase of the opioid activity (in particular the Bêta-endorphin). However, the rates of the plasma beta-endorphin concentrations in autistic children are contradictory. We have therefore studied in autism the relationship between the behavioural pain reactivity and the verbal and non verbal communication disorders. This study suggests that the apparent decrease of the behavioural pain reactivity in autistic children can be explained by a different way to express pain, specifically in relation with the communication and symbolisation disorders and other cognitive disorders (learning disabilities; own body image disorders; difficulties for mental representations of sensations and emotions; difficulties in understanding causes and effects relations), rather than a real endogenic analgesia.

Key words: autism, pain, cognitive disorders, language disorders

INTRODUCTION

Clinical observations show an apparent reduction of response to pain, even analgesia in some autistic children (absence of nociceptive reflexes like for instance absence of reflex of withdrawal of hand from fire, absence of protection of painful cutaneous areas or absence of position analgesic, unnoticed fractures, etc.) (C. Guillbert and coll., 1985 [5] ; S. Willemsen-Swinkels and coll., 1995 [15]). (The hypothesis of a link was then established between an increase of central opioid activity (the beta-endorphins in particular) and the reduction of response to pain observed in autistic patients. The beta-endorphins (BE) belong to the endomorphin family (endogenous opioid peptides) that has an effect on controlling pain and a central analgesic action. The increase of action of BE in autism has also been brought up on the following claims:

There is a similarity between autistic disorders and the symptoms of opioids dependency and animal behaviour after injections of BE (C. A. Sandman et coll., 1991) [12] ;

Preliminary studies suggested a therapeutic effect of endogenous antagonists of BE (naloxone, naltrexone) on the major autistic disorders, among which self-injurious behaviours and behavioural stereotypes.

But the double blind therapeutic trials did not confirm these results or prove the effectiveness of BE antagonists (S. Willemsen-Swinkels and coll., 1995 [15] ; C. A. Sandman and coll., 1991) [12] . Finally, studies that carried out dosages of plasma BE or in cerebrospinal fluid of autistic patients show inconsistent and contradictory results (for facts on the subject, see S. Willemsen-Swinkels et coll., 1996) [16] . It is important to underline that the results of BE dosages in the blood are difficult to interpret with regard to the central analgesic activity of the opioids since BE can't go through the blood-brain barrier and are foremost considered in the periphery as *stress* neuro hormones.

In order to understand the question of a possible analgesia in infantile autism, we have carried out a study on pain reactivity in eighty autistic children put in three different states of observation (parental evaluation, health care team evaluation, evaluation during blood drawing procedure). This was achieved within the framework of two INSERM research contracts (CRE 931009 et PARERCA, responsible: S. Tordjman).

RESEARCH METHODOLOGY

This longitudinal study was carried out, over a four-year period, on four evaluations, each one being performed over the same period (the same month) every eight months. Autistic patients were recruited within medical institutes (Medical and Educational Institutes, and day hospitals) and diagnosed according to the following classification criteria: the DSM-IV (American classification, 1994) [1] , the ICD-10 (OMS classification, 1993) and the CFTMEA (the French classification of mental disorders in children and adolescents, 1993) [10] . The study population included 52 boys (average age in years = standard deviation: 11.9 = 4.1) and 28 girls (11.4 = 4.5). The autistic patients, free of neuro-encephalopathic affliction, all showed an intellectual deficiency (global IQ ranging from 40 to 58) on the Wechsler scales.

One of the difficulties was to develop a pain reactivity evaluation tool adapted to autism, in particular to non-verbal communication disorders up to a total absence of language. We then created a nominal scale that can be used on subjects with or without verbal language: Pre-Linguistic Behavioral Pain Reactivity Scale or PL-BPRS. The study of the psychometric qualities of the pre-linguistic behavioral pain reactivity scale highlights good internal and external validities (internal validity: validity of content and structural validity, external validity: the concurrent validity was tested by comparing the PL-BPRS scale results to those of the "Child Pain Gustave Roussy" scale), as well as inter-judge loyalty and sensitivity (S. Tordjman and coll., 1999) [14] . The observations focused on behavioral pain reactivity as opposed to sensitivity to pain as apparent reactions to pain stimuli were only taken into account. Besides, detection of pain reactivity was only attained in daily life situations when the pain stimulus occurred by accident (to bang oneself, to cut, burn or prick oneself, , etc), not when it was triggered by the child itself (as in the case of self injurious behaviors).

Results and Discussion

The parents, as well as the health care teams, reported the three following types of observations:

- The child shows sudden other injurious behaviours aimed at people (bites, hits those around him) or things (throws objects, breaks them) and less frequently self injurious behaviours (bites himself, bangs his head against the walls) straight after or within the minutes following a stimulus that usually triggers pain and that occurred accidentally (burns, cuts, etc).
- The child's behaviour change alarms the people around him : he starts to moan, cry or he falls into an abnormal state of prostration. But parents or health care teams are unable to locate the pain. Some parents explain that, on a regular basis, they are confronted to situations where their child seems to be in pain (repeated cries, moaning) and where they have to go over all the possible causes for this state of distress (toothache, stomach ache, earache, etc.). In doubt, they end up giving him an analgesic that often manages to soothe the child. We have also been able to observe an increase of autistic withdrawal without further sign associated to it in cases of unnoticed fractures, when the child showed no attitude analgesic.
- The child expresses his pain (screams, cries) when facing a pain *stimulus* (like, for instance, a boiling hot shower) but endures this *stimulus* without even trying to interfere with the pain situation or its causal agent.

These Situations Suggest Several Hypotheses

- Following a pain *stimulus*, the autistic child would endure nociceptive *stress* and would live a state of ill-being but would be unable to identify, discriminate, elaborate a representation of the feeling of pain nor the nature of the pain *stimulus*. He would therefore be unable to interfere with the pain situation. The pain could correspond to an unpleasant stimulation which we don't know the exact nature of within the felt qualification: are we really in presence of the painful affect? Or could it be instead a physiological response to *stress* working upon the autonomic nervous system?

- The autistic patient would be able to elaborate a representation of the sensation of pain but would find it difficult to establish relations between cause and effect (relation between sensation painful felt and the stimulus responsible for it).
- The autistic child would be able to identify the painful sensation and establish relations between cause and effect but would be overcome by *stress* and thrown into an almost catatonic state of prostration preventing all reactions. Or he could not have acquired the behavioural response usually expected because of his learning disorders. We would then be in presence of a corresponding clinical picture that can be summed up, in appearance, to an increase of autistic withdrawal. We also know that the withdrawal that implies decommissioning and, at most, disembody (escape from body) can be found again in the child suffering from unbearable pain organic (A. Gauvain-Piquard et M. Meignier, 1993) [4]. We have ourselves observed a defensive withdrawal in a child aged around one who suffered esophageal burns, in all probability painful. This could raise the question of a link between autistic withdrawal and depression.

In order to be tested, these different hypotheses require subsequent studies including even more detailed observations from clinicians (child psychiatrists, clinical consultants, psychotherapists with training as psychoanalysts, various health care professionals) in collaboration with cognitivists, neuro-pediatrics, neurologists and neurophysiologists.

In addition, the same study revealed the existence of co-evolution between pain reactivity (in particular withdrawal reflex in response to burns) and autistic disorders. We have compared this normalization of reactivity to burns with the changing profile of the severity of autistic disorders assessed on ADOS scales (Autism Diagnostic Observation Schedule, P.C. Dilavore et coll., 1995) [2]. The results showed that the normalization of reactivity to pain assessed on these scales was consistent with an improvement in game scores on one hand, and in non-verbal communication scores on the other hand. The interpretation of this significant co-evolution between the normalization of reactivity to burns and the improvement in the capacity to play must take into account that the capacity to play, according to ADOS scales, corresponds to "pretend" games, therefore to access to symbolization and socialization. Yet, we might think that the improvement in the capacity of symbolization allows the autistic child to imagine the painful sensation and, as a result, to better respond to it. Similarly, the improvement in socialization plays a part in the learning abilities of the autistic child, learning process that allows the acquisition of socially adapted pain reactivity behaviours. Thus, the verbal and emotional expression of pain will differ according to cultural contexts and countries. Far from being inborn, it is a matter of social and cultural education (in Anglo-Saxon countries, for instance, the cry of pain will be expressed by "ouch" as opposed to "aie").

The co-evolution between the normalization of reactivity to burns and the improvement of non-verbal communication seems to indicate that the behavioural response to burns lies within a communication dimension. This co-evolution can be explained if we consider on one hand that the non-verbal communication encompasses the expression of sensations and emotions on the level body, and that, on the other hand, pain integrates sensorial, emotional and cognitive factors. In addition, we still have to compare this normalization of reactivity to burns with tracking of the stages of the "Self Body" restoration as presented in the clinical table used in the study (G. Haag et coll., 1995 [6] ; G. Haag et coll., sent to press [8]).

Finally, within the same study, the blood drawing situation led us to notice a paradoxical dissociation in autistic patients between the absence of exteriorized behavioural responses to pain reactivity (absence of emotional expression, absence of withdrawal reflex of the forearm from the needle) and the existence of important neuro-vegetative responses (reactive tachycardia to the needle as well as significantly higher levels of plasma norepinephrine in autistic children than in normal controls they were paired with in relation to age, sex and Tanner puberty stages). These abnormally higher neuro-vegetative responses to *stress* in autistic children confirm the results we previously obtained relative to responses to stress of the hypothalamic-pituitary axis in infantile autism (S. Tordjman and coll., 1993) [13].

The overall results show the existence of abnormally high biological responses to *stress* in infantile autism, on the hypothalamic-pituitary axis level (ACTH and BE) as well as on the sympathic nervous system axis level (Norepinephrine). It also suggests that this mechanism would be triggered by the difficulty created through the *stress* tension managing to release itself via exteriorized behaviours. It would be interesting to find out if the absence of withdrawal reflex is linked to a more or less important hypertonic reaction observed locally or rather on the whole body. We can ask ourselves if the paradoxical dissociation that was found in this research between external behavioural responses and internal vegetative responses would not see eye to eye with the Freudian notions of the destiny of pulsing excitations (endosomatic excitations) either directed, by a "specific action", outside the body to an existing object or an object in the process of being, or deviated to vegetative responses called internal changes (S. Freud, 1895) [3].

CONCLUSIONS

All our results suggest that the observation of an apparent decrease in pain reactivity in infantile autism would not be related to a mechanism of endogenous analgesia. Instead, it would come from a different mode of expression of pain in connection with symbolization problems, starting with primary symbolization that conditions the development of body image in the sense of "Self body" (G. Haag, 2000) [7], verbal and non-verbal communication disorders and other cognitive disorders: learning and body image disorders, problem of representation of sensations and emotions, difficulties to establish relations between cause and effect. A link between the improvement in pain reactivity behaviours and the progress in body creation, as shown in G. Haag and collaborators' grid, still needs to be established.

Last highlighting of a significant co-evolution between the severity of autistic disorders (non-verbal communication and symbolization disorders) and the response to pain abnormalities (to burns in particular) gives the opportunity to open up new angles regarding the monitoring of autistic patients. Within this longitudinal study, the "behavioural reactivity to pain" variable has indeed proved to be a good indicator of the evolution of infantile autism, a better one than autistic behaviours like behavioural stereotypes or auto-aggressive behaviours.

Finally, this study gives the opportunity to show, through the dissociation found in autism between exteriorized behavioural responses of reactivity to pain (absence of emotional expression or nociceptive reflex) and internal neuro-vegetative responses (heart rate and catecholamines increase), that the absence of behavioural pain reactivity does not mean absence of pain perception.

The myth of insensitivity to pain in autism, or more exactly of a diminished sensitivity to pain, can be compared with the same theory developed several years ago for babies (E.O. Poznanski, 1976) [11]. The baby's denial of pain was based on the idea of her neurological and psychological immaturity as well as on the recognition of the semiology characteristic of this age, as a consequence of the absence of verbal language. We might think that, like for babies, researches on autism would benefit from more in-depth clinical observations on direct signs of pain, emotional reactions and tonic-drive reactions that follow the pain *stimuli*. These researches would prevent concluding too hastily to a reduction in pain sensitivity, or even an analgesia in autistic children in relation with an increase of core opioids activity. They could help us better understand the mechanisms involved in the existence of a different mode of expression of pain in these children.

REFERENCES

[1] Amercian Psychiatric Association (1994), Diagnostic and Statistical Manual of Mental Disorders (DSM-IV, 4eme ed.), Washington DC.

[2] Dilavore P.C., Lord C., Rutter M. (1995), "The Pre-Linguistic Autism Diagnostic Observation Schedule", in *Journal of Autism and Developmental Disorders*, 4 : 355-379.

[3] Freud S. (1895), *"Entwurf einer Psychologie, Outline fo a scientific psychology"*, in *The birth of psychoanalysis*, Paris, PUF, 1973.

[4] Gauvain-Piquard A., Meignier M. (1993), *Pain of the child*, Paris, Calmann-Levy.

[5] Gillberg C., Terenius L, Lonnerholm G. (1985), "Endorphin activity in childhood psychosis", in *Archives of General Psychiatry*, 42, 781-783.

[6] Haag G, Tordjmann S., Duprat A., Cukierman A., Druon C., Jardin F., Maufras du Chatellier A., Tricaud J., Urwand S. (1995), "Presentation of a diagnostic grid of the progressive stages of infantile autism as observed in treatment", "in *Child Psychiatry*, XXXVIII (2), 495-527.

[7] Haag G., 2000, "Reflection on a form of primary symbolization in the creation of Moi body and spatial, geometric and architectural corollary representations", in *B. symbolization materials*, Lausanne, Delachaux et Niestle, 75-88.

[8] Haag G, Tordjmann S., Duprat A., Jardin F., Maufras du Chatellier A., Tricaud J., Urwand S., ., "Presentation of a diagnostic grid of the progressive stages of infantile autism as observed in treatment", in *International Journal of Psychoanalysis*, going to press.

[9] Lord C., Rutter M., Goode S., Heemsbergen J., Jordan H., Mawhood I., Schopler E. (1989), "Autism Diagnostic Observation Schedule", in *Journal of Autism and Developmental Disorders*, 19, 185-212.

[10] Mises R., Quemada N. (1993), "French Classification of Mental Disorders of the Child and Adolescent", in CFTMEA, CIM-10 - Chapter V of the CIM-10 (OMS), CTNERHI Vanves, Paris, PUF, 103-224.

[11] Poznanski E.O. (1976), " Children's reactions to pain : a psychiatric's perspective", in *Clinical Pediatrics*, 15, 1114-1119.

[12] Sandman C.A., Barron J.L., Chiez-DeMet A., Demet E.M. (1991), "Brief report : Plasma b-endorphin and cortisol levels in autistic patients", in *Journal of Autism and Developmental Disorders*, 21, 83-87.

[13] Tordjman S., Anderson G., MacBride A., Hetzig M., Snow M., Hall I., Ferrari P., Cohen D.J. (1997), "Plasma beta-endorphin, Adrenocorticotropin Hormon and Cortisol in autism", in *Journal of Child Psychology and Psychiatry*, 38(6), 705-716.

[14] Tordjman S., Antoine C., Cohen D.J., Gauvain-Piquard A., Carlier M., Roubertoux P., Ferrari P. (1999), "Study of the relationships between self-injurious behaviours and pain reactivity in infantile autism", in *L'encephale*, XXV, 122-134.

[15] Willemsen-Swinkels S., Buitelaar J.K., Nighof G.J., Van Engeland H. (1995), "Failure of Naltrexonero reduce self-injurious and autistic behavior in mentally retarded adults: double blind controlled studies", in *Archives of General Psychiatry*, 52, 766-773.

[16] Willemsen-Swinkels S., Buitelaar J.K., Weijnen F.G., Thijssen J.H., Van Engeland H. (1996), "Plasma beta-endorphin concentrations in people with learning disability and self-injurious and/or autistic behavior", in *British Journal of Psychiatry*, 168, 105-109.

INDEX

A

B

D

E

F

G

H

I

J

K

L

M

N

O

P

S

T

Y